TREATMENT PLANS AND INTERVENTIONS
FOR DEPRESSION AND ANXIETY DISORDERS

THE CLINICIAN'S TOOLBOX™

A Guilford Series

EDWARD L. ZUCKERMAN, Series Editor

Treatment Plans and Interventions for Depression and Anxiety Disorders

ROBERT L. LEAHY

STEPHEN J. HOLLAND

The Guilford Press

New York   London

Published by The Guilford Press
A Division of Guilford Publications, Inc.
72 Spring Street, New York, NY 10012
www.guilford.com

Library of Congress Cataloging-in-Publication Data
Leahy, Robert L.
    Treatment plans and interventions for depression and anxiety disorders / Robert
L. Leahy, Stephen J. Holland
       p. ; cm. — (The clinician's toolbox)
    Includes bibliographical references and index.
    ISBN 1-57230-514-2 (pbk. & CD-ROM)
    1. Depression, Mental—Treatment 2. Anxiety—Treatment. I. Holland,
Stephen J. II. Title. III. Series.
    [DNLM: 1. Depressive Disorder—therapy. 2. Anxiety Disorders—therapy. 3.
Cognitive Therapy. WM 171 L434t 2000]
RC537 .L43 2000
616.85'2706—dc21
                                                  99-059385

For Helen
—R. L. L.

For Jen
—S. J. H.

About the Authors

Robert L. Leahy, PhD, received his doctorate from Yale University and completed a post-doctoral fellowship at the Center for Cognitive Therapy at the University of Pennsylvania, Philadelphia, where he worked with Aaron T. Beck. Dr. Leahy is a clinical associate professor of psychology in psychiatry at the Cornell University Medical College, New York, New York; founder and director of the American Institute for Cognitive Therapy in New York City; and editor of the *Journal of Cognitive Psychotherapy.* He is also on the Executive Committee of the International Association for Cognitive Psychotherapy and the Academy of Cognitive Therapy. The author of *Cognitive Therapy: Basic Principles and Applications* and *Practicing Cognitive Therapy: A Guide to Interventions,* he is currently completing a book on a cognitive therapy model of resistance, to be published by The Guilford Press in Fall 2000.

Stephen J. Holland, PsyD, maintains a full-time private practice in Washington, DC. Previously, he was affiliated with the American Institute for Cognitive Therapy in New York City. He has taught classes for doctoral students at Columbia University in New York, and the American School of Professional Psychology, as well as for professional audiences. His publications include chapters on cognitive-behavioral therapy, brief psychodynamic therapy, and theoretical integration.

Contents

List of Figures, Tables, and Forms

FIGURES

TABLES

FORMS

Series Editor's Note

I am delighted to offer this book to my fellow clinicians because it is unique and practical. There are hundreds of books on therapy of the common disorders, but this book pulls together all the pieces a clinician needs to do effective therapy for seven of the most common disorders. No other book integrates symptoms, theory, interventions, patient education, and data collection so well for so many diagnoses. The authors label these elegant collections "treatment packages" and provide the following for each disorder:

- A symptom list to reinforce comprehensive data collection and evaluations
- An explanation of how the symptoms are understood in a cognitive-behavioral treatment approach
- A diagnostic flow chart
- Materials to support comprehensive treatment planning
- Descriptions of empirically supported techniques relevant to that disorder (even more detailed descriptions of these cognitive and behavioral methods are presented on the accompanying CD-ROM)
- Reproducible patient education handouts and homework forms to increase adherence, to improve outcome, and (of course) to meet the requirements of ethical therapy; these are also available on the CD-ROM so that readers can reproduce and modify them for their own practices
- Reproducible therapist record and assessment forms (also on the CD-ROM)
- Tips for troubleshooting common problems in therapy for that disorder
- A session-by-session protocol for treating the disorder
- Current information on medications (on the CD-ROM)
- A detailed case example for the disorder, which brings to life the integration of all these aspects of therapy

In offering these treatment packages, the authors do more than teach the theory and methods required (although they do those very well). They also offer practical strategies for obtaining treatment approval from managed care organizations, and they gather in one place the resources to implement the treatments in full for all seven disorders. All of this information is necessary to the proper practice of psychotherapy, and here it is all made accessible. What could be more practical?

The authors go beyond just collecting material; they have integrated them into a comprehensive and comprehensible resource for all clinicians. To put it simply, this is the way therapy skills ought to be taught, learned, and implemented.

EDWARD L. ZUCKERMAN

Preface

DESCRIPTION OF THE BOOK

This book has been written with practicing clinicians in mind. Our goal is to provide a hands-on guide to the best research-based cognitive-behavioral treatments for anxiety and depression, and to do so in a form that will allow busy clinicians to adopt these treatments readily in their own practices.

Cognitive-behavioral treatment protocols now exist for all of the major anxiety disorders and for major depression. Empirical studies have shown that these protocols effectively reduce the symptoms of most patients. One problem with these research protocols, however, is that their formats (e.g., sessions lasting an hour or longer, meetings more than once a week) are often not practical for most private practices or outpatient clinics.

In putting together the treatment plans and interventions described in this book, therefore, we have relied on our experience as full-time clinicians, as well as our experience in training graduate students and other professionals, to adapt these research-based treatments to the realities of the typical outpatient setting, including the demands of managed care.

The results are treatment plans and interventions for depression and for each of the major anxiety disorders. Each package includes a description of the disorder; instructions for assessing patients; assessment forms; detailed descriptions of the therapeutic interventions used to treat the disorder; a session-by-session treatment plan; sample symptoms, goals, and interventions to be used in writing reports for managed care companies; and informational handouts and homework forms that can be given to patients.

We have tried to make this book useful for clinicians of various theoretical backgrounds and levels of experience. For therapists already trained in cognitive and behavioral approaches, the book can offer a handy reference to the most recent treatments for specific disorders, in addition to providing a variety of forms that can be used with patients. For therapists trained in other orientations, the book can provide an introduction to the kind of short-term treatments now expected by many patients and third-party payers. It is our belief that the treatment techniques described in the book need not be incompatible with other theoretical orientations. Finally, graduate students may find in this book a useful introduction to cognitive-behavioral therapies.

The first chapter introduces some of the basic assumptions of cognitive-behavioral therapy and offers suggestions for obtaining treatment authorization from managed care companies. Following are chapters for specific disorders: depression; panic disorder and agoraphobia; generalized anxiety disorder; social phobia; posttraumatic stress disorder; specific phobia; and obsessive–compulsive disorder.

The CD-ROM that accompanies the book is designed to provide a quick reference to the treatment packages. Users may access key information, including session-by-session guidelines; lists of interventions for each disorder; and sample symptoms, goals, and interventions for use in writing treatment reports. The CD-ROM also allows users to print the various forms and handouts for use with their patients. In addition, it includes expanded appendices on behavioral techniques and on cognitive concepts and techniques, which provide detailed instructions for how to carry out the interventions described in the book.

THE TREATMENT PACKAGE APPROACH: ADVANTAGES AND CAUTIONS

Using structured, research-based treatment packages presents a number of advantages. The plans and interventions included in these packages are empirically based, so clinicians can know that they are offering a treatment that is likely to work. In addition, the gains made by patients using these packages have been found to be durable. For some disorders, the evidence suggests that patients actually continue to improve after treatment has terminated.

The packages are also practical; treatment is laid out step by step. Moreover, they are short-term; dramatic changes in symptoms can be achieved in a relatively brief period of time. They are compatible with managed care and with the resources available to many patients. In addition, treatment is specific for each disorder, while drawing on a limited number of basic techniques. Finally, patients with multiple Axis I diagnoses may be served by combining elements from each of the appropriate treatment packages.

Despite all the advantages of these treatment packages, some cautions must also be noted. First, they cannot be used like cookie cutters. For most patients, following the steps of these treatment plans and interventions will yield good results. Other patients will present problems that hinder treatment, ranging from life crises to characterologically based resistance. In such a case, the therapist will need to use clinical judgment to adapt a package to the needs of the patient, while staying mindful of the techniques that are essential to successful treatment of the specific disorder.

Length of treatment is a touchy subject. To the extent possible, we have based the length of the treatment packages on the amount of therapeutic contact provided in the best research protocols, while limiting all packages to 20 sessions or fewer. We are aware that some managed care companies consider 20 sessions excessive and seek to have people treated in 8 or even fewer sessions. We do not believe that this is supported by current research. Certainly some patients can be treated quite briefly (and we include case examples of fewer than 20 sessions). However, recent outcome studies for depression and social phobia have found that 16 sessions of treatment (after assessment) produces significantly better outcomes than 8 sessions (Barkham et al., 1996; Scholing & Emmelkamp, 1993a, 1993b). For some of the disorders covered in this book, the best recent research protocols provide 30 to 40 hours of therapist contact. In addition, patients with severe symptoms, comorbid Axis I conditions, and/or personality disorders often require longer than standard treatment.

We do not claim that cognitive-behavioral approaches are the only effective treatments for anxiety and depression. They are, however, the most extensively researched. We also do not pretend that these treatment packages encompass all that can be offered to patients. Once their most troubling symptoms have remitted, patients often find that they are able to address long-standing issues in their lives. These issues are typically related to the original symptoms in some way. It is our conviction that patients who have the psychological capacity and the desire to work on such issues should have the opportunity to do so. Although we see many patients in brief therapy, we both routinely work with some patients for periods of up to several years. We incorporate elements of psychodynamic, systems, and humanistic approaches in our long-term work.

One last caution is in order. These treatments can appear simple, and, conceptually, they are. However, applying them to real patients is a skill that requires time to master. Clinicians who have not had training and experience doing cognitive-behavioral therapy should seek consultation when first attempting to use these treatment packages.

In summary, we believe that the treatment plans and interventions presented in this book are essential tools for any therapist. We have sought to present them in a form that will be helpful to busy clinicians struggling with the demands of outpatient practice in a managed care world. It is our belief that these treatment packages, skillfully applied, will provide effective treatment for most patients with depression and anxiety disorders. However, the packages must be used with sensitivity and good clinical judgment.

Writing this book has been a rewarding experience. The process of preparing it has helped us to be more effective with our own patients. We hope that others find it useful as well.

CHAPTER 1

Treatment in a Managed Care Context

The purpose of this book, as we have noted in the Preface, is to provide a user-friendly guide to short-term cognitive-behavioral treatments for depression and anxiety disorders. For each disorder, we have taken the best research-based treatments and adapted them for use in typical outpatient settings. The results are treatment packages that include step-by-step instructions, along with assessment instruments, informational handouts, and homework forms for patients.

One of the advantages of using the cognitive-behavioral treatments described in this book is that because they are short-term and empirically validated, they are particularly well suited for practice in a managed care context. These treatment techniques have been shown in studies using real patients to provide effective relief for depression and anxiety disorders, and to do so in relatively few sessions. Since managed care exists by definition to control costs, therapies that are brief and effective will of course be favored.

However, the synergy between managed care and cognitive-behavioral therapy is more basic than the fact that these treatments work and work fast. The managed care industry has adopted a number of the basic assumptions that underlie cognitive-behavioral approaches to mental disorders. Understanding these assumptions (even if you don't necessarily agree with them) will help both in dealing with managed care reviewers and in applying these treatments to patients.

Three key assumptions shared by managed care and cognitive-behavioral approaches are as follows:

1. **Symptoms are the problem.** Rather than viewing symptoms as signs of "deeper" issues that must become the target of treatment, cognitive-behavioral approaches focus on patients' symptoms as the problems to be solved. Therefore, the disorders to be treated are defined by patients' symptoms and the impairments in daily functioning they cause.
2. **Symptom relief is the goal.** Because symptoms are viewed as the problem, the goal of therapy is the reduction or elimination of those symptoms. In order to show that treatment has been effective, there must be some means of measuring changes in symptom severity and improvements in functioning.

3. **Treatment interventions must have scientific evidence of effectiveness in reducing symptoms.** Cognitive-behavioral researchers develop treatment techniques based on their theoretical understanding of the disorder being addressed. However, they do not consider these techniques valid until they have been shown in clinical studies to reduce symptoms effectively. Often researchers will compare the effectiveness of different cognitive-behavioral techniques to determine which technique or combination of techniques is most effective.

In summary, cognitive-behavioral researchers (and most managed care reviewers) assume that patients' symptoms dictate the goals, which in turn dictate the empirically validated treatment techniques to be used.

The assumptions outlined above influence who gets approved for treatment by managed care companies, what types and lengths of treatment are approved, and even what questions are asked on treatment reports. The rest of this chapter provides suggestions on how to use an understanding of these assumptions to increase the likelihood of getting treatment approved. Each of the remaining chapters in the book describes a cognitive-behavioral treatment package for a specific disorder. The chapters follow the basic logic of symptoms leading to goals leading to interventions; as such, they guide you through the process of working with patients, from assessment to theoretical formulation to implementation of treatment. Topics covered in each chapter include the following:

- A description of the disorder and related features
- A cognitive-behavioral conceptualization of the disorder
- A brief review of the outcome literature supporting the use of specific interventions
- Detailed instructions for assessing and treating patients, including patient handouts and homework forms
- Hints for troubleshooting common problems in therapy
- A case example
- Sample symptoms, goals, and interventions to be used in writing treatment reports
- A detailed session-by-session plan of treatment options

GETTING APPROVAL FOR TREATMENTS: GENERAL CRITERIA

Getting approval from managed care companies, particularly for the kinds of treatments described in this book, need not be a nerve-wracking experience, provided you understand what reviewers are looking for. Although you may still encounter unreasonable restrictions on treatment from some companies, following the recommendations in this chapter should increase the likelihood of getting a favorable response.

Virtually all companies require that two basic criteria be met before a treatment plan will be approved: (1) medical necessity and (2) appropriate treatment. Let us look more closely at what these entail.

Medical Necessity

"Medical necessity" is determined by the patient's symptoms. In order for treatment to be considered medically necessary, the patient must meet criteria for a mental disorder as defined by the *Diagnostic and Statistical Manual of Mental Disorders*, fourth edition (DSM-IV; American Psychiatric Association, 1994), which include evidence of distress or impairment in social, occupational, or educational functioning. Reviewers check whether the specific symptoms and mental status described on a treatment report are consistent with the diagnosis shown. They also check the Global Assessment of Functioning (GAF) score on Axis V to see whether it indicates sufficient impairment to justify treatment.

Appropriate Treatment

"Appropriate treatment" involves both the goals of treatment and the interventions used to reach those goals. Goals must relate to the reduction of the patient's symptoms or to amelioration of impairments, and they should be specified in terms that can be measured.

When evaluating interventions, reviewers typically consider two questions: (1) Does the level of care match the severity of the patient's symptoms? (2) Is the treatment approach appropriate for the symptoms? "Level of care" has to do with the intensity of treatment—that is, whether the patient should be hospitalized, placed in a partial hospitalization or day treatment program, or seen in an outpatient setting. If the patient is seen on an outpatient basis, level of care also involves how often the patient is seen. Many companies will not approve sessions more than once a week unless the patient is clearly in crisis and/or unable to carry out routine daily functions, such as work or child care. Meeting more than twice a week is unlikely to be approved unless the patient is actively suicidal or homicidal and an argument can be made that intense outpatient treatment will prevent hospitalization.

The treatment approach must also be judged appropriate for the patient's symptoms. For example, a treatment plan for a patient with a bipolar disorder that includes intensive psychotherapy but no medication is likely to be questioned. The treatment techniques described in this book, because they are empirically validated and specific to each disorder covered here, will almost always be considered appropriate treatment.

THE INITIAL TREATMENT REPORT

Each managed care company has its own form for filing treatment reports. However, the key elements are the same for all reports and cover the three key areas discussed above: symptoms, goals, and interventions. Symptoms are assessed in most treatment reports by questions related to the patient's DSM-IV diagnosis, presenting problem, and mental status. Virtually all treatment reports request specific goals. Interventions are assessed by questions related to frequency of visits, type of therapy provided, and medication. Some reports request the specific types of interventions to be used for each goal listed. Outlined below are guidelines for completing the sections found in a typical treatment report.

Symptoms

Diagnosis

Be sure that the diagnosis is accurate and complete. Underdiagnosing a patient may result in fewer sessions' being approved or in questions' being raised when additional sessions are requested.

Axis I. List all Axis I diagnoses for which the patient meets criteria. The presence of comorbid conditions may complicate treatment, and the reviewer should be aware of this from the start. Be aware that some companies will not cover treatment of certain disorders—for example, sexual dysfunctions. Some companies require that any patient with a primary or secondary diagnosis of substance abuse or dependence be evaluated and treated by a clinician with special certification in substance abuse treatment (e.g., a certified alcoholism counselor). This may result in the original clinician's losing the patient, even if this clinician has experience in treating substance abuse or dependence. In general, "V-code" diagnoses will not be covered. Marital/couple therapy is also not covered by most companies. However, if one of the partners has an Axis I diagnosis, some companies will cover conjoint therapy with the spouse participating, as long as the treatment goals relate to the symptoms of the partner who is the identified patient.

Axis II. Some companies do not cover treatment of Axis II personality disorders unless there is also an Axis I diagnosis. Treatment goals should therefore be targeted to Axis I symptoms. However, the patient should be given an Axis II diagnosis if one is appropriate, because the presence of a personality disorder will have an impact on the course of treatment. On initial treatment reports, most companies will accept "diagnosis deferred on Axis II," especially if you have had only one evaluation session. An Axis II diagnosis can be added on subsequent treatment reports.

Axis III. List all medical conditions.

Axis IV. List all current stressors.

Axis V. Be sure to rate the patient accurately on the GAF Scale. Most companies have a maximum score, above which treatment will not be considered medically necessary; this is typically about 71. Conversely, if the GAF score is too low, a reviewer may question whether partial or full hospitalization will be more appropriate. In addition, be sure to indicate the highest prior GAF score, if this is requested. Many companies only cover treatment intended to return the patient to a "baseline" level of functioning. If the highest GAF score is too low, this may indicate a chronic condition, for which psychotherapy is less likely to be covered.

Presenting Problem

The section on the presenting problem should cover three areas: (1) precipitating events or stressors; (2) specific symptoms; and (3) impairments in life functioning.

Precipitating Events. Briefly list the events that have resulted in the patient's seeking treatment at this time. Protect the patient's confidentiality by giving only enough detail to indicate the level of stress. Any known history of physical or sexual abuse or other trauma should be noted here.

Specific Symptoms. This is not a place for creative writing. Get out the DSM-IV, or the tables listing sample symptoms in this book, and simply list the criteria (other than the DSM-IV criterion pertaining to distress or impairment; see below) that the patient meets for each disorder. Remember, reviewers are going to check off these symptoms to make sure the patient meets the diagnosis. You might as well make their job easy.

Impairments. Indicate how the specific symptoms interfere with the patient's functioning. Be sure to note any impairments in work, school, parenting, marital, or social functioning.

Mental Status

Some treatment reports provide a checkoff list for evaluating mental status. Others request a brief written mental status report. The key elements of a mental status report, based on the guidelines in Kaplan and Sadock (1988), are as follows:

Appearance. Describe the patient and note anything unusual in his or her appearance (e.g., marked obesity, poor grooming, unusual clothing or makeup).

Attitude. Describe the patient's attitude toward you as the therapist (e.g., cooperative, guarded, belligerent, seductive, etc.).

Consciousness. Is the patient alert, or is there some impairment in consciousness (e.g., drowsy, clouded, unconscious)?

Orientation. Is the patient aware of (1) person (who he or she is, who other people present are); (2) place (where he or she is); and (3) time (date, day of week)? If the patient is oriented in all three areas, this is often abbreviated as "oriented times three" or "oriented × 3."

Memory. Note any deficit in immediate, short-term, or long-term memory.

Psychomotor Activity. Describe any abnormalities in the patient's movement (e.g., agitation, retardation, nervous tics, etc.).

Speech. Note anything unusual in the rate, tone, or volume of speech (e.g., slow and halting, rapid, pressured, barely audible, high-pitched).

Mood. Briefly describe the patient's mood, either as the patient reports it or by observation (e.g., anxious, depressed, calm, angry).

Affect. "Affect" refers to the manner in which the patient's mood is expressed. Normal affective response is described as "full range," indicating that the patient is able to express a variety of emotions. Common variations in affect include "restricted" (ability to express only one or a few emotions); "blunted" (emotions are present, but their expression is muted); "flat" (lack of emotion); "labile" (rapid swings between emotions); and "inappropriate" (emotion does not match the situation or content of what is being discussed).

Perception. Indicate any abnormalities of perception, such as visual or auditory hallucinations, depersonalization, or derealization.

Thought Content. Indicate any abnormalities of expressed ideas, such as delusions, persecutory ideation, or ideas of reference. Also note any suicidal or homicidal ideation.

Thought Process. The thinking of patients who can stay on topic is described as "goal directed." Variations in thought include "circumstantial thought" (excessive detail), "tangential thought" (going off topic), "loose associations" (jumping from one topic to another with no apparent logic), and "perseveration" (returning to the same topic repeatedly).

Judgment. "Judgment" refers to the patient's ability to make sound decisions in social situations and to understand the likely consequences of behavior. Judgment is typically described as "poor," "fair," or "good."

Insight. "Insight" refers to the degree to which the patient is aware that he or she has a problem or is ill.

The mental status report should support the diagnosis. For example, a patient who is depressed may be expected to have depressed mood. In addition, such a patient may or may not have psychomotor retardation, halting speech, constricted affect, and suicidal ideation.

Goals

Whenever possible, treatment goals should be stated in terms that are observable and measurable (e.g., specific countable behaviors, scores on assessment instruments, client reports). Goals may cover the following areas:

1. **Completion of tasks required as part of treatment.** Examples: (a) completing exposure to all avoided situations; (b) engaging in one pleasurable/rewarding activity daily; (c) acquiring assertion skills.
2. **Relief of specific symptoms.** Examples: (a) eliminating intrusive memories of

trauma; (b) reducing self-critical ideation; (c) reporting anxiety below 2 on a scale from 0 to 10 in business meetings.

3. **Reduced impairment.** Examples: (a) bringing grades up to prior level (A's and B's); (b) resuming all household activities; (c) beginning to date; (d) finding appropriate employment.

4. **Cognitive change.** Examples: (a) stating less than a 10% belief in assumption of need for perfection; (b) modifying schema of worthlessness.

5. **End-state goals.** These are goals that will indicate that treatment has been successfully completed. Examples: (a) eliminating all depressive symptoms (Beck Depression Inventory score under 10 for 1 month); (b) engaging in all previously avoided activities; (c) eliminating panic attacks.

Interventions

Treatment Frequency and Type; Specific Techniques

Some treatment forms request only basic information about the treatment: frequency and length of sessions, type of therapy (e.g., cognitive-behavioral, psychodynamic, systems), and format (individual, conjoint, family). Others request more specific information about the types of interventions to be used to meet each goal. In such cases, the specific techniques described in the treatment packages in this book can be listed. Sample goals and corresponding interventions can be found in the chapters for each disorder, as well as on the CD-ROM.

Medication

Most treatment forms request information regarding what medication, if any, the patient is receiving. If the patient is not taking medication, it can be helpful to indicate that the patient has been educated regarding the advantages and disadvantages of medication (which should always be done). It may also be helpful to give a rationale for why medication has not been chosen as an option. Symptoms in the mild to moderate range, lack of suicidal or homicidal ideation, and good initial response to psychotherapy are generally acceptable reasons to proceed without medication. However, expect that if the patient does not show improvement, reviewers may request that the patient receive a medication evaluation.

Sample Treatment Report

Table 1.1 shows a sample treatment report based on the case of Sam, who is described in more detail in Chapter 5 of this book.

REQUESTS FOR ADDITIONAL SESSIONS

Few managed care companies these days will authorize 20 sessions on the basis of an initial treatment report (although it does happen and is more likely to happen if the treat-

TABLE 1.1. Sample Treatment Report: The Case of Sam

Symptoms

Diagnosis

Axis I	300.23 Social phobia
	296.21 Major depressive disorder, single episode, mild
Axis II	None
Axis III	None
Axis IV	New job
Axis V	Current: 55
	Highest: 80

Presenting Problem

Patient recently took new job that requires public speaking. Patient has long-standing fear of public speaking and has avoided it in the past. He has responded by becoming very anxious and depressed in last month. Specific symptoms: Intense fear of anticipated speech, avoidance of public speaking, stomach cramps, muscle tension, insomnia, fatigue, impaired concentration, depressed and anxious mood, loss of appetite, weight loss, and feelings of worthlessness and guilt. These symptoms interfere with work functioning.

Mental Status

Patient is a 26-year-old white male. Appears stated age. Well groomed. Cooperative. Alert and oriented × 3. Memory intact. Movement normal. Speech soft. Mood depressed and anxious. Affect constricted. Thoughts goal-directed. No psychotic symptoms. Denies suicidal or homicidal ideation. Insight and judgment good.

Goals and Interventions

Treatment goals	*Interventions*
Reducing physical anxiety symptoms	Relaxation
Eliminating ideation of worthlessness and guilt	Cognitive restructuring
Engaging in one rewarding non-work-related activity/day	Activity scheduling
Reducing fear of public speaking	Cognitive restructuring, imaginal exposure
Seeking opportunities to speak	Public speaking group
Stating reduced belief (10%) in assumption of need for perfection	Developmental analysis, cognitive restructuring
Returning to normal level of work functioning	Relaxation, cognitive restructuring, exposure
Completing speaking assignment with anxiety level of 2 or less on a scale of 0–10	All of the above
Eliminating anxiety and depressive symptoms (BDI score 10; SCL-90-R score in normal range)	All of the above

Medication

None. Patient has been educated regarding costs and benefits of medication. Does not wish to consider medication at this time. Symptoms are mild and of brief duration.

Frequency of Sessions/Expected Duration of Treatment

One 45-minute session per week; 16–20 sessions.

Note. BDI, Beck Depression Inventory; SCL-90-R, Symptom Checklist 90—Revised.

ment report is well written). This means that you will probably be filing subsequent treatment reports requesting additional sessions. In evaluating such a report, reviewers generally look for two things: (1) evidence that the patient is making progress, and (2) the continued presence of symptomatology that makes additional treatment necessary. If the patient has not progressed, reviewers are likely to question the efficacy of the treatment and may suggest alternative treatment or disallow further sessions. If the patient no longer has symptoms, the reviewers will obviously consider treatment no longer medically necessary. Outlined below are things to consider when writing requests for additional sessions.

Progress Made in Treatment

Most treatment forms ask for some accounting of the progress the patient has made since the prior report. Progress should be described in relation to the symptoms (including impairments), goals, and interventions included on the initial treatment report (see below for specific suggestions regarding each of these). Remember, if you cannot document that your patient is making some progress, you may have trouble getting additional sessions.

You should also note any conditions that have interfered with progress in treatment. If the patient has been subject to a new stressor that has exacerbated his or her condition, this should be noted. For example, a depressed patient who has been laid off from his or her job since the last treatment report may reasonably be expected to have a temporary increase in symptoms. Most managed care companies will make allowances for such occurrences. In addition, if the patient is resistant to treatment in some way, this should be noted, along with the steps that are being taken to address the resistance.

Changes in Symptoms

Diagnosis

If any additional diagnoses have become apparent during your work with the patient (e.g., a comorbid anxiety disorder in addition to depression, an Axis II personality disorder that complicates treatment), be sure to add the appropriate diagnostic codes. Conversely, if the patient no longer meets criteria for one of the original diagnoses, or if the level of severity has changed (e.g., on a diagnosis of major depression), this should be noted. The GAF score should also reflect any progress that has been made.

Presenting Problem

List all specific symptoms and impairments that the patient continues to have. If some symptoms or impairments remain but have lessened in intensity or frequency, note that. As before, these should correspond to DSM-IV criteria for the patient's diagnoses. Even if some symptoms have remitted, additional treatment is likely to be approved if other symptoms are still present and there continues to be some impairment in functioning. Be sure to list symptoms and impairments for any additional diagnoses that are included, including any Axis II diagnoses.

Mental Status

Note any changes in mental status. As before, the mental status report should support the current diagnosis or diagnoses and the progress made in treatment. For example, if a depressed patient no longer has suicidal thinking, psychomotor retardation, or constricted affect, these changes should all be reflected in the mental status.

Changes in Goals

Note which goals from the original treatment report have been fully or partially met. Add goals related to any new diagnoses, specific symptoms or impairments, or life stressors. If it was not included in the first treatment report, it may be advisable to add the acquisition of relapse prevention skills as a goal.

Changes in Interventions

Treatment Frequency and Type; Specific Techniques

Note any changes that have been made in treatment frequency or type, as well as in specific treatment techniques employed. Be sure to give the rationale for these changes and to describe the patient's response to them.

Medication

Note any changes in the patient's medication or dosage, along with the rationale for the change and the patient's response.

Justification for Continued Treatment

Some forms request reasons for continued treatment. The explanation should be brief and summarize what has been included on the rest of the form. Progress that the patient has made should be noted, along with any new stressors, followed by a description of remaining symptoms and impairments. If a change in the patient's condition or life circumstances has necessitated new treatment goals, these should be highlighted. The need for continued treatment should be based on the continued presence of symptoms and on the need to prevent relapse.

TELEPHONE APPROVALS

Some insurance plans require that approval be obtained by phone rather than by written treatment report. For some clinicians, this can be especially anxiety-provoking (after all, rejection in person is harder to take than rejection by letter). However, the same principles apply in obtaining approvals via telephone as in submitting written reports. Reviewers want evidence that the treatment is medically necessary and appropriate, and, on subsequent approvals, that the patient is making reasonable progress while continuing to require treatment.

Two key principles to keep in mind when talking to reviewers by phone are: (1) Be courteous; and (2) be professional. Taking an adversarial stance is not likely to help. What will help is being prepared. Before calling, you should have thought through (and possibly written out) all of the information that would be required on a written treatment report. This will enable you to answer the reviewer's questions clearly and succinctly. Although reviewers are often expected by the managed care company to deny some portion of the requests they receive, they are less likely to target you for rejection if it is clear that you know what you are talking about and your diagnosis and treatment plan are sound. It has been our experience that describing a cognitive-behavioral treatment plan with specific techniques and an expectable short-term course makes approval more likely.

REQUESTS FOR EXTENDED TREATMENT

Managed care companies vary in the degree to which they are willing to approve sessions beyond a typical course of 16 to 20 sessions. For those companies that will consider longer treatment, we have found that the following indications make approval more likely:

1. More severe symptoms and impairments.
2. Suicidal or homicidal ideation.
3. A life crisis that has arisen during the course of treatment.
4. Clearly specified goals for continued treatment.
5. Evidence of progress between treatment reports.
6. Utilization of adjunctive treatments, such as medication or support groups.

This information must, of course, be accurate and must be supported by session notes.

CHAPTER 2

Depression

DESCRIPTION AND DIAGNOSIS

In this chapter, we identify the characteristics of major depression and present a treatment package for it. For the treatment of bipolar disorders, we refer the reader to other publications—specifically Goodwin and Jamison (1991), Basco and Rush (1996), and Leahy and Beck (1988).

Symptoms

A major depressive episode consists of a variety of symptoms. Five or more of these nine symptoms must persist for at least 2 weeks: depressed mood; suicidal ideation; feelings of guilt or worthlessness; loss of interest and pleasure; sleep disturbance; decrease or increase in weight; psychomotor retardation or agitation; tiredness or loss of energy; and inability to concentrate or indecisiveness.

Prevalence and Life Course

The lifetime prevalence of major depressive disorder (MDD) is estimated at between 10% and 25% for women and between 5% and 12% for men. Greatest risk for MDD occurs for individuals between 18 and 44 years of age, and lowest risk is for those aged 65 and over. Age cohorts born after World War II are at greater risk for MDD as well as other disorders (e.g., substance abuse) (see reviews by Clark, 1995, and Roy, 1995).

Rates for attempted suicide are higher for females, but completed attempts are higher for males, who prefer more lethal methods of suicide (e.g., guns and hanging as compared to medication overdose or wrist cutting). The highest suicide risk is for the separated, divorced, and recently widowed, and the lowest risk is for single and married individuals. Living alone and living in an urban environment confer greater risk than cohabiting or rural residence. Those individuals whose families show a history of suicide, alcoholism, and depression, or who perceive that they do not have good social support, are at greater risk.

Genetic/Biological Factors

Although heritability rates are greater for bipolar disorders than for unipolar MDD, there is some evidence of biological inheritance of a predisposition to MDD. The concordance for monozygotic twins for MDD is about 50%, whereas the concordance for dizygotic twins is about 35% (Kaeler, Moul, & Farmer, 1995). Kendler, Kessler, Neale, Heath, and Eaves (1993) estimate heritability for MDD at .39, indicating some biological predisposition, but reflecting the likelihood that other factors (such as life events, developmental history, and coping skills) are more prominent. Studies of adopted twins who are depressed show that the rates of MDD in biological and adoptive parents reflect a small effect of heredity.

Coexisting Conditions

MDD depression has high comorbidity with other disorders, including panic disorder, agoraphobia, social phobia, generalized anxiety disorder, posttraumatic stress disorder, and substance abuse. As suggested above, marital conflict is an excellent predictor of depression, with some clinicians recommending marital therapy as the treatment of choice for patients presenting with depression associated with marital discord (Beach, Sandeen, & O'Leary, 1990). Physical illness, especially in the elderly, is correlated with depression. Several different types of physical conditions are associated with depression (Akiskal, 1995). These may be pharmacological (steroid use, amphetamine/cocaine/alcohol/sedative withdrawal), endocrine (hypothyroidism and hyperthyroidism, diabetes, Cushing's disease), infectious (general paresis, influenza, hepatitis, AIDS), or neurological (multiple sclerosis, Parkinson's disease, head trauma, cerebrovascular disorder). (See Akiskal, 1995, for a more complete list.) In addition, MDD is highly correlated with personality disorders, although the diagnosis of a personality disorder may be uncertain until the depression is alleviated.

Differential Diagnosis

In addition to the diagnosis of MDD, there are several DSM-IV disorders of related interest. Dysthymic disorder is a milder form of depression, with symptoms for most days over at least a 2-year period. MDD may be superimposed on dysthymia, resulting in a diagnosis of "double depression"—that is, MDD and dysthymia. Atypical depression is characterized by mood reactivity (mood responds to pleasurable events), significant weight gain or increase of appetite, hypersomnia, heavy feelings in arms and legs, and/or sensitivity to rejection. Bipolar I disorder refers to the presence of at least one manic episode in the past, and usually also to the presence of one or more depressive episodes. (The past or present existence of a manic episode is necessary for the diagnosis of bipolar I disorder. A manic episode is characterized by elevated mood, grandiosity, decreased need for sleep, pressured speech, flight of ideas, distractibility, increased goal-directed activity or psychomotor agitation, and/or engagement in pleasurable but risky behaviors.) Bipolar II disorder is similar to bipolar I disorder, except that a past or present hypomanic episode (a milder form of a manic episode) is required. Finally, cyclothymic disorder consists of the presence of frequent (but less severe) symptoms of hypomania and depression. A diagnostic flow chart for major depression (Figure 2.1) distills this information.

UNDERSTANDING DEPRESSION IN COGNITIVE-BEHAVIORAL TERMS

In this treatment package, we emphasize Beck's cognitive model of depression and operant (behavioral) models that may be utilized as part of a general cognitive-behavioral treatment plan. We also review interpersonal factors and consequences in depression, since these are important and can serve as targets for intervention.

Behavioral Factors

Behavioral models view depression as a loss, decrease, or as absence of rewards, or the inability to obtain rewards. Similarly, stressful life events or aversive consequences for the individual, whether these are single dramatic events or daily hassles, are predictive of depressive episodes. For example, depression may be the result of a reduction of positive behavior, behavior that has become less rewarding, lack of self-reward, use of self-punishment (e.g., self-criticism), skill deficits, lack of assertion, poor problem-solving skills, exposure to aversive situations, sleep deprivation, noncontingency of behavior and outcomes, and/or marital or relationship conflict (Nezu, Nezu, & Perri, 1989; Lewinsohn, Antonuccio, Steinmetz, & Teri, 1984; Lewinsohn, Munoz, Youngren, & Zeiss, 1986; Rehm, 1990).

According to Lewinsohn's model, depression is often the result of passive, repetitious, unrewarding behavior—for example, staying home and watching television removes an individual from opportunities for other rewards. The goal of behavior therapy is gradually to increase the frequency and intensity of rewarding behavior through the use of techniques such as "activity schedules" and "reward menus" (the latter are lists of behaviors that were previously rewarding or could become rewarding in the future). The emphasis is on *acting better before feeling better.*

A related behavioral factor contributing to depression is that behavior that was once rewarding is no longer rewarding. This may be due to greater demands or standards in the environment (i.e., it takes more of the same behavior to get the same level of reward). Consequently, the individual may need to increase the intensity of previously rewarded behavior. Furthermore, if rewarding agents in the environment are no longer available or no longer providing rewards, the therapist may need to assist the patient in identifying alternative sources of rewards.

Lewinsohn, Coyne, and others have correctly identified maladaptive interpersonal behaviors as a source of depression. According to Coyne's (1989) interpersonal reward model, depressed individuals begin the cycle by complaining, often obtaining reassurance and attention as a result of their complaints. Coyne has proposed that these individuals

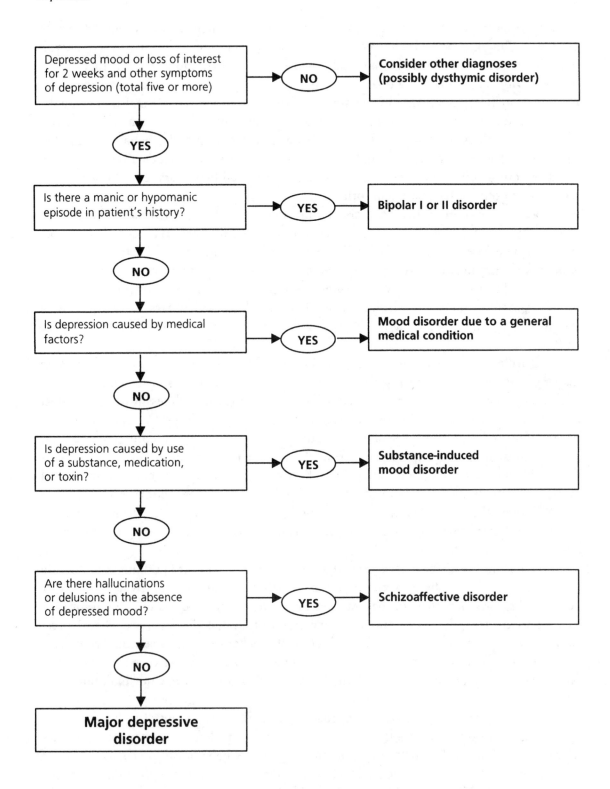

FIGURE 2.1. Diagnostic flow chart for major depression.

initially receive positive reinforcement from others for their complaining. However, continued complaining and self-preoccupation lead others to reject the depressed individuals, which results in a decrease in social reward and support, and thus in further confirmatory evidence of the individual's negative self-concept. As they increase their complaining and reject the help and reassurance provided, others view them as personally aversive and either withdraw from them or punish them through criticism. This negative response by others adds further to their depression. Consequently, behavioral models that emphasize the interpersonal nature of depression focus a patient's attention on decreasing complaining and increasing positive interpersonal behaviors (e.g., "Rather than complain to others, try rewarding others").

Absent or inappropriate social skills and assertion skills are also useful behavioral targets for therapy. Many depressed patients need to learn appropriate social behaviors (e.g., in some cases, fundamentals of hygiene and appearance are important goals). As Alberti and Emmons (1974) indicated some time ago, poor assertion skills may result in the inability to obtain rewards, greater feelings of helplessness, and (in some cases) more aggressive and nonrewarding behavior directed toward others. Consequently, a therapist may often include assertion training as part of a treatment plan for depression.

D'Zurilla and his colleagues (e.g., D'Zurilla, 1988) have argued that depression may result from the lack of problem-solving skills or behaviors, and hence in the persistence of mundane problems that contribute to feelings of helplessness. A therapist can assist a patient in developing problem-solving skills by helping the patient identify frustrations as "problems to be solved" rather than as issues to be complained about. The therapist may programmatically train the patient in problem definition ("What is the problem you are trying to solve?"), collecting information ("What resources do I have?", "How have others solved similar problems?"), brainstorming possible solutions ("How many different ways could this problem be solved?"), setting up an experiment to implement a possible solution, executing the plan, evaluating the outcome, and revising the plan if necessary.

As Bandura (1977) proposed years ago, behavior is often best maintained by the use of self-reward. This is because the individual is always available to reward himself or herself, whereas others may not be available or inclined to reward the individual for positive behavior. The self-control model of depression (Rehm, 1977) proposes that depression is the consequence of deficits in self-control mechanisms (e.g., self-direction, self-reward). The therapist may assist the patient in identifying self-reward as a goal of therapy, since positive behaviors may be quickly extinguished if they are not maintained by self-reinforcement.

To summarize, the behavioral approach (and, to some extent, the interpersonal approach; see below) suggests that a variety of behavioral deficits and excesses characterize depression, and that depression has distinctive behavioral precursors. All of those factors are listed in Table 2.1. Behavioral interventions for depression target the characteristic deficits and excesses of behavior; we describe specific behavioral techniques later in this chapter, in Appendix A, and in the CD-ROM accompanying this book.

TABLE 2.1. Behavioral Deficits and Excesses in, and Precursors of, Depression

Deficits	Excesses	Precursors
Social skills	Complaining	Marital or relationship conflicts
Assertiveness	Negative or punitive behavior toward others	Arguments
Self-reward	Self-criticism	Relationship exits
Rewards from others	Punishments from others	Daily hassles
Sleep deprivation		Negative life events (e.g., loss of job, divorce, death of close relative)
Problem-solving skills		Early loss of parent
Rewarding and pleasurable experiences		Parents with negative attributional style
Self-control and self-direction		Lack of nurturance from parents
Ability to reward others		Noncontingency of behavior and rewards

Cognitive Factors

The Three Levels of Cognitive Distortions

Several cognitive models of depression—notably Beck's—propose that the cognitive, motivational, and vegetative symptoms of depression are either caused by or maintained by three types of distortions at different levels of cognition: distorted automatic thoughts, maladaptive assumptions, and negative schemas.

Distorted Automatic Thoughts. According to Beck, the depressed individual suffers from a negative view of self, experience, and future. That is, the client believes "I am a failure," "Nothing in this experience is worthwhile," and "The future will be filled with failure." The content of the patient's view is negative because it is supported by distorted "automatic thoughts." These types of thoughts include labeling, fortunetelling, personalizing, all-or-nothing thinking, discounting positives, catastrophizing, and mind reading (for a full list, see Form B.2 in Appendix B). Thus, when an event occurs—for example, a conflict at work—it is processed through these automatic thoughts in an excessively negative fashion (e.g., "I am a failure" [labeling] or "It's terrible that this happened" [catastrophizing]). The consequence of this pervasive negativity is that the individual becomes depressed; this contributes to his or her negativity and to the lack of motivation to pursue rewarding behaviors.

Maladaptive Assumptions. Persons and her colleagues (Persons & Miranda, 1991, 1992) have demonstrated that vulnerability to future depressive episodes is predicted by the patient's endorsement of "maladaptive assumptions." As indicated in Form B.3 of

Appendix B, maladaptive assumptions are the rules or guiding principles that underlie automatic thoughts and that include "should" or "must" statements—for example, "I should succeed at everything I try," or "I must be accepted by everyone." These assumptions also include "if–then" statements—for example, "If I don't succeed on this, then I am a failure," or "If someone doesn't love me, then I am unlovable." These underlying assumptions are "maladaptive" in that they are rigid, punitive, and almost impossible to live up to. Consider the following: A patient, Bob, predicts that he will do poorly on an exam. This would qualify as the type of automatic thought called "fortunetelling"—that is, a negative expectation for the future. The thought can become problematic for Bob because of the assumption underlying the thought, such as "I must do well on everything in order to be worthwhile." What will it mean to Bob if he does do poorly on the exam? He thinks it means he is not worthwhile. And so he is vulnerable to depression whenever he falls short of his expectations. Because underlying maladaptive assumptions confer greater risk for depression, the therapist can seek to modify both distorted automatic thoughts and these underlying cognitive vulnerabilities.

Negative Schemas. Beck (1976) has proposed that when an individual is confronted with loss or failure, early maladaptive negative concepts of the self and others are activated. These "schemas" (see Table B.1 of Appendix B) constitute the deepest level of thinking. They reflect core beliefs about the self, such as that the self is unlovable, helpless, vulnerable to abandonment, controlled by others, ugly, and/or incompetent. In the example above, Bob predicts that he will do poorly on the exam because he believes that he is basically incompetent and prone to failure. Getting "better" in cognitive therapy is not only a matter of feeling better, but also of thinking and acting differently by modifying the core negative schemas that underlie distorted automatic thoughts and maladaptive assumptions.

Table 2.2 presents common examples of distorted automatic thoughts, maladaptive assumptions, and negative schemas in depression. Appendix B discusses these three types of cognitive distortions further and provides more examples of them. Specific cognitive techniques for dealing with these distortions are provided in Table B.3 of Appendix B and in the CD-ROM accompanying this book.

Other Cognitive Models

Seligman's (1975) earlier behavioral model of depression stressed that the noncontingency of behavior and consequences can lead to a belief in the self's helplessness—that is, "No matter what I do, it doesn't matter." Seligman and his colleagues later revised the noncontingency model to include cognitive components explaining individual differences relevant to the depressive syndrome—namely, the tendency of depressed individuals to explain their helplessness by referring to stable, internal causes of failure (lack of ability) and the belief that their failure will generalize to other situations. Later, however, Abramson, Seligman, and Teasdale (1978) proposed a reformulated model of learned helplessness. According to the reformulated model, self-critical depression and helplessness are consequences of a particular pattern of explanations, or "attributions," that the

TABLE 2.2. Examples of the Three Types of Cognitive Distortions in Depression

Distorted automatic thoughts

Labeling: "I'm a failure."

Dichotomous (all-or-nothing) thinking: "Nothing I do works out."

Fortunetelling: "My life won't get better."

Personalizing: "My depression is entirely my fault."

Maladaptive assumptions

"If I don't pass the exam, it means that I'm a failure."

"I'm weak because I have problems."

"If I'm depressed now, then I'll always be depressed."

"People will think less of me if I'm depressed."

"My value depends on what people think of me."

"I don't deserve to be happy."

Negative schemas

Undeserving: "People have treated me poorly because I don't deserve better treatment."

Failure: "I'm doomed to fail."

Unrelenting standards: "I can only succeed and gain approval if I'm perfect."

Approval: "People will reject me if I'm imperfect. I need their approval to be worthwhile."

individual makes for his or her failure. Depression results from the tendency to attribute failure to internal–stable qualities (e.g., lack of ability) as opposed to internal–unstable qualities (e.g., lack of effort). The individual who believes that he or she can try harder (more effort) is less likely to feel helpless, hopeless, self-critical, and depressed. Furthermore, attributing failure to external task difficulty ("Everyone does poorly on biochemistry") as opposed to internal deficits ("I'm no good at biochemistry") may lead to giving up on the task, but not to getting depressed and self-critical. Seligman's learned helplessness model, and recent advances such as Abramson et al.'s (Abramson, Metalsky, & Alloy, 1989) hopelessness model, have resulted in a considerable number of studies largely supporting these cognitive models of motivation and depression. The attribution model may be incorporated into a cognitive-behavioral treatment program by helping patients attribute their failure to lack of effort, task difficulty, or bad luck, and to attribute their successes to ability, perseverance, and other permanent qualities about themselves. Another aspect of attributional training is to help a patient evaluate a goal as an *alternative* rather than a necessity—that is, to help modify the idea that the particular goal *must* be attained.

Other cognitive models view depression as the failure to use self-enhancing or egoistic thinking, failure to use mitigating excuses, excessive self-focus, rumination, and passivity. Thus, those with depression are seen as differing from those without depression because they do not engage in ego-boosting, or even distorted, positive illusions that enhance their self-esteem. Similarly, depressed individuals are less likely to discount their negative illusions or to offer situational explanations for failure that do not imply personal responsibility. Self-focus models view depression as increased self-preoccupation, which is seen as a general process that increases negative affect. Supportive evidence on this topic indicates that depressives are more likely to ruminate about their negative feelings, asking rhetorical questions that have no answers, and that they are less likely to take an instrumental, proactive, and distracting approach to their negative affect.

Interpersonal Factors and Consequences

Although not considered a cognitive-behavioral approach, the interpersonal theory of depression, derived from Harry Stack Sullivan's (1953) social–psychodynamic model of psychopathology, has considerable relevance to depression. Klerman, Weissman, Rounsaville, and Chevron (1984) have proposed that depression is the result of dysfunctions in interpersonal relationships, such as interpersonal conflict and termination of valued relationships. According to this model, problems in childhood relationships (such as loss of a parent, lack of nurturance, or disrupted communication patterns), as well as current interpersonal difficulties (such as marital conflict or termination, lack of social support, or the lack of intimacy), may precipitate or exacerbate depression. The therapist therefore assesses the interpersonal context of the depression, such as problems in grief, interpersonal disputes, role transitions, and interpersonal deficits.

The therapist provides the patient with the diagnosis (i.e., depression), encourages the patient to adopt the "sick role" (i.e., the role of a person with an illness), and enters into an agreement with the patient that the two of them will discuss the patient's feelings and interpersonal relationships as related to the depression. As in the cognitive-behavioral model, there is considerable emphasis on conscious or preconscious thinking; on the here and now; and on a short-term, active, and relatively structured format of therapy. However, interpersonal psychotherapy differs from cognitive-behavioral therapy in that the former does not logically dispute the patient's negative thinking, nor is there emphasis on homework. Furthermore, interpersonal therapists would suggest that they place greater emphasis on the interpersonal context of depression, although one might argue that the cognitive-behavioral therapist does address social skills (e.g., Lewinsohn et al., 1986), communication patterns, and mutual problem solving (see Epstein, 1997; Leahy, 1996).

Specific techniques utilized in interpersonal psychotherapy include nondirective exploration (e.g., open-ended questioning), encouragement of affect (e.g., acceptance of painful affect, relating affect to interpersonal problems, eliciting suppressed affect), clarification, communication analysis, behavior change techniques, and the use of the transference. Klerman et al.'s (1984) *Interpersonal Psychotherapy of Depression*, as well as an excellent article by Markowitz and Weissman (1995) are useful references for the therapist who wishes to employ interpersonal psychotherapy. In recent years, experienced cognitive-behavioral clinicians appear to be emphasizing the interpersonal context of depression (e.g., Safran & Inck, 1995). We recognize the unique and important contribution of interpersonal psychotherapy to the field.

Marital or couple conflict is often either a cause or a consequence of depression.

Fifty percent of individuals seeking treatment for depression manifest such conflict (Rounsaville, Weissman, Prusoff, & Herceg-Baron, 1979), and 50% of couples seeking marital/couple therapy have at least one depressed member (Beach, Jouriles, & O'Leary, 1986; see Prince & Jacobson, 1995, for a review). Weissman (1987) has found that individuals in conflicted marriages are 25 times more likely to be depressed than individuals in nondistressed marriages. Depressed spouses/partners complain more, are less likely to reward others or to be rewarded themselves, show deficits in communication and problem solving, and are more likely to express negative affect. Furthermore, depressed individuals are more likely to elicit negative responses or withdrawal from their spouses/partners.

Because of the high concordance of depression and marital/couple conflict, the clinician may consider individual or couple therapy as the treatment for patients presenting with both problems. Excellent descriptions of behavioral and cognitive approaches to marital/couple therapy may be found in Baucom and Epstein (1990), Beach et al. (1990), and Prince and Jacobson (1995). The general approach involves assessment of areas of relationship distress; increasing the awareness, frequency, and contingency of rewards between spouses/partners; assertiveness training; scheduling of "pleasure days" where rewards can be dramatically focused; problem-solving training; communication training, focusing on the roles of both listener and speaker; identification and modification of dysfunctional thoughts and assumptions; use of time out to decrease aggressive interactions; sexual therapy where necessary; and training in acceptance of problems and self-care.

During the last decade, there has emerged considerable evidence that marital/couple therapy is useful in treating depression for patients with relationship conflict (Beach & O'Leary, 1986; Beach, Arias, & O'Leary, 1986). The advantage of such therapy over individual cognitive-behavioral therapy or medication is that both the individual's depression and the supportive environment (the marital/couple relationship) are significantly modified. Since depression is so highly correlated with relationship conflict, the clinician should always consider whether conjoint therapy should be the treatment of choice or whether it should be used in addition to individual therapy or medication. It is beyond the scope of this volume to describe the marital/couple therapy interventions available, but the reader is referred to the work of Baucom and Epstein (1990), Dattilio and Padesky (1990), Beck (1988), Jacobson and Margolin (1979), and Christensen, Jacobson, and Babcock (1995).

Outcome Studies for Cognitive-Behavioral Treatments

Numerous outcome studies attest to the efficacy of cognitive-behavioral therapy and/or tricyclic antidepressant medication in the treatment of major depression; cognitive-behavioral treatment is generally found to be equivalent or superior to medication. Across a number of studies, the mean percentage change is 66% for cognitive-behavioral therapy (Williams, Watts, MacLeod, & Matthews, 1997), with a number of studies demonstrating that most patients maintain their improvements 12 months later. Cognitive-behavioral therapy is as effective as medication in the treatment of severe depression (DeRubeis, Gelfand, Tang, & Simons, 1999).

ASSESSMENT AND TREATMENT

Rationale and Plan for Treatment

As we have stressed in Chapter 1, the advantage of the cognitive-behavioral approach is that it links symptoms to therapeutic goals to specific interventions. The specific symptoms of depression include low level of behavior, lack of pleasure and interest, withdrawal, self-criticism, and hopelessness (among others). Accordingly, the goals of treatment are to increase behavioral levels, to increase pleasurable and rewarding behaviors, to increase and enhance social relations, to improve self-esteem and decrease self-criticism, and to assist the patient in developing short-term and long-term positive perspectives. Various behavioral and cognitive interventions are utilized to achieve these goals: activity scheduling, reward planning/pleasure predicting, and graded task assignment (in order to increase behavioral level and increase pleasurable and rewarding behaviors); social skills training, assertiveness, and self-monitoring of complaining (to increase and enhance social relations); identifying, challenging, and modifying negative automatic thoughts, assumptions, and self-schemas (to improve self-esteem and decrease self-criticism); and identifying short-term and long-term goals, developing problem-solving strategies, carrying out and revising plans, and identifying and challenging dysfunctional thinking associated with hopelessness (to assist the patient in developing short-term and long-term positive perspectives). A behavioral assessment allows the clinician to evaluate the behavioral deficits and excesses associated with depression (e.g., low activity level, lack of self-reward, complaining, and rumination). In addition, the clinician can evaluate interpersonal problems that may contribute to the depression (e.g., frequent arguments, loss of relationships, lack of assertion, and other negative aspects of relating). Finally, a cognitive assessment provides an evaluation of typical distorted automatic thoughts, maladaptive assumptions, and negative schemas that may be targeted for cognitive disputation.

As Beck (1996) correctly indicates, cognitive therapy is not defined by the techniques that are employed, but rather on the emphasis that the therapist places on the role of thoughts in causing or maintaining the disorder. As cognitive-behavioral therapists, we view the behavioral model as a useful part of "cognitive" (Beckian) therapy. Behavioral assignments for patients are excellent (even necessary) vehicles for examining and testing the patients' cognitive distortions. For example, consider the use of self-reward as a simple intervention. In assigning this task, a therapist might ask the patient what he or she thinks about rewarding himself or herself. One typical response might be to "discount the positives": "It shouldn't be a big deal for me to do that [e.g., go to a museum]. Anyone can do that, so why should I reward myself?" Or negative self-schemas might emerge from the assignment: "I don't deserve to reward myself. I'm worthless." Or even fears of self-reward might emerge. One intelligent, articulate, highly accomplished young woman feared self-reward: "I'll become conceited if I say good things about myself. Then people will reject me."

A patient's distorted automatic thoughts clearly emerge with behavioral assignments. For example, with graded task assignments, the patient's fortunetelling ("I won't experience any pleasure") or negative filtering ("I didn't enjoy the lunch with Tom"—although the activity schedule might indicate many other activities with high pleasure ratings) can be examined. Similarly, thoughts indicating low frustration tolerance may emerge ("It'll be too hard to do that" or "I can't stand failing"). With assertion assignments, the therapist can examine the patient's maladaptive assumptions about assertion ("If I get rejected, it's awful; it means I'm unlovable," or "I shouldn't have to ask for those things. My spouse should know what I need"). Maladaptive assumptions about entitlement or about the need to ventilate ("I need to express my feelings; I should always be authentic") can be examined via assigning the task of decreasing complaining.

Another important component of behavioral assignments in cognitive therapy is to help the patient learn to choose which behaviors to engage in. For example, a depressed patient who sits at home ruminating (thereby getting more depressed) can be asked to consider alternatives to ruminating—for example, going to a museum. The patient can then be asked to calculate a cost–benefit ratio for sitting at home ruminating versus going to the museum. These "choice calculations" are helpful in motivating patients by getting them to focus on how their negative predictions are determining their choices. Behavioral assignments are thus used to collect information about thoughts.

We find that cognitive therapy works best with the integration of these many useful behavioral interventions. Patients often get a boost of hopefulness from behavioral assignments and can often convincingly see the difference between their distorted beliefs and reality. Simply having abstract debates with patients about how good reality is will prove far inferior as a strategy to helping the patients test out their cognitive distortions by engaging in behaviors that "act against the thoughts."

The steps in our treatment plan for depression are listed in Table 2.3. In addition to behavioral and cognitive interventions as listed in this table, we review below several other types of interventions (problem-solving skills, basic health maintenance, etc.) that may be included, depending on a patient's need.

TABLE 2.3. General Plan of Treatment for Depression

Assessment
    Cognitive, behavioral, and interpersonal assessment
    Tests and other evaluations
    Evaluation of suicidal risk
    Consideration of medication

Socialization to treatment

Establishment of goals

Behavioral activation and other behavioral interventions

Cognitive interventions

Inoculation against future depressive episodes

Phasing out therapy

Assessment

Forms 2.1 and 2.2 provide guidance for therapists in the assessment of depression. Form 2.1 permits a detailed assessment of cognitive, behavioral, and interpersonal factors that are playing a role in a patient's depression. Form 2.2 provides space for recording the patient's scores on various assessment instruments, for noting other relevant aspects of the patient's history (substance use, previous mood episodes), and for recording treatment recommendations.

Cognitive, Behavioral, and Interpersonal Assessment

Form 2.1 allows a therapist to determine the particular cognitive, behavioral, and interpersonal deficits and excesses that characterize a depressed patient. Under "Cognitive Assessment," space is provided for recording certain key statements made by the patient; from these, the specific distorted automatic thoughts, maladaptive assumptions, and negative schemas exhibited by the patient can be determined. Life events that may have caused the patient to develop his or her negative schemas, and strategies the patient is using to compensate for or to avoid these schemas, are also recorded. Under "Behavioral Assessment" and "Interpersonal Assessment," space is provided for recording examples of the particular behavioral (low levels of behavior, social withdrawal, inadequate self-reward, etc.) and interpersonal (frequent arguments, loss of relationship, lack of assertiveness, etc.) factors that are affecting the patient's depression.

Tests and Other Evaluations

The following self-report and interview measures may be used to evaluate baseline symptoms and problems: the Beck Depression Inventory (BDI, Beck, Ward, Mendelson, Mock, & Erbaugh, 1961); the Beck Anxiety Inventory (BAI; Beck, Epstein, Brown, & Steer, 1988); the Hamilton Rating Scale for Depression; the Symptom Checklist 90—R (SCL-90-R; Derogatis, 1977); the Global Assessment of Functioning (GAF) Scale (American Psychiatric Association, 1994); the Structured Clinical Interview for DSM-III-R, Axis II (SCID-II; First, Spitzer, Gibbon, & Williams, 1995); the Hopelessness Scale (Beck, Weissman, Lester, & Trexler, 1974); and the Locke–Wallace Marital Adjustment Test (Locke & Wallace, 1959). Form 2.2 provides space for recording scores on all of these instruments. It also enables the therapist to record the patient's medication, alcohol and other drug use; to record (at intake only) the history of previous depressive episodes and any manic or hypomanic episodes; and to note treatment recommendations.

In addition to completing Forms 2.1 and 2.2, the therapist should do the following as part of the assessment of any depressed patient:

- Consult with the patient's physician
- Evaluate suicidality (see below)
- Evaluate the need for medication (see below) and consult with a psychopharmacologist if necessary

FORM 2.1. Cognitive, Behavioral, and Interpersonal Assessment of Depression

Patient's Name: _____ Today's Date: _____

Cognitive Assessment

Describe a situation in which you feel sad or depressed: _____

_____

_____

_____

Complete the following sentence: "I would feel sad because I am thinking . . . ": _____

_____

_____

_____

_____

"And this would bother me, because it would mean . . . ": _____

_____

"I would feel less depressed if . . . ": _____

_____

Typical distorted automatic thoughts of this patient:

Mind reading:

Fortunetelling:

Catastrophizing:

Labeling:

Discounting positives:

Negative filtering:

Overgeneralizing:

Dichotomous thinking:

(cont.)

Personalizing:

Blaming:

Unfair comparisons:

Regret orientation:

What if?:

Emotional reasoning:

Inability to disconfirm:

Judgment focus:

Low frustration tolerance:

Underlying maladaptive assumptions of this patient:

Underlying negative schema (specify):

Hypothesized earlier childhood or life events:

Compensatory strategies:

Avoidant strategies:

(cont.)

Behavioral Assessment

Specify examples of each that apply, indicating, if possible, frequency, duration, intensity, and situational determinants:

Low level of behavior:

Withdrawal from others:

Rumination:

Social skill deficits:

Inadequate self-reward:

Inadequate reward in environment:

Exposure to aversive situations:

Inadequate challenge and novelty:

Poor problem-solving ability:

Lack of resources (e.g., financial):

Loss of past rewarding activities:

Interpersonal Assessment

Specify examples of each that apply:

Frequent arguments:

Loss of relationship:

Lack of assertion:

Not rewarding to others:

Punitive to others:

Frequent complaining:

Rejects support from others

Few contacts with others:

Deficient or inappropriate appearance/grooming:

FORM 2.2. Further Evaluation of Depression: Test Scores, Substance Use, History, and Recommendations

Patient's Name: _____ Today's Date: _____

Therapist's Name: _____ Sessions Completed: _____

Test data/scores

Beck Depression Inventory (BDI) _____   Beck Anxiety Inventory (BAI) _____

Global Assessment of Functioning (GAF) _____   Symptom Checklist 90—R (SCL-90-R) _____

Structured Clinical Interview for DSM-III-R, Axis II (SCID-II) _____   Hopelessness Scale _____

Hamilton Rating Scale for Depression _____   Locke–Wallace Marital Adjustment Test _____

Substance use

Current use of psychiatric medications (include dosage) _____

_____

Who prescribes? _____

Use of alcohol/other drugs (kind and amount) _____

_____

History (intake only)

Previous episodes of depression:

    Onset   Duration   Precipitating events   Treatment

Previous manic/hypomanic episodes (if any):

    Onset   Duration   Precipitating events   Treatment

Suicidal intent: None   Weak   Moderate   Strong

Recommendations

Medication evaluation or reevaluation:

Increased intensity of services:

Behavioral interventions:

Cognitive interventions:

Interpersonal interventions:

Marital/couple therapy:

Other:

- Evaluate the need for electroconvulsive therapy (ECT)
- Evaluate the need for substance abuse counseling or detoxification if the patient has substance abuse or dependence
- Evaluate the need for hospitalization

Evaluation of Suicidal Risk

As noted in the list above, evaluation of suicidal risk is part of the assessment of the patient, but this problem is so important and the link between assessment and intervention is so strong that we place special emphasis on it here. A clinician working with depressed patients should realize that all such patients should be evaluated for suicidal risk. The therapist should ask each patient about the presence of current and past suicidal ideation and behaviors, including passive suicidal behaviors (e.g., failure to take required medication, avoid dangerous traffic, or excessive driving speed). Patients are at greater risk if they talk spontaneously about suicide, threaten suicide, leave suicide notes, obtain methods (e.g., harboring pills, purchasing a gun), or have made previous attempts. Living alone, excessive alcohol or drug use, chronic physical illness, old age, recent losses, hopelessness, and the presence of a mood disorder are the best predictors. The therapist should ask the patient directly about the wish to live and wish to die; reasons for living and dying; frequency and intensity of suicidal thoughts, and ability to control such thoughts; passive attitude toward (acceptance of) suicidal wishes; deterrents to suicide (e.g., guilt, hope of improvement, religious concerns); availability of methods; and plans, verbalization, and motive (e.g., to escape pain, to punish others, to gain attention, to manipulate others, or to join someone who has died). Form 2.3 provides guidance in the evaluation of suicidal risk.

Our experience is that a therapist who takes an active and directive role in handling suicidality is much more capable of helping a patient. We insist, as a prerequisite for treatment, that each patient agree to a "no-suicide contract" in which the patient solemnly promises the therapist that, under any condition, the patient will not harm himself or herself while under the care of the therapist, and that the patient will call and consult with the therapist before any harmful actions are taken. We believe that *it is the responsibility of the patient to prove to the therapist that the patient can be trusted in an outpatient setting.* Thus the burden of proof is on the patient to assure the therapist that no harmful action will be taken. If the therapist believes that the patient is unreliable or unwilling to make this contract, then we recommend hospitalization in order to protect the patient during this critical time.

Although a few patients may refuse this contract (and therefore refuse treatment), our experience with this directive approach has been overwhelmingly positive. We indicate to a suicidal patient that suicide would be an extreme measure to take at a time when the patient is most irrational and hopeless and least capable of making life-and-death decisions. Our recommendation is that the patient can now examine all the reasons for his or her hopelessness and can learn to apply the techniques of therapy and medication to resolve the problem.

FORM 2.3. Evaluation of Suicidal Risk

Patient's Name: _____ Today's Date: _____

Therapist's Name: _____

Evaluate for current suicidal ideation and behavior and for any past incidence of suicidal plans, intentions, or behavior.

Question	Current	Past
Do you have any thoughts of harming yourself? [If yes:] Describe.		
Have you ever felt indifferent about whether something dangerous would happen to you and you took a lot of risk—like you really didn't care if you died or hurt yourself? [If yes:] Describe.		
Have you ever threatened that you would hurt yourself? [If yes:] Whom did you say this to? Why?		
Have you ever tried to hurt yourself on purpose? [If no, go on to p. 3 of form]		
Exactly what did you do to try to hurt yourself?		
How many times have you tried this? When? Describe.		
Did you tell anyone before or after your attempt? Had you threatened to hurt yourself or talked about it before? [If yes:] Describe.		

(cont.)

Questions	Current	Past
Had you planned to hurt yourself, or was it spontaneous?		
What was your state of mind when you attempted to hurt yourself? Were you depressed, spaced out, anxious, relieved, angry, excited? Were you using alcohol, medication, other drugs?		
Did you call someone at that time, or were you discovered by someone? What happened?		
Did you go to a doctor or to the hospital? [If yes:] Which doctor/hospital? [Obtain release of information.]		
Did you feel glad that you were alive? Embarrassed? Guilty? Sorry you didn't kill yourself?		
Did you want to hurt yourself soon after your attempt?		
Was there any event that triggered your attempt? [If yes:] Describe. [If no, go to next page of form]		
What were you thinking after this event that made you want to hurt yourself?		
If something like that happened again, how would you handle it?		

(cont.)

Question	Current	Past
Has any family member or close friend ever hurt himself or herself?		
How would you describe your current [past] desire to live? None, weak, moderate, or strong?		
How would you describe your current [past] desire to die? None, weak, moderate, or strong?		
[If current or past desire to die:] What would be the reason for wanting to die or harm yourself? Hopelessness, depression, revenge, getting rid of anxiety, being with a lost loved one again, other reasons?		
[If current or past desire to die:] Have you ever planned to hurt yourself? What was that plan? Why did you [did you not] carry it out?		
Are there any reasons why you would not harm yourself? Explain.		
Do you have more reasons to live than reasons to die?		
[If not:] What would have to change so that you would want to live more?		
Do you own a weapon?		

(cont.)

Question	Current	Past
Do you live on a high floor or near a high bridge?		
Are you saving medications for a future attempt to hurt yourself?		
Do you drive excessively fast?		
Do you ever space out, not knowing what is going on around you? [If yes:] Describe.		
Do you drink more than three glasses of liquor or beer a day? Do you use any medications? Other drugs? Do these substances affect your mood? [If yes:] How?		
Have you written a suicide note? Have you recently written out a will?		
Do you feel there is any hope that things can get better?		
What are the reasons why things could be hopeful?		
Why would things seem hopeless?		
Would you be willing to promise me that you would not do anything to harm yourself until you have called me and spoken with me?		

(cont.)

Question	Current	Past
Is your promise a solemn promise that I can rely on, or do you have doubts about whether you can keep this promise? [If doubts:] What are these doubts?		
Can I speak with [loved ones or a close friend] to be sure that we have all the support that we need?		
[Does this patient need to be hospitalized? Increase frequency of treatment contact and level or type of medication? ECT?]		

Therapist: Summarize dates, precipitating factors, and nature of the patient's previous suicide attempts, if any: _____

_____

_____

If the patient is willing to promise that he or she will contact and speak with the therapist before engaging in any self-harmful action, have him or her sign this statement:

I, _____, promise that I will not do anything to harm myself until I have called and spoken to you, my therapist. I also agree that you may speak with a loved one or close friend of mine to be sure that you and I have all the support we need.

_____
Patient's Signature

_____
Therapist's Signature

_____
Date

Consideration of Medication

All patients presenting with depression should be given the option of antidepressant medication as part of their treatment. The patient information handout on depression (see below), as well as the recommended readings, will provide a patient with information about medication for depression. Various antidepressant medications are available, including tricyclics, monoamine oxidase inhibitors (MAOIs), selective serotonin reuptake inhibitors (SSRIs), lithium, and bupropion; some of these are more easily tolerated than others. A full history of medication trials, as well as dosage, length of time on medications, and side effects, should be obtained from each patient. The physician prescribing the medication should have a full medical history available to avoid contraindications. If another biological member of the patient's family has responded well to a specific class of medications, then that medication class is more likely to be effective. Our experience is that medications are especially helpful in increasing motivation, energy, appetite, concentration, and the ability to gain distance from negative thoughts—especially with the severely depressed. For patients who do not respond positively to medication and therapy, and whose depression is severe and unrelenting, ECT is an alternative treatment with rapid efficacy in many cases. The physician should review the costs and benefits of ECT, which is far more effective today than it was twenty years ago. However, many patients undergoing ECT report memory losses that they find disturbing.

Socialization to Treatment

The patient should be told that his or her diagnosis is depression as soon as the initial evaluation is completed. Each patient should be given the patient information handout on depression (see Form 2.4), and should be required to begin reading one of two books by David Burns—either *Feeling Good: The New Mood Therapy* (Burns, 1980) or *The Feeling Good Handbook* (Burns, 1989). We find it helpful to indicate to patients that we utilize several models in our conceptualization of depression. Specifically, we indicate that depression is due to decreases in rewards and increases in negative events, to skill deficits, and to lack of assertion (behavioral models); to negative biases in thinking and unrealistic standards of perfectionism and approval seeking (cognitive models); to conflicts and losses in personal relationships (interpersonal model); and to biological factors affecting brain chemistry and familial predisposition toward depression (biological model). We emphasize that these models are not mutually exclusive, and that interventions from each model will be utilized (see Form 2.4).

Part of the socialization of the patient is to provide the patient with a case conceptualization and treatment plan. Although we are providing our readers with a "prototypical" guideline for a treatment plan later in this chapter, we recognize that each treatment plan must be tailored for each individual patient. For example, some depressed individuals do not present with behavioral deficits, and some do not present with self-criticism or hopelessness. However, the conceptualization should include an outline of behavioral excesses and deficits; patterns of life problems; typical distorted automatic thoughts, maladaptive assumptions, and negative schemas; and examples of how the pa-

FORM 2.4. Information for Patients about Depression

What Is Depression?

Depression has a variety of symptoms, such as loss of energy, loss of interest in activities and in life, sadness, loss of appetite and weight, difficulty concentrating, self-criticism, feelings of hopelessness, physical complaints, withdrawal from other people, irritability, difficulty making decisions, and suicidal thinking. Many depressed people feel anxious as well. They often feel worried, nauseated, or dizzy, and sometimes have hot and cold flashes, blurred vision, racing heartbeat, and sweating.

Clinical depression varies from mild to severe. For example, some people complain of a few symptoms that occur some of the time. Other people, suffering from severe depression, may complain of a large number of symptoms that are frequent, long-lasting, and quite disturbing.

Clinical depression is not the same as grieving after the loss of a loved one through death, separation, or divorce. Feelings of sadness, emptiness, low energy, and lack of interest are normal during grief; anger and anxiety can also be part of the normal grief process. Clinical depression differs from normal grief, however, in that clinical depression sometimes may occur without a significant loss. In addition, depression may last longer than grief and includes feelings of self-criticism, hopelessness, and despair.

It would be an unusual person who said that he or she never felt "depressed." Mood fluctuations are normal and help inform us that something is missing in our lives and that we should consider changing things. But clinical depression is worse than simple fluctuations in mood. Because there are various degrees of depression, the severely depressed patient may wish to consider a number of treatments in combination.

Who Gets Depressed?

Depression is not something that happens to people who are "unusual" or "crazy." It is everywhere. Along with anxiety (which occurs more frequently than depression), it is the common cold of emotional problems. During any given year, a large number of people will suffer from major depression: 25% of women and 12% of men will suffer a major depressive episode during their lifetime. The chances of recurrence of another episode after the initial episode are high.

The reason for the sex difference in prevalence of depression is not entirely clear. Possible reasons may be that women are more willing to acknowledge feelings of sadness and self-criticism openly, whereas men may "mask" or hide their depression behind other problems, such as alcohol and drug abuse. In addition, women are often taught from an early age to be helpless and dependent. Women may also control fewer sources of rewards than men do, and their achievements may be more often discounted.

What Are the Causes of Depression?

There is no one cause of depression. We view depression as "multidetermined"—that is, a number of different factors can cause it. These factors can be biochemical, interpersonal, behavioral, or cognitive. Depression may be caused in some people by factors in one of these areas, but it is just as likely to be caused by a combination of factors from all these areas. Biochemical factors can include your family's

(cont.)

genetic predisposition and your current brain chemistry. Conflicts and losses in interpersonal relationships can be factors in causing depression, as can behavioral factors, such as increases in stress and decreases in positive, enjoyable experiences. Cognitive factors include various distorted and maladaptive ways of thinking. Let us look at the behavioral and cognitive factors in a little more detail.

How Does Behavior Affect Depression?

The following is a more specific list of behavioral factors involved in depression.

1. **Loss of rewards.** Have you experienced significant losses in your life recently—for example, loss of work, friendships, or intimacy? There is considerable research evidence that people who suffer significant life stresses are more likely to become depressed—especially if they lack or do not use appropriate coping skills.

2. **Decrease of rewarding behavior.** Are you engaged in fewer activities that were rewarding for you in the past? Depression is characterized by inactivity and withdrawal. For example, depressed people report spending a lot of time in passive and unrewarding behaviors, such as watching television, lying in bed, brooding over problems, and complaining to friends. They spend less time engaged in challenging and rewarding behaviors, such as positive social interactions, exercise, recreation, learning, and productive work.

3. **Lack of self-reward.** Many depressed people fail to reward themselves for positive behavior. For example, they seldom praise themselves, or they are hesitant to spend money on themselves. Many times depressed people think that they are so unworthy that they should never praise themselves. Some depressed people think that if they praise themselves, they will become lazy and settle for less.

4. **Skill deficits.** Are there any social skills or problem-solving skills that you lack? Depressed people may have difficulty asserting themselves, maintaining friendships, or solving problems with their spouses, friends, or work colleagues. Because they either lack these skills or do not use the skills they have, they have greater interpersonal conflict and fewer opportunities to make rewarding things happen for them.

5. **New demands.** Are there new demands for which you feel ill prepared? Moving to a new city, starting a new job, becoming a parent, or ending a relationship and trying to find new friends can cause significant stress for many people.

6. **Being in a situation where you feel helpless.** Depression may result from continuing to stay in a situation in which you cannot control rewards and punishments. You feel sad or tired, lose interest, and feel hopeless because you believe that no matter what you do, you cannot make things better. Unrewarding jobs or dead-end relationships can lead to these feelings.

7. **Being in a situation of continual punishment.** This is a special kind of helplessness: Not only are you unable to get rewards, but you find yourself criticized by others and rejected. For example, many depressed people may spend time with people who criticize them or hurt them in various ways.

Although each of the factors of stress and loss described above may make you prone to depression, they do not necessarily have to result in depression. Certain ways of thinking can increase your chances of becoming depressed, however. You are more likely to become depressed if you think that you are entirely to blame, that nothing can change, and that you should be perfect at everything. These *interpretations* of stress and loss are the "cognitions" or thoughts that you have about yourself

(cont.)

and your environment. Cognitive therapy is specifically focused at identifying, testing, challenging, and changing these excessively negative views of life.

How Does Thinking Affect Depression?

Certain ways you think (your cognitions) can cause depression. Some of these are described below:

1. **Dysfunctional automatic thoughts.** These are thoughts that come spontaneously and seem plausible; however, they reflect distorted perceptions and are associated with negative feelings such as sadness, anxiety, anger, and hopelessness. Examples of some types of these thoughts are the following:

Mind reading: "He thinks I'm a loser."
Labeling: "I'm a failure," "He's a jerk."
Fortunetelling: "I'll get rejected," "I'll make a fool of myself."
Catastrophizing: "It's awful if I get rejected," "I can't stand being anxious."
Dichotomous (all-or-nothing) thinking: "I fail at everything," "I don't enjoy anything," "Nothing works out for me."
Discounting positives: "That doesn't count because anyone could do that."

2. **Maladaptive assumptions.** These include ideas about what you think you *should* be doing. They are the rules by which depressed people think they have to live. Examples include the following:

"I should get the approval of everyone."
"If someone doesn't like me, that means I'm unlovable."
"I can never be happy doing things on my own."
"If I fail at something, then I'm a failure."
"I should criticize myself for my failures."
"If I've had a problem for a long time, then I can't change."
"I shouldn't be depressed."

3. **Negative self-concepts.** People who are depressed often focus on their shortcomings, exaggerate them, and minimize any positive qualities they may have. They may see themselves as unlovable, ugly, stupid, weak, or even evil.

What Is Cognitive-Behavioral Treatment of Depression?

The cognitive-behavioral treatment of depression is a highly structured, practical, and effective intervention for patients suffering from depression. This type of therapy treats depression by identifying and addressing the behaviors and thinking patterns that cause and maintain depression. This therapy focuses on your present, here-and-now thoughts and behaviors. You and your therapist will look at how actions, or lack of actions, contribute to your feeling bad or good. There are actions you can take to start feeling better. You and your therapist will also look at the negative and unrealistic ways of thinking that may make you feel depressed. Therapy can give you the tools to think more realistically and feel better.

In cognitive-behavioral therapy, you and your therapist will first identify your symptoms and how

(cont.)

mild or severe they are. You will be asked to fill out forms or standardized questionnaires that can scientifically measure your symptoms. These may include the Beck Depression Inventory, the Symptom Checklist 90—Revised, the Locke–Wallace Marital Adjustment Test, or other questionnaires. In the initial meetings, you will be asked to select goals you wish to attain—such as increasing self-esteem, improving communication, reducing shyness, or decreasing hopelessness and loneliness. You and your therapist will monitor your progress in therapy by referring to your initial measures of symptoms and your movement toward the goals that you establish.

How Effective Is Cognitive-Behavioral Therapy for Depression?

Numerous research studies conducted at major universities throughout the world have consistently demonstrated that cognitive-behavioral therapy is as effective as antidepressant medication in the treatment of major depression. Within 20 sessions of individual therapy, approximately 75% of patients experience a significant decrease in their symptoms. The combination of cognitive-behavioral therapy with medication increases the efficacy to 85% in some studies. Moreover, most patients in cognitive-behavioral therapy maintain their improved mood when checked 2 years after ending therapy. In cognitive-behavioral therapy, we hope not only to reduce your symptoms, but to help you learn how to keep those symptoms from coming back.

Are Medications Useful?

Various medications have been found to be effective in the treatment of depression. These include Prozac, Paxil, Zoloft, Effexor, Tofranil, Wellbutrin, Elavil, Nardil, Parnate, lithium, and several other medications. It takes 2 to 4 weeks for you to build up a therapeutic level of the medication in your system. Some medications may have negative side effects. Some of these side effects may be temporary and decrease over time, or they may be handled with combinations of other medications. In some cases, patients with severe depression may wish to consult their physician about the possibility of electroconvulsive therapy (ECT).

What Is Expected of You as a Patient?

Cognitive-behavioral treatment of depression requires your active participation. During the initial phase of therapy, your therapist may request that you come to therapy twice per week until your depression has decreased. You will be asked to fill out forms evaluating your depression, anxiety, and other problems, and to read materials specifically addressing the treatment of depression. In addition, your therapist may ask you at later points, or on a weekly basis, to fill out forms evaluating your depression and other problems that are the focus of therapy. Your therapist may also give you homework exercises to assist you in modifying your behavior, your thoughts, and your relationships. Although many patients suffering from depression feel hopeless about improvement, there is an excellent chance that your depression may be substantially reduced with this treatment.

tient has avoided situations or compensated for his or her negative schemas (see J. S. Beck, 1995; Leahy, 1985, 1996; Young, 1990). The treatment plan may outline behavioral, cognitive, interpersonal, marital/couple, and biomedical interventions that are considered relevant.

A further part of the socialization of patients is to indicate what therapy will be like and what we expect of them as patients. The patient handout we use to introduce the patient to cognitive-behavioral therapy can be found in Appendix B (see Form B.1). We also find it useful to review with each patient reasons why he or she might be reluctant to do homework in therapy, or assumptions that the patient might have about the necessity of uncovering early life events in a psychodynamic process.

Establishing Goals

Setting goals is important with all patients, but especially so with depressed patients who feel hopeless. A clinician can help such a patient identify goals for the next day, few days, week, month, and year, continually linking the patient to a proactive position toward the future. The therapist asks the patient to state goals that he or she wishes to accomplish in therapy (e.g., changes in depression, anxiety, procrastination, self-esteem, assertion, problem solving, marital conflict, etc.). Scores on several of the self-report scales mentioned earlier—for example, the BDI and SCL-90-R—can be used as symptom targets or goals for the patient to review periodically to assess progress. Shorter-term goals can include increasing behavioral activity, seeing friends, increasing exercise, or getting work done. Longer-term goals can include taking courses, obtaining credentials, losing weight, or changing one's job. The therapist and the patient can agree to review these goals periodically.

Behavioral Activation (Reward Planning and Activity Scheduling)

Increasing the rewarding and productive behavior of a depressed patient is one of the first goals of therapy. Behavioral activation, which combines reward planning and activity scheduling, is a means of achieving this goal. As a first step, the clinician provides the patient with the Patient's Weekly Activity Schedule (Form 2.5) in order to monitor the activities he or she is involved in for each hour of the day, and to note the amounts of pleasure and mastery (feelings of accomplishment and effectiveness) actually experienced during each activity. This allows the patient and therapist to review how the patient's time is being used; whether the patient generally plans activities; whether many or most current activities are monotonous, ruminative, asocial, and/or unrewarding (this will usually be the case); and which of these activities are associated with the highest and which with the lowest degrees of pleasure.

Next, the therapist reviews with the patient activities that were once enjoyable but that the patient is engaging in less often, or activities that the patient thinks he or she might enjoy but has never tried, and urges the patient to begin planning more of those activities and fewer low-reward activities (watching TV, lying in bed, ruminating, etc.). Lewinsohn's lists of pleasurable and unpleasurable activities may be used to focus on

FORM 2.5. Patient's Weekly Activity Schedule

Patient's Name: _____   Date: _____

Instructions: For each hour of the week, fill in what you *actually did* and ratings for how much pleasure and mastery you *actually experienced.* To rate pleasure, use a scale where 0 = "no pleasure" and 10 = "the most pleasure you can imagine," with 5 indicating a moderate amount of pleasure. For example, fill in "talked with friend, 6" in the box for Tuesday at 10 A.M. if you rate yourself as experiencing that amount of pleasure from talking with a friend at that day and hour. To rate mastery (the feeling of effectiveness or accomplishment you get from an activity), use a similar 0–10 scale, and write the rating as the second number after the activity (e.g., "talked with friend, 6/5").

Hour	Monday	Tuesday	Wednesday	Thursday	Friday	Saturday	Sunday
6 A.M.							
7							
8							
9							
10							

(cont.)

FORM 2.5. Patient's Weekly Activity Schedule (p. 2 of 3)

Hour	Monday	Tuesday	Wednesday	Thursday	Friday	Saturday	Sunday
11							
12 noon							
1 P.M.							
2							
3							
4							
5							
6							

(cont.)

FORM 2.5. Patient's Weekly Activity Schedule (p. 3 of 3)

Hour	Monday	Tuesday	Wednesday	Thursday	Friday	Saturday	Sunday
7							
8							
9							
10							
11							
12 midnight							
1–6 A.M.							

what could be increased and decreased (see Lewinsohn, Mermelstein, Alexander, & MacPhillamy, 1985; MacPhillamy & Lewinsohn, 1982). The patient is then assigned to schedule some of these activities for each day, and to use the Patient's Weekly Planning Schedule (Form 2.6) to predict the amount of pleasure and mastery he or she expects to obtain from each. Finally, the patient actually engages in the activities and again uses Form 2.5 to record his or her actual ratings for mastery and pleasure. Appendix A of this book also provides a discussion of behavioral activation.

The therapist can introduce a cognitive component into the behavioral activation process by having the patient compare expected and obtained pleasure readings (as a check on negative fortunetelling); helping the patient to see that pleasure varies with activities, and that he or she can thereby control the amount of pleasure achieved; and having the patient examine the automatic thoughts associated with various activities. For example, depressed patients will often have discounting thoughts ("This wasn't as good as it used to be") or low-frustration-tolerance thoughts ("I can't stand doing this"). These negative thoughts associated with negative activities may be addressed in therapy. Some patients, driven by their desire to appear unconstrained and spontaneous, may resist scheduling pleasurable activities. They may believe that they are not being authentic or free, and that in order to be themselves, they have to act in accordance with their true feelings. Therapists may address this resistance by reviewing the evidence that the patients' strategy—of doing what they feel like doing—has been working. We also find it useful to use physical exercise analogies. We may say to patients, "In order to get into better shape, would you only exercise when you felt like it? Have you ever begun to exercise even though you didn't feel like it? Precisely what would happen if you exercised and you didn't feel like it?" Patients' discounting thoughts that activities are not as enjoyable as they once were (prior to the depression) may be examined as well: "Is it possible that positive activities take a while to kick in? Perhaps when you are depressed, these activities are not as enjoyable as they once were, but they may be more enjoyable than doing nothing."

Other Behavioral Interventions

We have emphasized behavioral activation (reward planning and activity scheduling) here because of its importance in increasing depressed patients' low levels of behavior, but many other behavioral interventions can and should be used with such patients as the need arises. Table 2.4 summarizes all the behavioral techniques that can be employed in the treatment of depression; some of these are described in more detail in Appendix A, and most are described in the CD-ROM accompanying this book.

Cognitive Interventions

The course of cognitive therapy begins with educating the patient about the various types of cognitive distortions. The patient is then helped to identify and categorize distorted automatic thoughts; to identify underlying maladaptive assumptions and negative schemas; and to use a wide variety of techniques to challenge his or her thoughts, as-

FORM 2.6. Patient's Weekly Planning Schedule: Predicting Pleasure and Mastery

Date: _____

Instructions: For each hour of the week, fill in what you *plan to do* and how much pleasure and mastery you *think you will experience.* To rate pleasure, use a scale where 0 = "no pleasure" and 10 = "the most pleasure you can imagine," with 5 indicating a moderate amount of pleasure. For example, if you predict that you will derive a pleasure rating of 6 if you exercise at 8 A.M. on Monday, then write "exercise, 6" in the box for Monday at 8 A.M. To rate mastery (the feeling of effectiveness or accomplishment you get from an activity), use a similar 0–10 scale, and write the rating as the second number after the activity (e.g., "exercise, 6/8").

Hour	Monday	Tuesday	Wednesday	Thursday	Friday	Saturday	Sunday
6 A.M.							
7							
8							
9							
10							

(cont.)

From *Treatment Plans and Interventions for Depression and Anxiety Disorders* by Robert L. Leahy and Stephen J. Holland. Copyright 2000 by Robert L. Leahy and Stephen J. Holland. Permission to photocopy this form is granted to purchasers of this book for personal use only (see copyright page for details).

FORM 2.6. Patient's Weekly Planning Schedule: Predicting Pleasure and Mastery (p. 2 of 3)

Hour	Monday	Tuesday	Wednesday	Thursday	Friday	Saturday	Sunday
11							
12 noon							
1 P.M.							
2							
3							
4							
5							
6							

(cont.)

FORM 2.6. Patient's Weekly Planning Schedule: Predicting Pleasure and Mastery (p. 3 of 3)

Hour	Monday	Tuesday	Wednesday	Thursday	Friday	Saturday	Sunday
7							
8							
9							
10							
11							
12 midnight							
1–6 A.M.							

TABLE 2.4. Summary of Behavioral Techniques for Depression

Technique	Example
Identifying goals	Help the patient to develop short-term and long-term behavioral goals that he or she wishes to accomplish.
Reward planning	Have the patient list positive behaviors enjoyed in the past or anticipated in the future.
Activity scheduling	Have the patient schedule rewarding activities, rating each activity for predicted pleasure and mastery, and then self-monitor actual activities.
Graded task assignment	Encourage the patient to self-assign increasingly demanding and challenging positive behaviors.
Self-reward	Help the patient to increase use of positive self-statements and identify tangible reinforcers that may be associated with positive behavior.
Decreasing rumination and excessive self-focus	Encourage the patient to develop distracting and active behaviors to replace passivity and rumination.
Social skills training	Help the patient to increase positive and rewarding behaviors toward others, such as complimenting and reinforcing other people; to increase self-reliability; to improve personal hygiene, appearance, approach behavior, etc.; and to decrease complaining and negative social behavior.
Assertiveness training	Help the patient to increase responsible positive assertion—reinforcing others, giving compliments, making requests, and knowing when to escalate assertion.
Problem-solving training	Train the patient in problem recognition, definition, identifying resources, generating possible solutions, developing plans, and carrying out solutions.

sumptions, and schemas. Table B.3 in Appendix B, and the CD-ROM accompanying this book, provide a fairly extensive list of cognitive techniques that are applicable to depression. Indeed, many of the behavioral interventions listed in Table 2.4 may be integrated with a cognitive orientation (e.g., activity scheduling can be treated as hypothesis testing).

As indicated earlier in this chapter, depressed patients show greater vulnerability to negative life events and recurrence of depression if they continue to have distorted automatic thoughts, to endorse maladaptive assumptions, and to maintain negative schemas. Therefore, all three of these types of cognitive distortions must be identified and challenged in therapy. Once a patient has been introduced to the concept of distorted automatic thoughts and has been shown how to identify and categorize these, the therapist works with him or her in sessions to challenge these thoughts, using many different techniques. Examples of these techniques include examining the costs and benefits of a thought; examining the evidence for and against a thought; using "vertical descent" (i.e., asking, "Why would it bother you if such and such were true? What would happen next? Why would that bother you?" and so on); applying the "double standard" (i.e., asking, "Would you apply the same standards to other people as you do to yourself? Why/why not?"); and many others (again, see Table B.3 in Appendix B and the CD-ROM for a full listing). As the patient is learning to do this, he or she can use the Patient's Daily Record of Dysfunctional Automatic Thoughts (Form 2.7) to record such thoughts and their accompanying emotions, to evaluate his or her confidence in the accuracy in these thoughts, and to record rational responses to the thoughts. (The Patient's Event–Mood–Thought Record in Appendix B [Form B.4] can also be used to record thoughts and emotions.) Maladaptive assumptions and negative schemas can and should also be challenged in many ways, but because they occur at deeper cognitive levels than automatic thoughts, the patient will usually need even more guidance from the therapist in addressing them. Table 2.5 illustrates how the maladaptive assumption "If someone doesn't like me, then I'm worthless" might be tested and challenged in therapy. Table 2.6 does the same for the negative schema "I'm a rotten person," which was endorsed by a depressed man who had been physically abused as a child by his father.

Troubleshooting Problems in Therapy

Hopelessness

In evaluating hopelessness, the therapist should ask the patient to specify exactly what he or she believes will not improve and why. For example, a woman whose severe depression and obsessiveness had not remitted for several years claimed that she would always be depressed, that she would never stop ruminating, and that she had missed all of her opportunities to have a meaningful relationship with a man. Specifically, she expected that her self-criticism, lack of concentration, and regrets would continue forever, thereby making life unbearable. Since this patient had been in therapy for several years and had tried some medications, it might have been easy for the therapist to buy into her hopelessness. However, following the cognitive model, the therapist decided to treat her hopeless predictions as hypotheses to be tested. For example, her idea that her mood would always be negative was tested in the session by identifying instances when her mood was better, when she laughed, and when she began to challenge a negative thought.

THERAPIST: Have you noticed some change in your mood during today's session?

PATIENT: Yes, I guess I felt a little bit better. But it was only for a few minutes.

THERAPIST: What if you were able to do some of these things on your own—perhaps a little bit every day—perhaps even every hour?

PATIENT: I guess I'd feel better than I do now.

FORM 2.7. Patient's Daily Record of Dysfunctional Automatic Thoughts

Patient's Name: _____ Date: _____

Time	Situation: Specify what happened, where, and who was involved.	Emotions: Specify emotion and rate its intensity (0–100%).	Automatic thoughts: Write automatic thoughts that preceded emotions; rate each for confidence in accuracy (0–100%).	Rational response: Write rational responses to automatic thoughts; rate each for confidence in accuracy (0–100%).	Outcome: Now rate present confidence in accuracy of original thought, and present intensity of emotion (0–100%).	
					Thought	Emotion

TABLE 2.5. Testing and Challenging a Maladaptive Assumption: "If Someone Doesn't Like Me, Then I'm Worthless"

Technique	Questions to test and challenge the assumption
Cost–benefit	What are the costs and benefits of this assumption? What are the costs and benefits of caring less about whether people like you? What would you be able to do, think, feel, and communicate if you cared less about whether people like you?
Semantic technique	How would you define "liking"? What is 100%, 50%, 20%, and 0% liking? How would you define "worthless" and "worthwhile"? What is 100%, 50%, 20%, and 0% worthless or worthwhile? Can you point to the particular part of someone (or behavior) that is totally worthless? Would anyone disagree with your definitions? What do you make of that?
Distinguishing behaviors from people	What are some worthwhile behaviors? Have you ever done a single thing that is worthwhile? Have you completely stopped engaging in worthwhile behaviors? Is there anyone that you know who does everything in a worthless way? If you do some things that are worthwhile, then how can you be worthless?
Examining evidence for and against the assumption	What is the evidence for and against the idea that you are worthless? What is the quality of the evidence? Would a good lawyer, defending you, think that this is good evidence?
Logical analysis	How does someone's not liking you make you worthless? If that person then likes you, then are you worthwhile? If one person likes you and another doesn't, are you worthless or worthwhile?
Double-standard technique	Do you know anyone who is liked by everyone? If not, then does that mean that everyone is worthless? Think of some people you admire and like. Does anyone dislike them? Would you consider them worthless? Why do you apply a different standard to yourself than you do to others?
Revision of assumption	Can you think of a more practical, less negative assumption? (Possible examples: "If someone doesn't like me, maybe we have different standards, styles, or tastes," "If someone doesn't like me, then maybe they don't know me very well.")

TABLE 2.6. Testing and Challenging a Negative Schema: "I'm a Rotten Person"

Technique	Questions to test the schema
Identifying examples of schema	What are some examples of how you view yourself negatively? If we assume that you have been looking for evidence that you are rotten, how has this distorted your view of yourself? Has this schema (concept of yourself) made you ignore and discount positive information about yourself?
Identifying avoidance and compensation strategies	Have you avoided certain things—work, relationships, or anything—because you thought you were rotten? Have you tried to compensate for the idea that you are rotten by being especially pleasing, nonassertive, or self-defeating?
Cost–benefit analysis	What are the costs and benefits of viewing yourself as a rotten person? What would change in your life if you thought better of yourself?
Activating early memories	Can you recall when you first thought this? [This patient replied, "When my father locked me in the basement."] If that happened today, would you think it reflected something about you or something about your father?
Imagery restructuring	Try to recall the memory of your father beating you and then locking you in the basement. Except now you're strong like you are today and you can fight back. Can you create an image of you fighting back against your father? What are some assertive things that you can say to him?
Writing letters to the source	Write an assertive, angry letter to your father—which you don't have to send him. Tell him that what he did was wrong, and describe how angry you are. Tell him that he'll never do this to you again.
Examining the evidence for and against the schema	What is the evidence for and against the idea that you are a rotten person? What is the most vivid memory or image that you have of something good that you did? [The patient was a veterinarian. He recalled saving a child's bunny.] If you saw a man taking care of a child's bunny, what thoughts would you have about him?
Rewriting a life script	Imagine if your father had been kind, loving, and supportive, and had never hit you or locked you in a basement. What kinds of things would you think about yourself today that are different?
Developing nurturant self-statements	Let's imagine that you have decided to take over because your father was such a lousy father. You are now taking care of this child—you. Write out as many loving, caring, supportive, and accepting statements as you can—to yourself.

Technique	Questions to test the schema
Seeing self from (benevolent) others' perspective	Are there any people who do not think that you are a rotten person? Make a list of those people who like you. List all the things that you can think of that they like about you. Ask them what they like about you. How does this reconcile with the idea that you are a "rotten person"?
Revising the schema	What would be a new, more positive, more realistic way of viewing yourself—including the good and bad things about you, and including your ability to grow and change?

THERAPIST: If you can feel better in a session because you challenge your thoughts, and if you notice that your mood changes with the activities that you pursue, perhaps those might be the keys to long-term change.

PATIENT: But I've had therapy before, and I've taken medications.

THERAPIST: You've had a different kind of therapy, and you have only just begun to pursue medication possibilities. Is it possible that changing your thoughts and changing your biochemistry could have an effect?

PATIENT: I guess it's possible. But there's no guarantee.

THERAPIST: That's right. There's no guarantee—either way. Why don't we see what happens?

Although this patient still maintained some hopelessness, she was more skeptical about her depression than before. In fact, her skepticism about therapy and medication was used as a reinforcement for challenging hopelessness.

THERAPIST: Just as you're skeptical about therapy, why not be skeptical about your hopelessness, too?

PATIENT: I never thought of it that way.

THERAPIST: There's always a different way to think about anything. Let's agree that you will maintain a healthy skepticism—a "wait and see" attitude.

The therapist and the psychopharmacologist worked together to coordinate this patient's therapy. Changes in medication were viewed as experiments, and self-critical and regretful statements were treated as hypotheses. The therapist told the patient that, along with her depression, she had an obsessive–compulsive personality structure, given to doubts, qualifications, and second-guessing. (Ironically, this was helpful to her as a lawyer, but it made her daily life difficult.) Rather than trying to change her style of thinking, the therapist indicated to her that she would probably have to accept a certain amount of doubt and qualification as part of her cognitive nature. Consequently, when she made decisions, she would *inevitably* have doubts, simply because she was extremely adept at seeing both sides of an issue. These doubts were not evidence that she made the wrong decision (as she almost always believed), but simply part of the "noise" of her style of thinking. This normalization of a problematic style proved immensely helpful to her, since she could now accept her obsessive doubting as coming with the territory (of being a brilliant lawyer) and did not imply anything negative about the "real world." After several months, her hopelessness lifted, her depression and regrets abated to a large extent, and (fortuitously) she became engaged. It is important to note that her depression and hopelessness lessened *before* the engagement, so this was not a Cinderella story.

Self-Criticism for Being Depressed

Many depressed patients criticize themselves for their depression; they say such things as "I shouldn't be depressed," or "I should have been able to solve my problems on my own." Such a patient is locked in a self-maintaining cognitive loop—"I'm depressed because I'm self-critical, I criticize myself for my depression, and I'm depressed because I'm depressed." It is essential to help the patient recognize that he or she did not choose to be depressed; that depression often has a biological component; that self-criticism does not help anyone snap out of it; that taking responsibility for depression means accepting the fact of depression and pursuing treatment; and that the hopelessness, avoidance, and procrastination exhibited by the patient are to a large extent symptoms of depression.

Noncompliance with Homework

Typical of depression is this belief: "Nothing will work, so why should I bother to carry out cognitive-behavioral homework assignments?" In such a case, the therapist should first elicit the patient's reasons for noncompliance (e.g., "I didn't think it would work," "I don't have the time," "I would be embarrassed to show you what I did," "Homework will just remind me of my problems," "I shouldn't have to do homework," or "I don't like being told what to do"). The noncompliance should then be directly addressed by taking each of the reasons for noncompliance and treating them as automatic thoughts to be evaluated:

- What are the costs and benefits of doing homework?
- What's a better alternative?
- What is the evidence for and against the idea that homework won't work?
- What homework would you assign yourself?
- What would you recommend to a friend in your position?
- How is your pessimism regarding homework similar to other thoughts you have about getting better?
- What reason would you have to believe that the therapist would think less of you if you didn't do the homework a specific way?
- Would you be willing to experiment with a little bit of homework?

Compliance may be increased by modeling the homework in the session, anticipating reasons not to do homework and having the patient examine or challenge these thoughts, asking the patient to do homework on reasons not to do homework, having the patient assign his or her own homework, and/or giving smaller or shorter assignments. As with all assignments, the therapist should offer a rationale for the homework and reinforce it when it is done.

Problem-Solving Deficits

Depression is viewed in some models as a deficit in problem-solving ability or in the use of problem solving (see D'Zurilla, 1988; Nezu & Nezu, 1989a, 1989b, 1989c). Life events or conflicts that are currently having an impact on the patient may be conceptualized as problems to solve. The patient may be trained in a specific problem-solving approach (Nezu & Nezu, 1989a, 1989b, 1989c; see Table 2.7).

Basic Health Maintenance

Educating patients in basic health maintenance (in cases where this seems necessary) may focus on elementary behavioral skills, such as maintaining hygiene, proper sleep habits, adequate diet, and attention to medical problems. With a severely depressed patient, inadequate bathing and inappropriate dress may lead to decrease in rewards in the environment. Insomnia is a frequent correlate of depression and may be treated with appropriate sleep hygiene. (Form 2.8 is a patient information handout on insomnia.) Many depressed patients forego adequate diet, either because of lack of appetite or lack of interest in maintaining their well-being. A therapist should not hesitate to encourage a patient to eat small amounts of food frequently, even if the patient lacks appetite. Finally, many depressed patients do not obtain proper medical evaluations, or, if they require medication for health problems (e.g., for hypertension or diabetes), they are often care-

---

TABLE 2.7. Problem-Solving Approach to Depression

 1. Identify problem to be solved.
 2. Examine costs and benefits of solving problem.
 3. List all resources and information available.
 4. Generate as many possible solutions, without evaluating these solutions.
 5. Rank order the most desirable to least desirable solutions.
 6. Develop a plan of action based on the best solution.
    a. Identify each step in the sequence.
    b. Identify resources available for each step.
 7. Schedule the first step(s).
 8. Evaluate the outcome.
 9. Revise the plan, if necessary.
10. Reward yourself for carrying out the steps.

FORM 2.8. Information for Patients about Insomnia

One of the more troubling experiences for depressed and anxious patients is insomnia. Some people experience difficulty falling asleep (onset insomnia or anxiety), while others wake several times during the early morning hours (early-morning insomnia or depression). Usually, as depression and anxiety lift, insomnia decreases and sleep is more restful. However, a number of cognitive-behavioral interventions may assist in the treatment of insomnia.

Before you attempt any interventions, you should record some baseline information about the number of hours per night that you sleep and the number of times that you wake. You can then compare your sleep over the next month or two with the baseline measure.

- **Develop regular sleep times.** Go to bed and get out of bed at about the same time, regardless of how tired you are. Also avoid naps.

- **Use your bed only for sleep and sex.** Insomnia is often the result of increased arousal preceding bedtime and while lying awake in bed. Many who have insomnia use the bed for reading, talking on the phone, and worrying; as a result, the bed is associated with arousal (anxiety). Read or talk on the phone in another room. If you have friends who call late at night, tell them not to call after a specific hour. Avoid anxiety arousal during the hour before bedtime (for instance, avoid arguments and challenging tasks).

- Sleep is often disturbed by **urinary urgency**. Reduce or eliminate liquid intake several hours before bedtime. Avoid all caffeine products, heavy foods, and liquor. If necessary, consult a nutritionist to assist in planning a change in diet.

- **Do not try to fall asleep**—this will only increase your frustration and anxiety. Paradoxically, a very effective way of increasing sleep is to practice giving up trying to fall asleep. You can say to yourself, "I'll give up trying to get to sleep and just concentrate on the relaxing feelings in my body."

- If you are lying awake at night for more than 15 minutes, get up and go in the other room. **Write down your negative automatic thoughts and challenge them.** Typical automatic thoughts are "I'll never get to sleep," "If I don't get enough sleep, I won't be able to function," "I need to get to sleep immediately," and "I'll get sick from not getting enough sleep." The most likely consequence of not getting enough sleep is that you will feel tired and irritable. Although these are uncomfortable inconveniences, they are not catastrophic.

- Your therapist can teach **systematic relaxation and breathing,** which will enhance your restfulness. Try to make your mind go blank. Count backward by threes from 100 or 1,000, as slowly as possible. Visualize a relaxing scene—for example, snow falling on a house in the woods at night.

- Because your disturbed sleep patterns have taken a long time to learn, it may take you a while to unlearn them. **Do not expect immediate results.**

less about compliance. In some cases, this lack of attention to health problems may reflect a subintentional suicide orientation and should be addressed accordingly. Similarly, potentially dangerous sexual behavior, illicit drug use, overuse of prescription medication, and hazardous driving may reflect a subintentional or even active suicidal orientation. A clinician should evaluate a patient for all of these risks.

Communication and Social Skills

As noted earlier, depression is often associated with deficits in social behavior. A clinician should note a patient's social skills in terms of appropriate greeting, attire, ability to listen, ability to reward others, responsibility in relationships, management of finances, and tendency to complain or punish others. Since any of these deficits may hinder the acquisition of interpersonal rewards, they may be addressed directly through the behavioral component of therapy. Assertiveness training is often useful with a depressed patient; it may be structured by having the patient develop a hierarchy of least to most difficult situations for assertion and practice these skills in behavioral rehearsal in the session and *in vivo* outside sessions.

Communication training is frequently indicated for patients whose interpersonal relationships are strained—especially married or cohabitating patients. Here the patient may be trained in active listening skills as well as in effective speaker skills, such as editing statements and clarifying feelings (see Baucom & Epstein, 1990; Leahy, 1996). Mutual problem solving is useful with married or cohabitating patients. This involves one partner's volunteering to raise the need for a problem-solving session and follow through in a structured format of acknowledging partial responsibility for the problem, brainstorming, and developing plans (Jacobson & Margolin, 1979). Furthermore, many patients need training in negotiation skills, whether in their personal relationships or in other relationships (especially at work). The excellent book *Getting to Yes*, by Fisher and Ury (1981), is a readable and invaluable guide to practical issues in negotiation.

Marital or Relationship Discord

Since marital or relationship problems are often the center of depression for many patients, the therapist may consider a conjoint format of therapy a more desirable approach. Beach et al.'s (1990) manual on marital/couple therapy, as well as Baucom and Epstein's (1990) outstanding text and Dattilio and Padesky's (1990) manual, are helpful in developing a conjoint therapy approach to depression. Cognitive-behavioral interventions involve training the partners in attending to, labeling, and reinforcing positives in each other; helping them develop reward menus for each other; helping them schedule pleasure days; teaching sensate focus; teaching positive assertiveness; training partners in communication skills (see above); identifying and modifying dysfunctional or irrational automatic thoughts, maladaptive assumptions, and negative schemas; and teaching the use of time-out procedures as well as self-instructions for anger. In addition, many couples are helped by learning to accept the problems that exist, rather than working too hard at trying to make everything right. These interventions are described in more detail in the references cited above, as well as in the excellent chapter by Christensen et al. (1995).

Inoculation against Future Depressive Episodes

Since many depressed patients are vulnerable to recurrences of episodes, each patient should be cautioned about the possibility of recurrence. Many patients may benefit from maintenance treatment with antidepressant medication after the initial episode has subsided. Other patients may benefit from preparation for future episodes. A clinician and patient may review the precipitating factors of current and/or previous episodes, to determine whether a pattern exists. For example, some patients are especially vulnerable to interpersonal losses, which may activate self-schemas such as helplessness and worthlessness.

The inoculation phase includes a list of typical signs of depression and coping strategies for each cluster of symptoms. For example, a patient who withdraws and becomes passive during the early phase of depression can be given a coping strategy of behavioral activation, contacting the therapist, and getting out of his or her apartment. Patients with suicidal histories are especially in need of inoculation therapy. Here they may be asked to return to their past suicidal ideation and practice how they would respond differently, now that they have had the benefit of therapy.

Phasing Out Therapy

Abrupt discontinuation of weekly therapy is less desirable than phasing back to less frequent, but regular, sessions—that is, biweekly, monthly, or every 3 months. During the phasing-out period, the patient should be encouraged to develop his or her own homework assignments, since continuation of homework is a good predictor of maintaining improvement. The patient should also be told that he or she may call the therapist and come back for therapy, if depression recurs. Self-monitoring may be enhanced by giving the patient a list of depressive or anxiety symptoms and copies of the BDI or BAI.

In this section, we have outlined the basic elements of a treatment plan for major depression. The clinician should determine the specific areas for intervention by evaluating the patient's individual presentation of depression. For example, many patients are able to overcome the vegetative symptoms of depression (e.g., loss of appetite and energy, sleep problems, and anhedonia) by using antidepressant medication. In these cases, it may be more helpful for the therapist to address issues of hopelessness, self-criticism, and underlying cognitive distortions (automatic thoughts, assumptions, and schemas) that contribute to the depressive vulnerability. Table 2.8 gives examples of specific targeted symptoms and the kinds of questions and interventions that might be helpful for these symptoms.

TABLE 2.8. Targeted Depressive Symptoms and Interventions

Symptom	Questions and interventions
Self-criticism	What are the costs and benefits of criticizing yourself? Of accepting yourself? Of trying to improve? Specifically, what are you saying about yourself? What standard are you using? How would you define "failure" and "success"? Do you engage in any behaviors that succeed? Even partly? How would you compare yourself to the biggest failure, the average person, and the perfect person? Would you be as critical of someone else who did what you do? Why/why not?
Inactivity	What alternatives are you considering? What are the costs and benefits of each alternative? (Use reward planning, activity scheduling, graded task assignment.) Do your moods vary with activity? With whom you're interacting? (Develop short-term and long-term goals.)
Lack of pleasure	Are there some activities that you enjoy more than others? (Consider medication, reward planning, activity scheduling, graded task assignment.) Are you discounting the activities that you engage in? Do you have "rules" that you apply to pleasure—for example, "I can't enjoy anything if I'm alone"?
Social withdrawal	What are the costs and benefits of interacting with people? Are you saying to yourself, "I'm a burden," or "I have nothing to offer"? When you are with people, are you assuming that they will reject you, or that they will see that you are depressed? Do you complain too much when you are with people? Could you focus on rewarding and empathizing with others? What do you predict would happen if you planned some activities with others?
Sadness	Are you ruminating and focusing on negative memories? Are you spending excessive periods of time alone, inactive? Try to recall pleasurable behaviors and experiences. Identify automatic thoughts and challenge them.
Indecisiveness	What are the alternatives? Are you considering too few alternatives? Weigh the costs and benefits of each. Are you assuming that you have to find a perfect solution? Do you criticize yourself if things do not work out exactly as planned? Examine the costs and benefits of trying to be absolutely certain versus trying to get on with your life. Are you using your emotions to guide you (e.g., "I feel lousy; therefore, there aren't any good alternatives")? What advice would you give a friend? If something doesn't work out, what is the difference between regret and learning from the experience?
Suicidality	What are some reasons for living? If you were not depressed, what would be some pleasurable and meaningful things that you could enjoy? What is the evidence for and against your hopelessness? Before you were depressed, what are some things that you enjoyed? (Establish suicide contract; consider commitment; enlist assistance of family members; reduce opportunities; eliminate weapons or large supplies of medications.)

(cont.)

TABLE 2.8 *(cont.)*

Symptom	Questions and interventions
Negative life events	Exactly what happened? What negative automatic thoughts did this generate? Are you fortunetelling, personalizing, catastrophizing, etc.? (Examine the evidence, look at the event on a continuum, divide up the responsibility, learn from the experience, etc.). What can you still do, even though this event occurred? How will you feel about it in a week, month, or year? If someone else had this problem, what advice would you give him or her? What are some new goals that you can focus on? What are some positive events that could occur in the future?

CASE EXAMPLE

Session 1

Assessment

Symptoms and comorbid conditions

Evaluation of suicidal risk

Medication evaluation

Nancy was a 34-year-old married female middle manager with a history of alcohol dependence, cocaine abuse, and depression. Her current episode of depression had begun 2 years prior to therapy, and she had been hospitalized for alcohol abuse 1 year prior to intake. Nancy complained of depression, anxiety, procrastination, hopelessness, insomnia, low self-esteem, loneliness, low sexual desire, lack of social skills, lack of assertiveness, and regrets. Her BDI score was high (28), and she had elevated scores on the SCL-90-R on depression, obsessive–compulsiveness, and interpersonal sensitivity. On the SCID-II she had elevated scores on obsessive–compulsive, self-defeating, histrionic, and borderline personalities, although clinical inquiry ruled out borderline personality disorder as a diagnosis. Her Locke-Wallace Marital Adjustment Test score of 124 revealed a high level of marital satisfaction, although she complained about her lack of sexual desire. The diagnosis was as follows: MDD, recurrent, and mixed personality disorder (histrionic and obsessive–compulsive), with alcohol dependence and cocaine abuse in remission. Nancy indicated that she had had thoughts of suicide in the past and was still having such thoughts, but that she never had any strong intent or plans to harm herself. Consequently, she was not viewed as presenting a serious suicidal risk.

Nancy had been taking nortriptyline (Pamelor, 75 mg) for the previous year and had tried several other antidepressant and anxiolytic medications. During the course of treatment, Nancy told her physician that she wished to discontinue medication so that she could pursue having a baby.

Session 2

Socialization to treatment

Review of diagnosis

Development of goal list

The therapist provided Nancy with a copy of David Burns's (1980) *Feeling Good: The New Mood Therapy* and explained to her the nature of cognitive-behavioral therapy. The therapist indicated how thoughts, feelings, and facts differ; stressed the importance of homework; and noted the emphasis on how one functions in the here and now. The therapist indicated that her evaluations indicated that Nancy was experiencing significant depression, but that it might be treatable by a combination of cognitive-behavioral treatment and medication. Nancy and her therapist agreed to the following goals: decreasing her depression, self-criticism, need for approval, and hopelessness, and increasing her self-esteem, self-help, energy level, assertiveness, and independence.

Sessions 3–4

Identifying and categorizing automatic thoughts

Insomnia treatment

Reward planning, activity scheduling, graded task assignments

The initial interventions focused on identifying and categorizing Nancy's distorted automatic thoughts, with the instruction that she should write down any of her thoughts when she felt especially low. She was given the Patient's Daily Record of Dysfunctional Automatic Thoughts (Form 2.7) to record these thoughts. Nancy's insomnia was treated by having her increase her exercise during the day, and eliminate naps on weekends, advising her to go to bed at the same time and get up at the same time, and instructing her to write down any negative thoughts about sleep disturbance. She was also given the patient information handout on insomnia (Form 2.8). Her behavioral level was increased by the use of reward planning, activity scheduling, and graded task assignment, with Nancy gradually increasing her level of activity by seeing friends, going to museums, increasing exercise, and pursuing reading.

Session 5–7

Social skills training

Reward planning, activity scheduling, graded task assignment

Nancy's social anxiety and concern about approval were addressed via a structured antiavoidance approach. She was instructed to track her rewards and compliments of others, to note her use of inquiry and empathy with colleagues at work, and to increase her assertiveness and limit setting with people. She continued with reward planning and activity scheduling, attempting to increase the frequency of activities associated with pleasure and

Monitoring and challenging negative thoughts

to decrease activities associated with sadness. She also continued to use the Patient's Daily Record of Dysfunctional Automatic Thoughts (Form 2.7) to monitor her negative thinking, and to challenge her thoughts by examining the evidence for and against her thoughts and by considering more positive alternative interpretations. In addition, she found the double-standard technique ("Would you think less of someone else who did what you do? Why/why not?") helpful.

Sessions 8–12

Behavioral activation and assertiveness

Identifying negative automatic thoughts, maladaptive assumptions, and negative schemas

Nancy continued with behavioral activation, graded task assignments, and assertiveness. Her therapist began to focus more on the content of her thinking when her mood changed by having her record her negative thoughts between sessions. Nancy's most common distorted automatic thoughts were "I'm not doing enough," "I'm lazy," "I'm worthless," "I'll lose my job," and "People won't respect me." Her maladaptive assumptions were "I should do anything to be liked," "I should be very successful," and "I should be more productive than other people at work." Her underlying self-schemas were that she was a failure, worthless, and unlovable, while her schemas of others were that they were rejecting and evaluating. She attempted to compensate for her low self-esteem by seeking approval, and she avoided rejection by not pursuing more challenging work.

Cognitive techniques for challenging thoughts, assumptions, and schemas

The therapist assisted her in identifying her automatic thoughts, categorizing them, and examining the evidence for and against her thoughts. Her assumptions were examined by using vertical descent ("What would happen if someone didn't like you?"), by examining the costs and benefits of her assumptions, by using the double-standard technique, and by assigning behaviors (e.g., assertion) that conflicted with her assumptions. Her self-schemas were examined by using the semantic technique ("How would you define 'failure' and 'success'?"); using the continuum technique ("Place yourself and others along a 100-point continuum of success and failure"); examining her discounting of positives; and evaluating how she had learned in her family from her father that great success was the only thing that mattered, and from her abusive mother that she was unlovable. In addition, Nancy and the therapist "diversified" her criteria of valuing herself by placing less relative emphasis on great prestige in a job and more emphasis on other factors, such as her relationship with her husband, her willingness to work hard and overcome problems,

Developing new schemas, assumptions, and thoughts

the ability to be a friend, her interests in cultural activities and learning, and her interpersonal warmth and caring. After 5 sessions, her BDI score was reduced to 8; it had dropped to 3 after 12 sessions, at which time therapy was phased back to once every 3 weeks.

Sessions 13–16

Phasing back treatment

Developing new schemas and assumptions

After therapy was phased back to once every 3 weeks, the emphasis was on daily records of dysfunctional thoughts and on assertiveness at work. As part of her improvement, Nancy described herself as having a "new persona"—as being someone who now valued herself for a variety of qualities, who did not overvalue others and their approval, and who was willing to be assertive. During the course of her treatment, her psychopharmacologist reduced her Pamelor to 20 mg, and eventually discontinued medication altogether because of Nancy's desire to have a child. Nancy terminated therapy after 16 sessions; her final BDI score was 3.

DETAILED TREATMENT PLAN FOR DEPRESSION

Treatment Reports

Tables 2.9 and 2.10 are designed to help you in writing managed care treatment reports for depressed patients. Table 2.9 shows sample specific symptoms; select the symptoms that are appropriate for your patient. (Readers may also wish to consult the *Clinician's Thesaurus* [Zuckerman, 1995] for a large collection of additional words and phrases.) Also, be sure to specify the nature of the patient's impairments, including any dysfunction in academic, work, family, or social areas. Table 2.10 lists sample goals and matching interventions; again, select those that are appropriate for the patient.

Session-by-Session Treatment Options

Table 2.11 is a detailed, session-by-session outline of treatment options for depression, which can be used in report writing as well as in the planning of therapy. Options for 16 treatment sessions are presented. Once again, choose those options that are appropriate for a particular patient.

TABLE 2.9. Sample Symptoms for Major Depression

Affective Symptoms
Depressed mood
Irritable mood
Anhedonia
Low motivation

Cognitive Symptoms
Feelings of worthlessness
Excessive guilt
Impaired concentration
Difficulty making decisions

Vegetative Symptoms
Lack of interest in usual activities
Loss of appetite or increased appetite
Weight loss or gain
Insomnia or hypersomnia
Psychomotor agitation or retardation
Fatigue
Low energy

Other Symptoms
Suicidal ideation (specify whether plan is present and whether there have been prior attempts)
Thoughts of death
Specify how long symptoms have been present
Specify whether there have been prior depressive episodes

TABLE 2.10. Sample Treatment Goals and Interventions for Major Depression

Treatment goals	Interventions
Eliminating suicidal ideation	Cognitive restructuring, removing access to means, setting up a contract to contact therapist
Engaging in one rewarding activity/day	Reward planning, activity scheduling, graded task assignment
Reducing negative automatic thoughts	Cognitive restructuring, distraction
Sleeping 7–8 hours/night	Relaxation, insomnia treatment plan
Engaging in one assertive behavior/day	Assertion training
Increasing social contacts (three/week)	Social skills training, reward planning, activity scheduling
Increasing self-reward for positive behaviors (one/day)	Reward planning, self-reward
Reporting a decreased belief in assumption of need for perfection (<10%) (or other assumptions—specify)	Cognitive restructuring, behavioral experiments
Modifying schema of worthlessness (or other schemas—specify)	Cognitive restructuring, developmental analysis
Eliminating impairment (specify—depending on impairments, this may be several goals)	Cognitive restructuring, problem-solving training, or other skills training (specify)
Eliminating all depressive symptoms (BDI score <10 for 1 month)	All of the above
Acquiring relapse prevention skills	Reviewing and practicing techniques as necessary

TABLE 2.11. Session-by-Session Treatment Options for Major Depression

Session 1

Assessment

  Ascertain presenting problems
  Inquire regarding all symptoms
  Assess for cognitive, behavioral, and interpersonal deficits (Form 2.1)
  Assess impairment in social, educational and occupational functioning
  Administer standard battery of intake measures (see Form 2.2)
  Evaluate for comorbid conditions (e.g., anxiety disorders)
  Evaluate for suicidal risk (Form 2.3)
  Evaluate substance use; evaluate need for counseling or detoxification if patient has
    substance abuse or dependence
  Assess need for medication

Homework

  Have the patient begin reading David Burns's *Feeling Good* or *The Feeling Good
  Handbook*

Session 2

Socialization to Treatment

  Inform patient of diagnosis
  Develop list of treatment goals
  Provide patient with information handouts on depression (Form 2.4) and on cognitive-
    behavioral therapy in general (Form B.1, Appendix B)
  Evaluate homework

Behavioral Interventions

  Identify behavioral targets (behavioral deficits and excesses) (see Table 2.1)
  Instruct patient in reward planning and activity scheduling (Forms 2.5, 2.6)
  Encourage patient to increase self-reward
  Encourage patient to decrease rumination time and passive/asocial behavior
  Evaluate need for patient to modify personal hygiene, grooming, diet, bingeing, etc.
  Evaluate/treat insomnia (provide patient with handout—Form 2.8)

Cognitive Interventions

  Train patient in relationship between automatic thoughts and feelings
  Train patient in categorizing distorted automatic thoughts (see Form B.2, Appendix B)
  Elicit and challenge automatic thoughts in session
  Evaluate reasons for and challenge hopelessness
  Establish no-suicide contract
  Challenge antipleasure thoughts

Medication

  Consider medication (if patient is not already using it)
  Evaluate side effects
  Evaluate need to increase dosage

Homework

  Have patient record thoughts and moods, categorize automatic thoughts, begin self-directed
    reward planning and activity scheduling, increase self-reward, and use graded task assignment

(cont.)

TABLE 2.11 *(cont.)*

Sessions 3–4

Assessment
   Evaluate homework
   Evaluate depression (BDI) and anxiety (BAI)
   Evaluate suicidality
   Evaluate any side effects from medication

Behavioral Interventions
   Teach and practice assertion skills in session
   Increase rewarding behavior toward others
   Increase positive social contacts—initiating contact, building support network
   Evaluate self-reward
   Introduce problem-solving skills (Table 2.7)

Cognitive Interventions
   Teach use of Patient's Daily Record of Dysfunctional Automatic Thoughts (Form 2.7)
   Use specific cognitive techniques to help patient challenge negative automatic thoughts (see
      Table B.3, Appendix B, for a full list)
   Identify and challenge underlying maladaptive assumptions (again, see Table B.3 for a list of
      techniques)

Medication
   Evaluate side effects
   Evaluate need to increase dosage
   If no improvement, either increase dosage, add another medication, or change class of
      medication (consider the need to taper or discontinue one class of medication when
      adding another class)

Homework
Have patient use Patient's Daily Record of Dysfunctional Automatic Thoughts (Form 2.7);
assign specific cognitive techniques for challenging automatic thoughts and assumptions; have
patient continue with graded task assignment, social skills training, reward planning, activity
scheduling, problem solving

Sessions 5–7

Assessment
   Evaluate homework
   Evaluate depression (BDI) and anxiety (BAI)
   Evaluate suicidality

Behavioral Interventions
   Continue to teach and practice problem-solving skills
   Train patient in communication skills (active listening, editing communication, empathy)
   Continue graded task assignment
   Continue assertion and social skills training

Cognitive Interventions
   Identify and challenge automatic thoughts that are particularly difficult for patient
   Continue identifying and challenging maladaptive assumptions
   Begin to identify and challenge negative schemas

Medication

Evaluate side effects

Evaluate need to increase dosage

If no improvement, either increase dosage, add another medication, or change medication class

Homework

Have patient practice using various techniques to challenge assumptions and schemas; continue graded task assignment, assertiveness, self-reward; and continue practicing communication and problem-solving skills

Sessions 8–12

Assessment

Evaluate homework

Evaluate depression (BDI) and anxiety (BAI)

Evaluate suicidality

Behavioral Interventions

Continue to teach and practice problem-solving skills

Continue to train patient in communication skills (active listening, editing communication, empathy)

Continue graded task assignment

Continue assertion and social skills training

Cognitive Intervention

Continue identifying and challenging difficult automatic thoughts and assumptions

Review old automatic thoughts (from previous sessions) and see if they still make sense to patient

Examine origin of schemas and evaluate how schemas have affected important experiences throughout life

Use empty-chair role plays to help patient challenge negative schemas and people who have been the source of these schemas

Help patient develop more realistic assumptions and schemas

Help patient develop positive self-statements and "bill of rights"

Medication

Evaluate side effects

Evaluate need to increase dosage

If no improvement, either increase dosage, add another medication, or change medication class

Homework

Have patient continue identifying and challenging automatic thoughts, assumptions, and schemas; develop list of new, adaptive assumptions and schemas; write out "bill of rights"; continue graded task assignment, assertiveness, and self-reward; and continue practicing communication and problem-solving skills

Session 13–16 (Scheduled Biweekly or Monthly)

Assessment

Evaluate homework

Evaluate depression (BDI) and anxiety (BAI)

Evaluate suicidality

Evaluate any side effects from medication

(cont.)

TABLE 2.11 *(cont.)*

Behavioral Interventions

    Continue to teach and practice problem-solving skills

    Continue graded task assignment

    Continue assertion and social skills training

Cognitive Interventions

    Help patient to continue developing more realistic assumptions and schemas

    Have patient continue work on positive self-statements and "bill of rights"

    Review old automatic thoughts (from previous sessions and from homework assignments) and continue challenging them

    Plan phase-out of therapy

    Have patient identify which interventions were helpful and which were not

    Have patient examine previous episodes of depression and describe how he or she will handle depression in the future

Homework

    Develop plans for how problems can be handled in future

    Have patient assign own homework

    Have patient indicate which problems he or she will work on once therapy ends

CHAPTER 3

Panic Disorder and Agoraphobia

DESCRIPTION AND DIAGNOSIS

Symptoms

Panic attacks consist of a frightening set of physical symptoms that may include heart palpitations, sweating, shakiness or trembling, shortness of breath, feelings of choking, chest pain, nausea, dizziness, feelings of detachment or unreality, fear of losing control (or fear of going insane), fear of dying, numbness or tingling, and hot or cold flashes. Panic attacks have a sudden onset and seldom last more than 30 minutes, with peak anxiety usually reached at 10 minutes. A person who has unexpected, recurring panic attacks, who is fearful of having additional attacks or worried about their implications, and who changes his or her behavior as a result is said to have panic disorder.

According to DSM-IV (American Psychiatric Association, 1994), many individuals with panic disorder may also show evidence of agoraphobia (from mild to severe). Agoraphobia is characterized by fear of being in such situations as open spaces, public places, bridges, or tunnels; traveling in buses, trains, automobiles, and airplanes; or of being in situations in which escape is blocked or help may be difficult to obtain. A person may either avoid these situations, endure them with great discomfort, or need the help of a companion (a "safety person") to enter them.

After the first panic attack, an individual may be overly focused on any physical sensations of anxiety and may develop anticipatory anxiety for situations that might arouse panic. Thus, many persons with panic disorder may present with few recent attacks, but may complain of the need to avoid situations (agoraphobia) and of their ruminative anticipations of further attacks. Traveling away from home; riding in trains, planes, cars, or elevators; walking down the street; and shopping in a store are frequently mentioned as distressing situations for these persons, because of their fear that a panic attack will occur, either "endangering" their lives or embarrassing them publicly. Because of the seeming generality and unpredictability of attacks, and the lack of control over them, many persons with panic disorder and agoraphobia find their lives greatly constricted by the need to avoid a variety of situations. The consequence for many is depression.

People with panic disorder (with or without agoraphobia) can also have panic attacks at home—in fact, panic often occurs in the hours directly after 1:30 A.M. A person may be wakened from sleep in a panic. Nocturnal panics occur between 1 and 4 hours after onset of sleep, with 54% of subjects labeling nocturnal panics as more severe than daytime panics (Barlow & Craske, 1988). These "nocturnal panics" differ from other panic attacks, in that they are not associated with physical activity and the patient is "relaxed" (lowered blood pressure, reduced respiration, and reduced heart rate; Barlow, 1988; Taylor et al., 1986).

Persons with both panic disorder and agoraphobia may seek various ways of adapting to their fears. Some will only live or work on the first or second floor of buildings, thereby avoiding the risk of being trapped in an elevator or a stairwell. Others arrange to do all their shopping by phone or accompanied by a family member (the "safety person"). Many of these individuals self-medicate with alcohol and sedative drugs, and present to a clinician with substance abuse or dependence as their primary diagnosis. In fact, the panic disorder and agoraphobia may not be obvious until after detoxification has begun.

Prevalence and Life Course

The lifetime prevalence of panic disorder, with or without agoraphobia, is between 1.5% and 3.8%; the female-to-male ratio is 2:1 (Eaton, Dryman, & Weissman, 1991). Onset of the first panic attack is generally in the early 20s, with few children under 16 manifesting a first panic attack and few individuals over 45 manifesting a first attack.

Genetic/Biological Factors

Panic disorder and agoraphobia have a moderate genetic loading. Biological signs include compensated respiratory alkalosis (this is related to the hyperventilation syndrome often accompanying panic disorder). In addition, individuals with panic disorder have elevated responses to lactate infusion and to CO_2 inhalation, although these are not sufficient biological markers to diagnose panic disorder. Panic is also related to dysregulation in the noradrenergic and serotonergic systems. Finally, a biological link for panic disorder is evident from the fact that certain medications (e.g., imipramine, fluvoxamine) inhibit panic attacks.

An evolutionary model of panic disorder and agoraphobia suggests that sensitivity to certain stimuli or conditions (being at great heights; being trapped in closed spaces, open fields, or public places; being left alone) may be biologically adaptive in the human species. For example, crossing an open field confers greater danger because of vulnerability to being sighted and attacked by predators. The response to this is flight or freezing—similar to the sympathetic and parasympathetic responses in panic disorder. However, since the individual's escape is blocked in contemporary life (e.g., on subways or in supermarkets), the anxiety escalates to a panic attack (Beck, Emery, & Greenberg, 1985; Marks, 1987).

Coexisting Conditions

Frequently coexisting with panic disorder are the following conditions: major depression, dysthymic disorder, social phobia, generalized anxiety disorder, obsessive–compulsive disorder, specific phobia, hypochondriasis, and substance abuse or dependence. Withdrawal from substances or alcohol may often precipitate panic attacks. Many patients with panic disorder and agoraphobia deny or refuse to report marital/couple conflict; they feel such a need to rely on their spouses or partners as their "safety persons" that they may have difficulty acknowledging relationship problems. However, couple conflict is not uncommon among these patients, since agoraphobia often strains the patience of a spouse or partner who has to care for a patient. Although one study found that suicidal risk was higher with panic disorder than with major depression, reanalysis of these data demonstrates that this higher incidence for panic disorder is attributable to either borderline personality disorder and/or concomitant substance abuse. Thus panic disorder per se is not a strong predictor of suicidal risk (see McNally, 1994).

Differential Diagnosis

Since many patients with panic disorder have initially contacted a physician because of their fear that they have a life-threatening illness, medical causes may already be ruled out by the time such a patient sees a therapist. However, because panic symptoms are similar to those of serious medical conditions, it is essential for the patient to have a thorough medical evaluation before psychological treatment commences. The clinician (and physician) will want to rule out the following physiological disorders that are accompanied by panic-like symptoms (this list is adapted from Wilson, 1987, pp. 13–14; see also Fyer, Mannuzza, & Coplan, 1995):

1. *Cardiovascular:* Arrhythmia, tachycardia, coronary heart disease, myocardial infarction (recovery from), heart failure, mitral stenosis, hypertension, postural orthostatic hypotension, stroke, transient ischemic attack, pulmonary embolism, pulmonary edema.
2. *Respiratory:* Bronchitis, emphysema, asthma, collagen disease, pulmonary fibrosis.
3. *Endocrine/hormonal:* Hyperthyroidism, hypoglycemia, premenstrual syndrome, pregnancy, pheochromocytoma, carcinoid tumors.
4. *Neurological/muscular:* Temporal lobe epilepsy, myasthenia gravis, Guillain-Barré syndrome.
5. *Aural:* Meniere's disease, labyrinthitis, benign positional vertigo, otitis media, mastoiditis.
6. *Hematological:* Anemia.
7. *Drug-related:* Antidepressant withdrawal, sedative or tranquilizer withdrawal, alcohol use or withdrawal, stimulant use, side effects of medications, caffeinism.

There is a controversy in the literature about the relationship between mitral valve prolapse and panic disorder. Mitral valve prolapse is usually diagnosed by echocardiogram.

Although most patients with this condition do not have panic disorder and most panic disorder patients do not have mitral valve prolapse, it is important in patients who do have mitral valve prolapse to evaluate whether the patients are overinterpreting their symptoms (e.g., dizziness and palpitations). (See McNally, 1994, for a discussion of mitral valve prolapse and panic.)

Panic disorder differs from other anxiety disorders in that the latter are more situationally bound or precipitated. For example, social phobia occurs only in social situations (e.g., eating in public or using a public restroom); specific phobia only occurs in the presence of the specific feared stimulus (e.g., touching a snake); and obsessive–compulsive disorder occurs only when the person is exposed to the stimulus that is the content of the obsession (e.g., exposure to dirt). About half of panic disorder patients present with personality disorders; avoidant and dependent personality disorders are the most common Axis II diagnoses (Chambless, Renneberg, Goldstein, & Gracely, 1992; Mavissakalian & Hammen, 1986; Reich, Noyes, & Troughton, 1987). In some cases, the personality disorder may partly result from the agoraphobic avoidance. For example, a person with agoraphobia may *become* dependent because of his or her need to be accompanied.

Consider the following as an example of differential diagnosis of anxiety disorders. A patient complains of fear of elevators and will not go into an elevator. The question that should be asked is this: Does the patient have a fear that the elevator will crash (specific phobia of elevators), or is the patient afraid that he or she will become so anxious as to have a panic attack and lose control (panic disorder and agoraphobia)? The treatment implications are different: for a specific phobia of elevators, we can rely on exposure to getting on elevators, whereas with panic disorder and agoraphobia we would recommend exposure to *panic attacks* as well as to elevators (see Barlow, 1988; Clark, 1986, 1989). A therapist can determine whether a patient suffers from specific phobia, social phobia, or panic disorder by determining the nature of the fear. An answer of "yes" to one of the following questions indicates the probable diagnosis.

Is the patient afraid of the stimulus (e.g., fear of snakes)?: Specific phobia.
Is the patient afraid of negative evaluation (independent of panic)?: Social phobia.
Is the patient afraid of internal sensations leading to loss of control?: Panic disorder.

A diagnostic flow chart for panic disorder with agoraphobia (Figure 3.1) illustrates the process of differential diagnosis in somewhat more detail.

UNDERSTANDING PANIC DISORDER AND AGORAPHOBIA IN COGNITIVE-BEHAVIORAL TERMS

A Cognitive-Behavioral Model

Currently, models of panic disorder integrate both behavioral and cognitive elements. Consequently, we have chosen to include discussions of both types of factors in this section, as well as a brief mention of interpersonal consequences. First, however, we outline

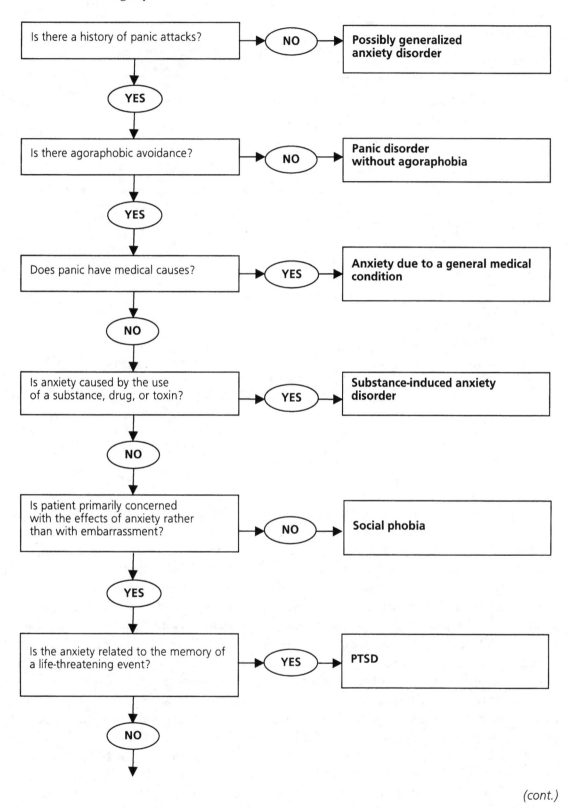

(cont.)

FIGURE 3.1. Diagnostic flow chart for panic disorder with agoraphobia.

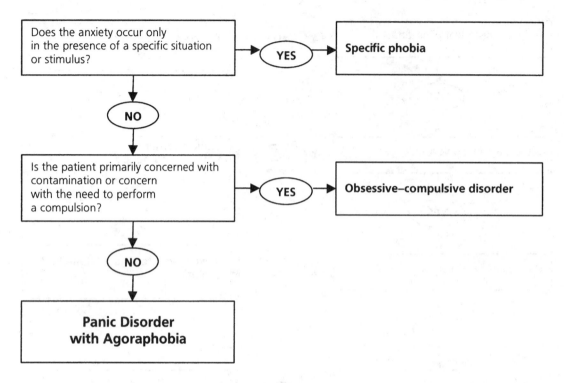

FIGURE 3.1 (*cont.*)

our own cognitive-behavioral model of panic disorder and agoraphobia. This model is based on the adaptive nature of fears in primitive environments (Barlow, 1988; Beck et al., 1985; Marks, 1987; see also Chapter 7 of this volume), as noted earlier. For example, avoiding open fields is adaptive for animals (such as humans) that are subject to predation, because they are at less risk on the periphery of the field. Heights (which often precipitate dizziness) are reasonable stimuli to avoid in the wild, because heights confer greater risk. The fear of being trapped can also be viewed as an "adaptive" fear. (See Marks, 1987, for an excellent discussion of innate fears.) These fears may have been retained in the species because of their potential adaptive value, but the "flight, fight, or freeze" response that the patient experiences as panic is not *currently* adaptive.

Our cognitive-behavioral model assumes that individuals with panic disorder may first experience panic or a high level of anxiety due to biological vulnerability, stress, or physical causes (such as illness). The resulting sensations of physiological arousal (e.g., hyperventilation, sweating, dizziness, or heart palpitations) lead to catastrophic misinterpretations (e.g., "I'm having a heart attack!" or "I'm going crazy!"), and thus to hypervigilance. On subsequent occasions, the individual misinterprets the sensations of physiological arousal as indications that catastrophic consequences will inevitably occur (these misinterpretations are "false alarms"), and experiences a full-blown panic attack as a result. Consequently, the individual develops anticipatory anxiety and avoids other situations that he or she associates with the risk of anxiety; this establishes agoraphobia. In some cases patients with agoraphobia use safety behaviors or magical thinking to cope. While these techniques can reduce anxiety, overall they reinforce the agoraphobia and so contribute to it. Form 3.1, a diagram illustrating this cognitive-behavioral model of panic disorder and agoraphobia, is intended for use as a patient handout. We now discuss in more detail the cognitive and behavioral factors that lead to and maintain these disorders, as well as interpersonal factors and consequences.

Cognitive Factors

The first panic attack is often identified with a stressful life event, such as taking on new responsibilities (e.g., a new job), moving, separation or loss, childbirth, physical illness, or relationship conflict. In many cases, however, the precipitating factor is not identified, and for most individuals this factor was not anxiety-provoking on previous occasions. As indicated earlier, the first panic attack is misinterpreted as catastrophic. Subsequent panic and agoraphobic avoidance are linked in an individual's mind with a variety of stimuli: crowded public places, open spaces, horizons, situations in which quick exit is blocked (e.g., elevators, trains, planes, automobiles, stairwells), traveling away from home, exercise or activity that raises the pulse, experiences associated with feelings of unreality (e.g., the use of Novocain by a dentist), waiting in line, changes in sunlight or darkness, heat, dehydration, heights, and sudden movements of the head (resulting in dizziness). Persons with panic disorder and agoraphobia report that their anxiety is reduced by going places with a "safety person," knowing all exits in a situation, sitting on the outside of an aisle near an exit, seeing that horizons that are broken by other structures, self-distraction, and wearing sunglasses (see Burns & Thorpe, 1977).

As noted above, the panic is exacerbated by a patient's cognitive distortions. These cognitive distortions focus on anticipatory anxiety ("I'll have a panic attack"), physical sensations ("My heartbeat means I'm having a heart attack"), and self-criticism ("I must be weak"). Cognitive therapy techniques—that is, identifying and challenging the patient's cognitive distortions—are useful in the treatment of panic and agoraphobia. A therapist who follows a strictly *behavioral* approach may overlook the importance of a patient's interpretations and distortions of events. Simple exposure to feared situations may not be sufficient in reducing panic or anticipatory panic if a patient's negative predictions and interpretations are not modified. Patients' cognitive distortions, as described in Appendix B, include distorted automatic thoughts (e.g., labeling, personalizing, catastrophizing), underlying maladaptive assumptions (i.e., "should," "if–then," or "must" statements), and dysfunctional schemas (e.g., deep-seated beliefs in the self's helplessness, abandonment, weakness, and inferiority, and in the correspondingly hurtful or rejecting qualities of others). The patient's response to his or her panic is an excellent opportunity to examine and modify the patient's more general cognitive distortions.

FORM 3.1. Cognitive-Behavioral Model of Panic Disorder and Agoraphobia for Patients

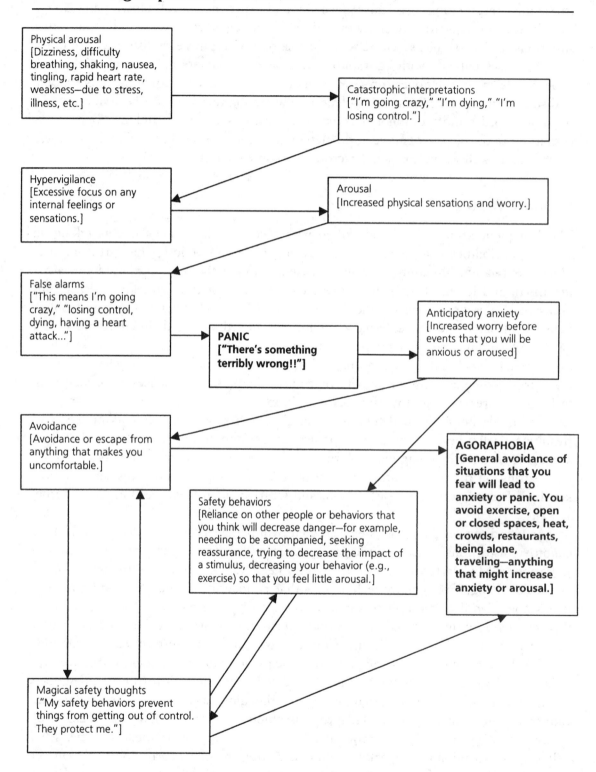

Table 3.1 gives some examples of the three types of these distortions in panic disorder and agoraphobia.

Behavioral Factors

From a behavioral view, agoraphobic avoidance is maintained because each time the individual avoids a situation, anxiety is decreased. This learned avoidance follows the principles of operant conditioning and stimulus generalization. Thus repeated reinforcement for avoidance results in a stronger tendency toward avoidance in the future, as well as greater tendency to generalize this avoidance to situations or stimuli similar to the most feared situation. For instance, an individual who begins to avoid crowded stores because of increased anxiety will later avoid going to any store or even going outside, where the anxiety may increase and lead to the feared panic attack. Similarly, the sensations of

TABLE 3.1. Examples of the Three Types of Cognitive Distortions in Panic Disorder and Agoraphobia

Distorted automatic thoughts

Fortunetelling: "I'll have an attack," "I'll lose control," "I'll faint."

Labeling: "There's something wrong with me."

Catastrophizing: "I can't stand being anxious," "I'll die from this."

Personalizing: "I'm the only one with this problem."

Mind reading: "People can see I'm panicking," "They know I'm neurotic."

Dichotomous (all-or-nothing) thinking: "Any anxiety is bad," "I'm always panicking."

Maladaptive assumptions

"I have to get rid of all of my panic and anxiety."

"I should never look foolish or out of control."

"If people know that I'm panicking, they'll reject me."

"I should never be weak."

"I should be in control of everything about me."

"If I don't know for sure what's going to happen, it will be bad."

"I should worry about panic so that I can prevent it."

"I should criticize myself for my weaknesses."

Dysfunctional schemas

Abandonment: "I'll be rejected and abandoned if I panic."

Biological integrity: "I'll become debilitated, pass out, and die if I panic."

Control: "I need to control everything about myself."

Humiliation: "People will make fun of me if I panic."

Specialness: "Panic is not consistent with my view of myself as successful and strong. This shouldn't be happening to me."

arousal initially associated with a panic attack are also avoided by the individual, resulting in a tendency to avoid situations that might increase arousal.

Interpersonal Factors and Consequences

We recommend focusing on the treatment of panic disorder and agoraphobia rather than depression when both are presented by a patient, because the depression is often secondary to the panic disorder and agoraphobia. As the patient gains greater flexibility in behavior and both anticipatory anxiety and panic subside, the depression may often abate. Furthermore, many of the cognitive techniques that address the patient's sources of anxiety are also relevant to the patient's depression.

Panic disorder and agoraphobia have substantial consequences for an individual's interpersonal life, as noted earlier. The fear of panic attacks in public places may dramatically curtail the patient's ability to socialize. For example, a single woman with a history of agoraphobia was unable to go to restaurants or theaters, or even to travel more than a few blocks from her house. Consequently, her opportunities to meet people or to develop relationships were diminished. As mentioned above, many individuals with agoraphobia will identify a "safety person" who can accompany them in case they have a panic attack and are unable to drive, to "escape" from public places, or to get medical attention. Because of their fear of a panic attack, some agoraphobia patients are hesitant to assert themselves with their significant others, to avoid risking abandonment and the resulting feelings of helplessness. Some agoraphobia patients fear being alone, since they may have a panic attack and fear that they will not be able to get help; consequently, they may cling to their spouses or partners and demand constant reassurance. In some cases, the agoraphobia makes it impossible for the patients to work outside the home or to work in jobs that require taking elevators or traveling.

Outcome Studies for Cognitive-Behavioral Treatments

Outcome studies for cognitive-behavioral treatments of panic disorder and agoraphobia are extremely favorable (75–90% efficacy; see Clark, 1996, for a summary). Follow-up 2 years after termination of treatment indicates maintenance of improvement in most cases. Furthermore, patients who have been in cognitive-behavioral treatment are far less likely to rely on psychotropic medication. In contrast, although approximately 80% of patients on medication (e.g., imipramine or alprazolam) show improvement, discontinuation of the medication results in substantial "rebound" of panic symptoms.

ASSESSMENT AND TREATMENT

Rationale and Plan for Treatment

Based on the cognitive-behavioral model described above and depicted in Form 3.1, the clinician must first assess the patient and diagnose panic disorder (with or without agoraphobia), differentiating it from social phobia, specific phobia, obsessive–compulsive disorder, or generalized anxiety disorder. The assessment of particular situations avoided or feared and the nature of the symptoms (e.g., hyperventilation, dizziness, heart palpitations) will prove useful in developing a hierarchy of feared stimuli and identifying the internal physical sensations that lead the patient to experience "false alarms." The symptoms of avoidance, anticipatory anxiety, autonomic arousal, dizziness, catastrophic thinking (e.g., "I'm choking," "I'm going crazy," or "I'll lose control"), and reliance on others or on superstitious behavior to gain "safety" are linked to specific goals in therapy. These goals include increasing the range of situations that the patient is willing to approach and stay in, decreasing apprehension, decreasing autonomic arousal, modifying breathing (to decrease dizziness), and developing more realistic assessments of internal sensations. In addition, since any anxious arousal may precipitate a panic attack, the clinician will work with the patient to decrease stressful responses to everyday problems. Finally, the therapist will assist the patient in relinquishing "safety" behaviors (e.g., the patient's reliance on others to accompany him or her, or the tendency to sit down, lie down, or seek physical support when uncomfortable). These goals are accomplished through a variety of interventions.

All patients with panic disorder should be assessed for substance abuse or dependence; in addition, medication should be considered as part of the treatment for many patients. Each patient is provided with an information handout on panic disorder and agoraphobia, as well as other readings relevant to anxiety. A list of feared situations, arranged in a hierarchy of least to most feared, is constructed as the basis for future imaginal and *in vivo* exposure. The therapist explains the cognitive-behavioral model of panic disorder and agoraphobia to the patient, stressing the evolutionary "value" of these disorders and indicating how fear is learned and generalized. The patient's "false alarm" interpretations of arousal are identified, and these cognitive distortions become targets for cognitive disputation. The ability to handle stress is enhanced through the use of problem-solving training, relaxation, and rebreathing exercises (which are also useful for exposure work), as well as through the application of cognitive therapy to the patient's unrealistic thoughts, assumptions, and schemas. Successful treatment of panic disorder may be accomplished in as few as 5 sessions, but may, in some cases, require 20 sessions.

The general plan of treatment for panic disorder and agoraphobia is outlined in Table 3.2.

Assessment

Forms 3.2 and 3.3 provide guidance for therapists in the assessment of panic disorder and agoraphobia. Form 3.2 permits a detailed assessment of the particular anxiety and avoidance symptoms exhibited by a patient, and facilitates the differential diagnosis of panic disorder agoraphobia from other anxiety disorders. Form 3.3 provides space for recording the patient's scores on various assessment instruments, for noting other relevant aspects of the patient's history (substance use, previous panic/agoraphobia episodes) for indicating treatment progress, and for recording treatment recommendations.

TABLE 3.2. General Plan of Treatment for Panic Disorder and Agoraphobia

Assessment
       Initial clinical evaluation of anxiety and avoidance
       Tests and other evaluations
       Consideration of medication

Socialization to treatment

Exposure
       Construction of a fear hierarchy
       Exposure (imaginal or *in vivo*) to hierarchy

Relaxation training

Cognitive interventions
       Panic induction (rebreathing, etc.)
       Challenging distorted automatic thoughts
       Challenging maladaptive assumptions
       Challenging dysfunctional schemas
       Coping with life stress

Phasing out treatment

Initial Clinical Evaluation of Anxiety and Avoidance

Form 3.2 allows a therapist to determine the specific characteristics of anxiety and avoidance that a patient is manifesting. The patient is asked to specify situations that he or she avoids; to give his or her reasons for avoiding these situations; to list symptoms experienced in these situations and to answer various questions about these symptoms; to give information about his or her use of substances, including caffeine, and medical conditions (a full medical checkup is also indicated for all patients with panic disorder); and to note any "safety" behaviors in which he or she engages. The answers to these questions will enable the therapist to determine whether the patient does indeed have panic disorder with or without agoraphobia (as opposed to social phobia or specific phobia), and they provide information that will prove useful in constructing the patient's fear hierarchy. (Note that the Initial Fear Evaluation for Patients [Form 7.1 in Chapter 7] can also be used in this context; however, Form 3.2 provides information that is more specific to panic disorder and agoraphobia.)

Tests and Other Evaluations

Patients with panic disorder and agoraphobia may be evaluated via self-report or interview questionnaires, such as the BAI, BDI, GAF, SCL-90-R, SCID-II, and Locke–Wallace (see Chapter 2); the Agoraphobia subscale of the Fear Questionnaire (Marks & Mathews, 1979; the Anxiety Disorders Interview Schedule—Revised (ADIS-R; DiNardo &

FORM 3.2. Initial Evaluation of Anxiety and Avoidance for Patients

Patient's Name: _____ Today's Date: _____

Which of the following situations do you avoid? (Circle each one.)

Restaurants	Stores	Malls
Subways	Buses	Airplanes
Elevators	Stairwells	Trains
Walking outside	Exercise	Bridges
Driving	Riding in a car	Viewing horizons
Being alone	Tunnels	Open fields
Sunlight	Heights	

Other situations avoided: _____

The three situations that I fear the most are:

1. _____
2. _____
3. _____

Do you avoid any of the following public situations because you might appear anxious? (Circle.)

Public speaking, eating, or drinking

Using a toilet or urinal not in your house

Undressing in a locker room

Parties

Family gatherings

Classrooms

Eye contact

Standing close to someone

Other situations: _____

I fear that in the situations circled in the lists above, I will become anxious and (check as many of the following that apply):

_____ I will have a heart attack or become physically ill.

_____ I will lose control and go insane.

_____ I will lose control and embarrass myself.

_____ I will not be able to get to a toilet in time.

_____ I will be harmed by someone.

_____ I am not afraid of my anxiety; I am afraid of the situation (for example, I am afraid the plane I am riding on will crash).

_____ I will collapse.

_____ People will see that I am anxious.

(cont.)

_____ Other: _____

_____ None of the above apply to me.

When did you start avoiding each of these situations?

Which of the following have you experienced in the situations you try to avoid? (Circle.)

Palpitations	Heart pounding	Chest pain or discomfort
Sweating	Trembling	Shaking
Shortness of breath	Smothering	Choking
Nausea	Dizziness	Light-headedness
Numbness	Tingling	Chills or hot flashes

Feeling that I myself am not real

Feeling that the situation is not real

Other: _____

During the past week, has there been any time when you experienced four of the symptoms listed above? (Circle.)

No   Yes   Which symptoms? _____

What would you say your average level of anxiety is during the last week? (Circle.)

None (0)   Slight (2.5)   Somewhat (5)   Very (7.5)   Extreme (10)

Do you ever wake up in a panic? (Circle.)   Yes   No

Do you worry about having anxiety or panic attacks? (Circle.)   Yes   No

What are some current stressors in your life?

How many coffees or caffeinated drinks do you have per day? _____

How much alcohol do you consume in a typical day? _____

Which medications do you presently take (include prescribed and over-the-counter drugs):

Name	Dosage	Frequency	Take for?	Prescribed by?
_____	_____	_____	_____	_____
_____	_____	_____	_____	_____
_____	_____	_____	_____	_____
_____	_____	_____	_____	_____
_____	_____	_____	_____	_____

(cont.)

Have you ever been diagnosed as having hyperthyroidism, Cushing's syndrome, hyperventilation, mitral valve prolapse? (Circle.)

What medical conditions do you have now?

Who treats each of these?

_____

_____

_____

_____

_____

_____

_____

_____

Which of the following do you do to make yourself feel safe when you are afraid of having a panic or anxiety attack? (Circle any that apply.)

Ask for reassurance

Take someone along when you go out

Repeat thoughts or words to yourself

Look around for signs of danger

Focus on physical sensations to see if you are OK

Clutch things for support

Sit down

Pace

Tense my body or hands

Take deep breaths (try to calm myself)

Other behaviors: _____

_____

FORM 3.3. Further Evaluation of Panic Disorder and Agoraphobia: Test Scores, Substance Use, History, Treatment Progress, and Recommendations

Patient's Name: _____ Today's Date: _____

Therapist's Name: _____ Sessions completed: _____

Test data/scores

Beck Depression Inventory (BDI) ____   Beck Anxiety Inventory (BAI) ____

Global Assessment of Functioning (GAF) ____   Symptom Checklist 90–Revised (SCL-90-R) ____

Structured Clinical Interview for DSM-III-R, Axis II (SCID-II) ____

Locke–Wallace Marital Adjustment Test ____   Fear Questionnaire (Agoraphobia subscale) ____

Other anxiety questionnaires (specify) _____

Substance use

Current use of psychiatric medications (include dosage) _____

_____

Who prescribes? _____

Use of alcohol/other drugs (kind, frequency, amount, consequences) _____

_____

History (intake only)

Previous episodes of panic/agoraphobia:

   Onset   Duration   Precipitating events   Treatment

Treatment progress (later evaluations only)

Situations still avoided: _____

_____

Situations approached that were previously avoided: _____

_____

Recommendations

Medication evaluation or reevaluation:

Increased hospitalization, day treatment, other:

Behavioral interventions:

Cognitive interventions:

Interpersonal interventions:

Marital/couple therapy:

Other: _____

Barlow, 1988); and/or the Mobility Inventory (Chambless, Caputo, Jasin, Gracely, & Williams, 1997). Form 3.3 provides space for recording scores on these instruments. It also enables the therapist to record the patient's medication, alcohol, and other drug use; to record (at intake only) the history of any previous episodes of panic and agoraphobia; to note (on later evaluations) which situations are still avoided and which the patient can now approach; and to indicate treatment recommendations.

Consideration of Medication

Although panic disorder may be treated effectively without medication, all patients should be given the option of medication as part of their treatment. Fluoxetine, sertraline, imipramine, alprazolam, and fluvoxamine have proven effective in inhibiting panic attacks. However, the use of medication should not preclude the use of cognitive-behavioral treatment, especially the use of behavioral exposure.

Socialization to Treatment

Educating the patient about the nature of panic is an essential component of therapy. As early as feasible in the evaluation, it is helpful to inform the patient that panic disorder is a diagnosis. The patient is also told that he or she mistakenly interprets the internal arousal as dangerous and then jumps to the conclusion that he or she is dying, going crazy, or losing control. We give patients a handout about cognitive-behavioral therapy in general (see Form B.1 in Appendix B); we use an information handout to educate patients about panic disorder and agoraphobia (see Form 3.4); and we recommend either *The Feeling Good Handbook* (Burns, 1989) or *Don't Panic* (Wilson, 1987) as bibliotherapy. Patients generally respond well to this socialization to the therapy process. Many of them have never been properly diagnosed as having panic disorder. (It was not uncommon 30 years ago for these patients to be diagnosed as schizophrenic.)

Exposure

Patients with panic disorder and agoraphobia almost always avoid situations where they expect to experience panic, or enter such situations with debilitating anxiety. The behavioral technique of exposure (which is fully discussed in Appendix A and the CD-ROM for this book) can be used to help such patients enter these situations and function in them without fear.

Construction of a Fear Hierarchy

Once the therapist explains the rationale for exposure procedures, discusses these procedures with the patient, and obtains his or her commitment to proceeding, the therapist helps the patient to construct a "fear hierarchy," which is a list of the patient's feared situations sequenced from least to most feared. The therapist asks the patient what situations are feared and/or avoided, requests him or her to rank-order these, and has the pa-

FORM 3.4. Information for Patients about Panic Disorder and Agoraphobia

What Are Panic Disorder and Agoraphobia?

Almost everyone feels anxious at times. But a panic attack involves such a high level of that it can feel as if you are having a heart attack, going insane, or losing control of yourself. During a panic attack, you may have physical symptoms such as shortness of breath, tingling sensations, ringing in your ears, a sense of impending doom, trembling, a feeling of choking, chest pain, sweating, and heart pounding. You should see your physician in order to rule out medical causes for these symptoms, such as hyperthyroidism, caffeine addiction, mitral valve prolapse, or other causes. A panic attack, however, can produce the same physical symptoms as these medical conditions. When a person has recurring, unexpected panic attacks, is afraid of having more or worried about their meaning, and makes changes in his or her behavior as a result, the person is said to have "panic disorder."

Many patients who have panic disorder also experience "agoraphobia." Agoraphobia is fear of places or situations where a panic attack may occur or from which escape might be difficult. For example, people with agoraphobia avoid being out alone, going to supermarkets, traveling in trains or airplanes, crossing bridges, being at heights, going through tunnels, crossing open fields, and riding in elevators. Many patients even experience panic when they are asleep, possibly because the large *decrease* in pulse rate during sleep elicits a compensating *increase* in pulse rate, resulting in feeling jolted out of sleep.

Some patients with agoraphobia experience anxiety in sunlight; others become anxious in dimming light. Heat is a major factor in panic disorder—there is a dramatic increase in panic disorder and agoraphobia during the summer, primarily because heat increases pulse rate, dizziness, and dehydration, and there are more opportunities to be outside (where an individual feels more vulnerable). The individual fears that in these situations, he or she will have a panic attack.

What Are the Causes of Panic Disorder and Agoraphobia?

According to some theories, many situations that can trigger panic attacks were truly dangerous earlier in human evolution. For example, being trapped in a tunnel could lead to suffocation or collapse; heights might be dangerous; in open fields, an individual was more susceptible to predators (such as lions or wolves); public places might have brought our ancestors into contact with hostile strangers. Many of the fears involved in panic disorder and agoraphobia are reminiscent of these earlier instinctive and adaptive fears. However, these situations are not dangerous today.

Research does demonstrate that panic disorder and agoraphobia have some genetic links, but they are not entirely inherited. In any given year, 30% to 40% of the general population will have a panic attack. However, most of these people will not interpret their panic as a signal of catastrophic danger, and thus will not go on to develop panic disorder or agoraphobia.

Initially, a panic attack is usually activated by a stressful situation, such as leaving home, marital/couple conflict, surgery, new responsibilities, or physical illness. These sensations of physical arousal (heavy breathing, sweating, dizziness, pounding heart, and so on) may be misinterpreted as signals of catastrophic danger—for example, a person may focus on the increase in heart rate and jump to the conclusion that he or she is about to have a heart attack. As a result, the person may develop "hypervigilance" (that is, an excessive focus on physical sensations), which can result in increased arousal (increased physical sensations and worry). This arousal triggers further catastrophic misinter-

(cont.)

pretations, which we call "false alarms" because they signal that danger is imminent when it really is not. A full-blown panic attack can result from such arousal and misinterpretations. Consequently, the person develops "anticipatory anxiety" (fear that panic attacks will continue to occur) and begins to avoid situations that give rise to such anxiety—especially if escape from these situations may be difficult or embarrassing, or if help may not be readily available. In fact, when avoidance and escape become the major coping mechanisms used to handle anxiety, the person has developed agoraphobia.

An individual with agoraphobia who does not avoid feared situations altogether usually enlists the aid of a "safety person"—that is, a person who accompanies the individual into these situations in case the anxiety becomes too great and the individual needs to escape. Even though reliance on the "safety person," avoidance, and other "safety behaviors" may mean that the individual has had no panic attacks in months, he or she often lives in fear of the next attack. The world becomes smaller and smaller as a result of the individual's fear and avoidance. Partly because of this constriction in their lives, and partly because they feel out of control and are unsure how to handle their problem, many people with panic disorder and agoraphobia also develop depression. Some of these people become so anxious and depressed that they self-medicate with alcohol, Valium, or Xanax.

What Are Some Common Misconceptions about Panic Disorder and Agoraphobia?

Some people incorrectly believe that panic disorder is a result of deep-seated psychological problems. Of course, anyone with or without panic may have deeper problems, but panic disorder and agoraphobia are not necessarily related to deeper psychological problems. You may become depressed, dependent, and self-critical because you have panic disorder—but panic, in itself, can be treated effectively without long-term therapy exploring your childhood experiences. People with panic disorder and agoraphobia often have unrealistic beliefs about anxiety, such as "All anxiety is bad" and "I have to get rid of my anxiety immediately." Some of these people misinterpret their anxiety as a sign of a dangerous medical condition. Others believe that because they have had panic attacks and agoraphobia for many years—and because traditional therapy has not been helpful for these problems—they can never improve. Cognitive-behavioral therapy, with or without medication, is often quite effective in the treatment of panic disorder and agoraphobia.

How Effective Is Cognitive-Behavioral Therapy for Panic Disorder and Agoraphobia?

Fortunately, there have been a number of studies examining the effects of cognitive-behavioral therapy for panic disorder and agoraphobia. These studies have been done at Oxford University in England, the University of Pennsylvania, the State University of New York at Albany, and other universities and medical schools. Over a course of 20 to 25 sessions, the efficacy rates ranges from 85% to 90%. Furthermore, once treatment is terminated, most patients who are tested 1 year later have maintained their improvement.

Medications for Panic Disorder and Agoraphobia

A number of medications have been found to be useful in the treatment of panic disorder and agoraphobia. These include antidepressants (such as Tofranil, Prozac, Zoloft, and monoamine oxidase inhibitors); Xanax and other medications for anxiety; and beta-blockers. These medications may help reduce

(cont.)

your arousal, but once you terminate the medication, your panic symptoms may return. Consequently, we recommend that even if you use medication for panic disorder and agoraphobia, you should also consider cognitive-behavioral therapy.

What Are Some of the Steps in Cognitive-Behavioral Treatment?

The cognitive-behavioral treatment of panic disorder and agoraphobia is organized around several goals: first, helping you to understand the nature of anxiety, panic, and agoraphobia; second, determining the range of situations that you avoid or fear; third, evaluating the nature of your particular symptoms, their severity and frequency, and the situations that elicit your panic; and, fourth, determining whether any other problems coexist with your panic—for example, depression, other anxieties, substance abuse, overeating, loneliness, or marital/couple problems.

Your therapy may include some or all of the following treatments: muscle relaxation training; breathing relaxation training and rebreathing training (especially if you hyperventilate); gradual exposure to situations that elicit panic; stress reduction; identification of your interpretation of physical stress symptoms; training in general cognitive therapy principles (that is, understanding how thoughts can lead to feelings such as fear, and learning how examining your thoughts and beliefs can help you feel better); assertion training (when needed); and training in the ability to recognize and reduce your panic symptoms when they occur. In addition, other problems that you may have (such as depression) may be addressed in the therapy.

What Is Expected of You as a Patient?

Cognitive-behavioral therapy is not a passive experience for patients. It requires your active involvement to work. You are expected to come to sessions weekly (sometimes more than once per week), to fill out forms that evaluate your problems, and to do self-help homework that you and your therapist plan and assign. As indicated earlier, most patients who participate in this treatment experience improvement in their panic disorder and agoraphobia—some experience rapid improvement. *Even if you experience rapid improvement, however, you should complete the full treatment package.* Premature dropout from treatment increases the likelihood that you will have relapses.

The course of treatment is planned for 12 sessions. The first few sessions are used for evaluation and explanation of the treatment. The last few sessions of the treatment are mainly for follow-up—these are scheduled twice a week and then once per month.

The treatment package that we use combines the excellent treatment techniques developed at Oxford University, the University of Pennsylvania, and the State University of New York at Albany. We view the treatment as a way in which you can learn how to help yourself. That is why doing homework in therapy is so important.

tient assign each situation a distress rating on a scale of 0 to 10 (these ratings are often referred to as "subjective units of distress" or "SUDs" ratings). Form 3.5 can be used with the patient to create a fear hierarchy in this manner.

When the fear hierarchy has been constructed, it is also useful to ask the patient whether—and, if so, how—the ratings of fear change if the patient is accompanied or alone. In particular, it should be indicated whether the patient is *more* frightened when accompanied by someone. As indicated earlier, most patients feel less frightened when accompanied by someone, since a "safety person" can help them out of feared situations. However, given the fact that panic disorder is often comorbid with social phobia, some patients would rather be alone, lest someone see their anxiety and judge them negatively. For a patient who relies on a safety person, it is useful to explore the patient's interpretations of what that person can do that the patient cannot do. Many patients believe that they will become so disoriented by their anxiety that they will not be able to get out of the situation (e.g., they will not be able to get out of a store), and therefore that a safety person will have to get them out. Other patients believe that they will require medical attention—that their anxiety will result in their physical collapse and fainting. Consequently, the safety person can get them to the hospital. Still others believe that if they are driving and they have a panic attack, the other person can take control of the driving and prevent a fatal accident. Since none of these feared events has probably happened, the therapist may inquire about the probability of these events happening, as well as how the patient can rescue himself or herself even if they do happen. In this way, construction of the fear hierarchy, and later exposure per se, can be used to identify and challenge cognitive distortions.

Exposure to the Fear Hierarchy

After the construction of the fear hierarchy, the therapist establishes a sequence of steps to be taken by the patient (see Appendix A). Initial exposure can consist of "imaginal exposure"; that is, the patient is asked to form a vivid image of the least feared situation. This feared situation can then be paired with relaxation (in some circumstances) and with cognitive coping statements regarding the physical sensations of anxiety. Form 3.6 is a list of coping statements that can be given as a handout to patients. In addition, the Patient's Imaginal Exposure Practice Form (Form A.1 in Appendix A) can be given to patients who are engaging in imaginal exposure. Once the patient has become comfortable with the image of the least feared situation, the next situation on the fear hierarchy is dealt with, and so on until the most feared situation on the hierarchy is imagined.

In vivo exposure—that is, exposure in the actual situation—can also be employed (and is in fact preferable to imaginal exposure whenever it is practicable; see Appendix A). The Patient's Panic Record (Form 3.7) is used whenever *in vivo* exposure is conducted. For example, one patient's anxious thought was that she would lose control of her car when crossing a bridge. She was instructed to write down her degree of anxiety, her prediction, and her confidence in the accuracy of this prediction before each time she crossed the bridge, and then to write down her actual degree of anxiety and the outcome of the situation after she had crossed the bridge. She was instructed to do this 10 times,

FORM 3.5. Patient's Hierarchy of Feared Situations

Patient's Name: _____ Today's Date: _____

Please rank your feared situations in order from least to most distressing. In the last column, note how upset each one makes you, from 0 (no distress) to 10 (maximum distress).

Rank	Situation	Avoided? (Yes/No)	Distress (0–10)
_____	_____	_____	_____
_____	_____	_____	_____
_____	_____	_____	_____
_____	_____	_____	_____
_____	_____	_____	_____
_____	_____	_____	_____
_____	_____	_____	_____
_____	_____	_____	_____
_____	_____	_____	_____
_____	_____	_____	_____
_____	_____	_____	_____
_____	_____	_____	_____
_____	_____	_____	_____
_____	_____	_____	_____
_____	_____	_____	_____
_____	_____	_____	_____
_____	_____	_____	_____
_____	_____	_____	_____

FORM 3.6. Coping Statements for Patients

Normalize your anxiety:

Anxiety is normal.

Everyone has anxiety.

Anxiety shows that I am alert.

Anxiety may be biologically programmed (this may be the "right response at the wrong time"—there is no danger that I have to escape from).

Take the danger away:

Anxiety is arousal.

I've been through this before, and nothing bad has happened.

Anxiety passes and goes away.

Challenge your negative thoughts:

I'm having false alarms.

I'm not going crazy or losing control.

These sensations are not dangerous.

People can't see my feelings.

I don't need to have 100% control.

Learn from the past:

I've made many negative predictions before that haven't come true.

I have never gone crazy, had a heart attack, or died from my anxiety.

Remember to keep breathing normally—this helps.

Plan acceptance:

I can sit back and watch my arousal.

I can accept that my arousal goes up and down.

I can observe my sensations increasing and decreasing.

I can accept my arousal and examine my negative thoughts.

FORM 3.7. Patient's Panic Record

Patient's Name: _____

Date/time/situation	Anxiety before entering situation (0–100%)	Predictions/thoughts and confidence in accuracy of them (0–100%)	Physical sensations while in situations	Rating of actual anxiety in situation (0–100%)	Outcome (what happened)

and then on each succeeding day to try a more difficult bridge. This graduated exposure was successful in overcoming her long-standing avoidance of bridges, which had greatly curtailed her movements for several years. (The Patient's *In Vivo* Exposure Practice Record—Form A.2 in Appendix A—can also be given to patients who are engaging in this form of exposure.)

Although *in vivo* exposure may seem "more difficult" than imaginal exposure, it can in fact be initiated fairly early in treatment. It can also be paired with cognitive techniques. For example, one of us (Robert L. Leahy) has a 10th-floor office. A 30-year-old male called to set up a session because of his fear of having a panic attack in elevators. He was on medical leave from his job in an office on a high floor in a skyscraper. Simply getting to Leahy's office was problematic for the patient, since he avoided elevators and he was afraid that his arousal in climbing the stairs to the office would precipitate a heart attack. The first meeting was used for *in vivo* exposure: Leahy met the patient in the lobby and walked with him up each flight of stairs, eliciting his catastrophic misinterpretations of his breathing—for example, "I'm breathing heavily. I won't be able to catch my breath. I'll have a heart attack." Similar thoughts were activated when the patient swam or walked more than two blocks from his apartment.

Relaxation Training

Relaxation training is useful in reducing the general level of arousal, although a sizable proportion of patients with panic disorder may experience "relaxation-induced attacks"—that is, relaxation exercises actually *increase* the likelihood of attacks. Why this is so is not entirely clear. However, it is plausible that there may be a "homeostatic" self-regulation of heartbeat in some patients, such that the lowering of heart rate during relaxation or sleep activates a self-correcting increase in arousal, which is experienced as panic. Because of the unexpected and uncontrollable nature of panic during relaxation or sleep, many patients are alarmed by these precipitants. We have found that inquiring about these specific "paradoxical panics" is helpful to patients, and that providing them with an explanation based on homeostasis (self-correction) allows them to decatastrophize the panic. See Appendix A for a full review of several types of relaxation procedures, or consult the CD-ROM that accompanies this book.

Cognitive and behavioral therapists may differ as to the advisability of either pairing relaxation with exposure or providing exposure without relaxation. The "strictly cognitive" approach argues in favor of exposure without relaxation, insofar as the goal is to allow the patient to understand that anxiety itself can be tolerated (e.g., see Wells, 1997). However, there are no empirical data to suggest that one approach to exposure is superior to the other. Consequently, the clinician may decide which approach seems most feasible.

A high percentage of patients with panic disorder are hyperventilators. When confronted with a phobic stimulus, they breathe rapidly, leading to further shortness of breath, and further exacerbating their desire to "catch" their breath (i.e., further hyperventilation). Chronic hyperventilators often sigh, take "deep breaths," and report themselves short of breath. Some researchers (Gorman, Liebowitz, Fyer, & Stein, 1989; Klein

& Klein, 1989) have interpreted the panic associated with hyperventilation as a "suffocation alarm" response. That is, such patients believe that they will be unable to catch their breath, and this triggers a sensation of suffocation, followed by hyperventilation. These hyperventilators may be instructed in breathing relaxation—slowing their breathing down, breathing into their stomachs—as a means of reducing their general risk of hyperventilation. Clark, Salkovskis, and Chalkley (1985) recommend providing patients with a tape that instructs them to breathe in for 2 or 3 seconds, then out for the same period of time; this is followed by a brief pause and then by a repetition of the in-and-out cycle.

The therapist can use the following breathing relaxation instructions (from Wilson, 1987, pp. 151–152): "Gently and slowly inhale a normal amount of air through your nose, filling only your lower lungs. Exhale easily. Continue this slow, gentle breathing with a relaxed attitude, concentrating on filling only the lower lungs." A patient may also be instructed to lie on a couch, place a small book on the stomach, and breathe so as to raise the book with each breath; this assures diaphragmatic breathing rather than shallow chest breathing. For more details and suggestions about breathing relaxation, see the discussion of this topic in the "Relaxation Training" section of Appendix A.

Cognitive Interventions

The following cognitive interventions are used in treating panic disorder and agoraphobia.

Panic Induction

The importance of hyperventilation in panic is demonstrated by David Clark's (1986) "panic induction" treatment. Although exposure is the central technique employed here, we consider Clark's model "cognitive" because the purpose of the exposure is to challenge the patient's belief that his or her physical sensations are dangerous. In fact, we have found that simply *describing* Clark's treatment has provided some patients with sufficient relief to end their panicking. Thus, "understanding" what is going on—and developing a less catastrophic interpretation—may be sufficient for some.

In Clark's treatment, it is assumed that the patient's hyperventilation is followed by catastrophic cognitions ("I'm having a heart attack," "I'll never catch my breath," or "I'm going to lose control and embarrass myself"). The patient is guided by the therapist into rebreathing, which induces panic symptoms. The therapist then instructs the patient in breathing into a bag, which then restores the proper CO_2 balance, thereby ending the "panic attack." This technique is remarkably useful for hyperventilators. It demonstrates, *in vivo,* that panic attacks are induced by overbreathing and can be terminated by simple behavioral means; panic attacks therefore become decatastrophized. Since the central fear for panic patients is the fear of the panic attack itself (not of, say, a subway, store, or open area), further exposure to these situations becomes more tolerable for these patients. We should warn our readers that some patients with asthma, cardiovascular, or pulmonary disorders should not be engaged in rebreathing exercises. Furthermore, not all panic patients are hyperventilators. However, Clark's treatment is highly successful in the treatment of patients with this symptom. See Appendix A and the CD-ROM for a discussion of rebreathing as a separate technique.

Other methods that induce a patient's feared sensations may also be adopted in treatment sessions. For example, many patients with panic disorder report cardiovascular sensations (which can be produced in sessions by having such a patient engage in vigorous exercise—e.g., running in place or using a stationary bicycle), audiovestibular sensations (which can be produced in sessions by spinning the chair), tension in the chest (which can be produced by tightening the chest muscles), and depersonalization (which can be induced by relaxation and meditation exercises). (See Barlow, 1988, and Barlow & Cerny, 1988.) One patient, who had a reflexive panic reaction to dimming lights (such as on an intermittently clouded day), was exposed in a session to recurrent dimming of lights in the therapist's office. This elicited the panic symptoms and allowed the patient and therapist to test out his catastrophic thought that he would "go crazy." His anxiety abated rapidly. *In vitro* (i.e., in-session) exposure to panic sensations or symptoms is a dramatic demonstration for patients of the fact that their panic symptoms are not dangerous, and in fact are both evocable and controllable.

Identifying and Challenging Distorted Automatic Thoughts

As indicated in Appendix B (see Table B.3) and in the CD-ROM that accompanies this volume, a wide variety of techniques can be useful in identifying and challenging the distorted automatic thoughts of a panic patient. Form 3.8 is a checklist of common dysfunctional automatic thoughts in panic disorder and agoraphobia. Once a patient has used this form to identify his or her top three automatic thoughts when anxious or panicking, the therapist can take these (beginning with the patient's most frequent automatic thought) and apply as many techniques for challenging automatic thoughts as are applicable in the situation. Let us consider the questions a therapist might ask to challenge this automatic thought: "I'm going to have a panic attack." (In the following list, the therapist's questions are in italics; the patient's answers are in roman with quotation marks.)

1. *What category does this thought belong to?* "Fortunetelling."
2. *What emotions or feelings do you have when you have this thought?* "Anxious, depressed."
3. *Rate your confidence in the accuracy of this thought, and the intensity of your feelings, from 0% to 100%.* "Thought: 90%. Feelings: anxiety, 90%; depression, 50%."
4a. *What is the evidence for and against this thought?* "For: I've had panic attacks in the past. I'm feeling anxious right now. Against: I've usually been wrong about my predictions. I'm usually not having panic attacks."
4b. *How would you evaluate the evidence? If you had to divide 100 points between*

FORM 3.8. Patient's Most Common Automatic Thoughts When Anxious/Panicking

Patient's Name: _____ Today's Date: _____

Directions: Check every automatic thought that you have when you start getting anxious or panicking. Then rank your top three thoughts, using 1 for the thought you have most often, and 2 and 3 for your next most frequent thoughts.

_____ I'll go insane.

_____ I'll lose control.

_____ I'll have a panic attack.

_____ I'll have a heart attack.

_____ I'll faint.

_____ I'll go into a coma.

_____ I'll be unable to escape.

_____ I'll be unable to get home.

_____ I'll be unable to get to the bathroom.

_____ I'll choke.

_____ I'll embarrass myself.

_____ I'll start yelling.

_____ I'll become violent.

_____ I'll start crying.

_____ I'll start shaking.

_____ I'll kill or harm myself.

_____ I'll never stop feeling this way.

_____ I'll vomit.

_____ I won't be able to breathe.

_____ I'll die.

Other thoughts: _____

_____

_____

the evidence for and against your thought, how would you divide these points? "I'd say 30 points in favor of having a panic attack, 70 against."

5. *What would happen if you had a panic attack?* "I'd get more anxious, I'd have difficulty breathing, I'd pass out, and I'd die."

6a. *Have you ever stopped breathing, passed out, or died?* "No."

6b. *What is the probability that you will die if you have a panic attack?* "Negligible, close to 0%."

7. *What could you do if you became short of breath?* (Let us assume that the patient has learned breathing relaxation, panic induction, and other exercises.) "I could breathe slowly, into my hands; I could run in place; I could breathe slowly into my stomach; I could sit down; I could raise my feet if I feel faint; I could distract myself with something else; I could leave the situation."

Challenging Maladaptive Assumptions

Assumptions are the general "rules" or "imperatives" that a patient has. These include "should" statements ("I shouldn't be anxious"), "if–then" statements ("If I'm anxious, people will reject me"), and "must" statements ("I must get rid of all of my anxiety"). Patients with panic disorder are often so focused on the discomfort of their anxiety that they have seldom spontaneously thought of examining and challenging these underlying assumptions. One goal in cognitive therapy is to slow down a patient's thinking so that maladaptive assumptions may be elicited and modified. Let us consider the questions a therapist would ask to challenge the following perfectionistic assumption: "I must eliminate my anxiety completely."

1. *How much do you believe this assumption?* "About 85%."

2a. *What are the costs and benefits of this assumption?* "Costs: Makes me anxious. Impossible to achieve. Makes me obsessive about my anxiety. I'm intolerant of any anxiety. Makes me feel out of control and self-critical. Benefits: Maybe if I try to get rid of all my anxiety, I'll be able to get rid of panic attacks. If I catch myself feeling anxious, maybe I can prevent it from escalating. Or maybe I can escape before it gets too bad."

2b. *How would you divide 100 points for the costs and benefits of your assumption?* "Well, I can see that the benefits are unrealistic. I know I can't get rid of all of my anxiety. It adds pressure to me. I'd say 80 points for costs, 20 points for benefits."

3. *What is the evidence for and against the idea that you could get rid of all of your anxiety?* "For: There are times when I'm not anxious. Against: My anxiety comes and goes. Everyone is a little anxious at times."

4a. *What do you think would happen if you did not eliminate your anxiety?* "Maybe I'd go crazy. Or my heart might just get worn out."

4b. *Have you gone crazy or had a heart attack?* "No."

5. *Do you know anyone else who has eliminated anxiety completely?* "No, everyone I know feels anxious some of the time."

6. *What would be the advantage of accepting anxiety as a natural part of life, just as you accept hunger and drowsiness as parts of life?* "I'd feel a lot less pressure about having anxiety. I'd feel less like a freak. I'd be less self-critical."

7a. *From 0% to 100%, how much do you believe right now that you should eliminate all your anxiety?* "Probably only 10%. But I sure wish I could."

7b. *Why did you decrease your belief in this assumption?* "I can see how unrealistic it is—you can't eliminate anxiety completely. A little anxiety now and then won't hurt me."

Challenging Dysfunctional Schemas

Schemas are the deep-level constructs that the patient uses in thinking about self and others. For example, is the patient primarily concerned about being special, unique, in control, invulnerable, loved, acceptable to everyone, and capable of perfect knowledge of the future? Does the patient view others as rejecting, abandoning, domineering, humiliating, rescuing, intolerant, or inferior? Panic means different things to different people. For a narcissistic patient, with a belief that he or she is uniquely superior, the existence of panic disorder is inconsistent with the patient's self-schema. If the patient views others as humiliating, then he or she has even more to be anxious about.

Although panic disorder can be effectively treated without addressing the patient's underlying schemas about self and others, the treatment of panic often leads the patient to an exploration of negative or otherwise dysfunctional schemas. For example, a 28-year-old male who had been suffering from panic disorder for 6 years, and who had previously abused alcohol as a means of self-medication, was successfully treated through the use of cognitive-behavioral techniques. During the course of the treatment, the therapist assisted him in examining his self-schemas of being "special" and needing to be "in control," as well as his fear that he would be humiliated. These schemas became apparent as the patient recounted his attempts to achieve perfection in his studies and in his work. The idea of having panic attacks was inconsistent with his view of himself as perfect and in control.

The patient recalled his childhood and adolescence. His father, an aristocratic refugee who socialized with internationally famous people, would insist that the son had to achieve "as much as Mozart." The narcissistic father demanded perfection in the son and would humiliate him whenever he disagreed with him or did not live up to his expectations. The patient's perfectionism, need to be special, and need to be in control were interpreted as attempts to avoid further humiliation with others—specifically, his colleagues. His schema about others was that they would be critical and intolerant of any of his weaknesses, just as his father had been.

The therapist helped the patient to examine the illogical nature of his father's expectations and the evidence that many of his colleagues had psychological problems that would dwarf his own. The therapist also engaged in "retrospective cognitive therapy" (Leahy, 1985), in which the therapist role-played the father and the patient role-played himself as an adolescent being assertive with his father. The patient's panic and general anxiety abated, and his work with colleagues became more productive and relaxed.

Coping with Life Stress

Many patients who panic are so focused on their physical sensations that they often overlook how life events are affecting them. Some patients feel trapped in relationships or jobs; other patients feel angry but have difficulty expressing their anger for fear of alienating a "safety person"; and other patients overrespond to simple life stressors. As part of the treatment of panic disorder and agoraphobia, the patient is also presented with a brief introduction to cognitive therapy of anxious and depressive thoughts in general. Those who panic often engage in catastrophizing or other kinds of dysfunctional automatic thoughts (e.g., fortunetelling, mislabeling, and selective filtering of information), as well as maladaptive assumptions about dealing with stressors (e.g., "I should be able to handle my problems on my own"). By addressing the patient's general cognitive distortions about everyday life stressors, the therapist can help reduce his or her overall level of anxiety.

Trouble-Shooting Problems in Therapy

Although the treatment package for panic disorder and agoraphobia appears to be relatively straightforward, patients with panic disorder (with or without agoraphobia) may present a number of problems. When we find that our patients are resistant to the prescribed treatment, we usually find that the cognitive components of therapy are quite helpful. Common problems with these patients are fear of intrapsychic processes, anxiety intolerance, noncompliance with homework, unrealistic expectations, and fear of the transference.

Fear of Intrapsychic Processes

Panic patients are often fearful of any experiences that may arouse anxiety. A patient may be fearful that therapy will lead to examination of psychological material that may threaten him or her. Just as the patient may fear that anxiety portends insanity, he or she may also fear that uncovering intrapsychic processes will lead to the discovery of "unconscious" material revealing either insanity or other unacceptable characteristics. This is especially true in panic patients presenting with an obsessive style of thinking regarding anxiety. The therapist can guide the patient to examine what evidence there is that self-reflection leads to insanity or loss of control. Since this fear may be recurrent throughout therapy, it is useful to indicate to the patient that his or her fears of examining his psychological processes have not been borne out.

Anxiety Intolerance

The panic patient may present with "emotional perfectionism"—that is, the belief that all anxiety is to be avoided and that no anxiety can be tolerated. The patient can examine the costs and benefits of this belief and the evidence for and against the belief that anxiety is intolerable and dangerous. We also find it helpful to indicate to the patient that anxiety is *useful information*; that is, it indicates that "things may not be working properly." One of the most interesting books on this subject is *The Meaning of Anxiety* by the existential psychoanalyst Rollo May (1950) who reviews the evidence that anxiety is an informative source of information about the self. For example, a 24-year-old male patient with emotional perfectionism found the discussion of May's book helpful because it led him to refocus from his symptoms of anxiety to the nature of conflicts in his everyday life. These conflicts included decisions about graduate school and career. As he began to recognize that he was "legitimately" anxious about making important decisions, he became more tolerant of his anxiety, and consequently less anxious.

Another way to approach intolerance of anxiety is to examine the patient's predictions about what will happen if he is anxious. Many panic patients believe that the onset of anxiety "always leads to panic" or that anxiety "will never go away." These dire predictions are easy to test by having the patients rate and record their anxiety over a period of time. Such a record will indicate that anxiety rises and subsides.

Noncompliance with Homework

There are numerous reasons for resistance to homework. For a patient with panic disorder, frequent reasons to resist include the belief that anxiety can only be faced if a "safety person" or therapist is there to rescue or direct him or her; that engaging in exposure to fearful situations will make matters worse; that writing down automatic thoughts will open up a "can of worms" of uncontrollable anxious thoughts; or that since all anxiety cannot be eliminated immediately, then things are hopeless. The therapist, in sessions, may examine how each of these thoughts or assumptions is characteristic of the agoraphobia that has developed. The therapist can submit each thought or assumption to cognitive evaluation: What are its costs and benefits? What is the evidence for and against it? Does this thought or assumption apply to other people as well? What is the evidence within therapy—is anxiety always dangerous? And, specifically, what will the "safety person" do that the patient cannot do himself or herself?

As with any treatment that involves exposure outside of sessions, homework noncompliance may result from the therapist's failure to engage in "rehearsal" of the exposure in the session *prior to assigning the exposure homework*. This "rehearsal" should involve specific instructions of exactly what the patient will do for homework—where, when, and for how long the exposure will occur. The therapist can ask the patient to imagine the situation he or she is afraid of, to activate mental images about the situation, and to determine his or her automatic thoughts. We find it very helpful to use a "stress inoculation" approach (Meichenbaum, 1974), in which the therapist role-plays the negative thoughts and the patient practices responding rationally. The therapist can also elicit any resistance thoughts prior to the exposure outside of sessions—for example, "What could be some reasons for not doing the homework?"

Finally, homework noncompliance may also be due to the fact that the therapy is moving too quickly—that is, the therapist is demanding more than the patient is ready for. A good rule to use is to reduce the amount and degree of homework, instead of eliminating homework altogether.

Unrealistic Expectations

Perhaps because cognitive-behavioral therapy has the reputation of solving problems rapidly, some patients have unrealistically positive expectations for therapy. Many cognitive-behavioral therapists find it helpful to examine these expectations up front with their patients, including the patients' expectations about and willingness to do self-help assignments. The information forms for patients that we provide in this treatment package may be helpful in dispelling some of these unrealistic expectations and providing the basis for a therapeutic contract and alliance that can moderate the patients' expectations.

Nonetheless, many patients with panic disorder have unrealistic expectations about psychological and physiological discomfort. We have already referred to these in regard to the all-or-nothing attitude toward anxiety and the intolerance of any anxiety. Some patients may have unrealistically negative expectations—especially patients with chronic problems that have been unsuccessfully treated in the past. Many of these patients have been "pathologized" by clinicians as "resistant," "psychotic," or "deeply disturbed." We find it helpful to inform these patients that the cognitive-behavioral approach to panic disorder is relatively new, that their other therapists may have been trained in another treatment modality developed at an earlier time, and that the treatment approach that we will use is quite different.

Fear of Transference

Just as panic patients are uncomfortable with uncontrollable anxiety, they are uncomfortable about uncontrollable relationships. Patients may be fearful that therapy will lead them into becoming dependent and trapped in their dependency; that their weakness will be exposed and that they will feel humiliated; that anxiety will get worse as they engage in introspection; or that they will become sexually aroused and attracted to their therapists and be unable to control these feelings and impulses. In fact, it is our belief that many such patients prefer a short-term, structured treatment approach because of some of these fears—especially the fear of becoming dependent. These automatic thoughts and assumptions can be examined in therapy, especially if the transference threatens continuation in treatment. We find it helpful to show how these fears parallel the general intolerance of unrealistic, uncontrollable, or anxious feelings—which is a general problem in panic disorder and agoraphobia. In some cases, the added credibility of the therapist due to the success in handling panic may be used in addressing more general relationship issues.

Phasing Out Treatment

Many patients report rapid improvement in their panic and agoraphobia after a few treatment sessions. We caution patients against premature termination, since the goal of therapy is not only the elimination of panic attacks, but also the acquisition of a variety of coping skills that will decrease the likelihood of relapse. Although our treatment package recommends 12 sessions, it may be possible to provide adequate treatment in fewer sessions. Phasing back to biweekly or monthly sessions for the last few sessions helps the patient practice functioning independently of therapy, thereby increasing the likelihood that improvement can be attributed to self-help rather than to the relationship with the therapist. During phase-out, the patient is encouraged to self-assign homework. Homework may focus on a review of typical difficult situations (those listed in the exposure hierarchy) and the cognitive distortions associated with these situations.

CASE EXAMPLE

Session 1

Assessment

Phyllis was a 29-year-old married woman who reported a 2-year history of anxiety, panic, worries, and agoraphobic avoidance. Her panic symptoms included heart palpitations, hyperventilation, feelings of derealization and depersonalization, and dizziness. On many occasions she avoided subways, trains, planes, long trips in cars, and crowded theaters. Although she did walk in the city on her own, she reported that at times she would become so anxious that she feared she would hyperventilate and collapse.

Assessment measures

Phyllis reported mild dysphoria (her BDI score was 11), and on the SCL-90-R she complained of nervousness, repeated unpleasant thoughts, suddenly being scared for no reason, feeling blue, worrying, feeling no interest in things, feeling fearful, heart pounding or racing, trouble falling asleep, fear of traveling on subways and trains, fear (trouble) getting her breath, avoidance of various places, feeling tense and keyed up, and having frightening thoughts and images. On the SCID-II, she had elevated scores on the scales assessing obsessive–compulsive and narcissistic personality traits. She reported no significant marital discord, no history of drug or alcohol abuse, and abstinence from caffeinated drinks and foods. Her parents had divorced when she was 5, and her grandmother had been a housebound agoraphobic for several

Anxiety evaluation

years. She reported such considerable anxiety about giving public speeches that she had made a career change *downward* to take a job as a secretary (for which she felt overqualified). This resulted in feelings of resentment toward her supervisors and self-criticism that she was not fulfilling her potential. She had the desire to avoid subways (especially the express train, with less frequent stops and therefore fewer opportunities for escape), trains, planes, and walking any considerable distance.

Although generally healthy, Phyllis reported gastroenterological problems, which had an onset 6 years prior to the beginning of the agoraphobic worries.

Phyllis described a panic attack on the subway in August of

the previous year when she felt dizzy, felt her heart racing, and was hot, she did not hyperventilate. At that time she worried that she might pass out. She described how during the last 2 years she would anticipate anxiety or panic attacks—ironically, often focused on hyperventilation, *even though she did not hyperventilate.* Her automatic thoughts regarding this were "I'll have trouble breathing," "I'll have to withdraw," and "I'll become an agoraphobic like my grandmother."

Diagnosis   The diagnosis was panic disorder with moderate agoraphobia, and comorbid social phobia. (Phyllis's therapy included treatment for the social phobia, but the present discussion focuses on treatment for her panic disorder and agoraphobia.) Although the SCID-II revealed several obsessive–compulsive personality traits, on inquiry she did not qualify for a diagnosis of obsessive–compulsive or narcissistic personality disorder. There were moderate stressors focused on the change in her job. Her marital relationship was good.

Session 2

Socialization to treatment   Phyllis was extremely ambivalent about therapy; she feared that therapy would lead her to label herself as very neurotic, or that she would uncover information about herself that would be upsetting to her. She believed that she should be able to solve all her problems without help, and that others would think less of her if they knew she was anxious.

Progressive muscle relaxation and breathing relaxation   Phyllis was trained in this session in the use of progressive muscle relaxation, and was asked to practice this daily at home. Breathing relaxation training was also initiated in this session, with the therapist modeling slow inhaling and exhaling, demonstrating that the goal of proper breathing would be to raise a small book placed on the abdomen. Phyllis was cautioned against shallow chest breathing and breathing too rapidly.

Providing feedback   The therapist provided Phyllis with feedback regarding the data from the intake forms and the clinical interview, including the diagnosis of the problem. She was given the general information handout for patients about panic disorder and agoraphobia (Form 3.4), as well as the Burns (1989) and Wilson (1987) books. She was also presented with a general outline of treatment options. Although medication was one option presented to her, she *Medication considered*   rejected this idea because of her belief that she should be able to solve her problems on her own. Because of her excellent compliance with homework as treatment progressed, the therapist eventually concluded that medication was unnecessary.

Session 3

Construction of fear hierarchy

A fear hierarchy was constructed by asking Phyllis to rate her feared situations from least to most feared (accompanied or unaccompanied). Her feared situation was traveling alone on a transatlantic flight (where escape would be blocked for hours and public humiliation in case of panic would be high). Her least feared situation was walking down the street accompanied by her husband.

One of Phyllis's feared and avoided situations was riding the subway, and this was listed in the middle range of her fear hierarchy. Riding the subway in the company of a friend made it somewhat less frightening. After construction of the fear hierarchy, the therapist suggested that they experiment by going down into the subway together at the end of the session. Phyllis accepted, and they prepared by reviewing the muscle relaxation and breathing relaxation techniques taught in the previous session. In addition,

Rebreathing

Phyllis practiced rebreathing (i.e., breathing into her hands cupped over her mouth). The therapist indicated that the purpose of this was to restore the proper balance of CO_2 and oxygen. Phyllis was asked to practice breathing relaxation and rebreathing techniques once per day and whenever she was anxious. Phyllis

In vivo exposure

and the therapist then went together to a subway entrance and down into the subway station.

Session 4

Cognitive and behavioral techniques used during in vivo *exposure*

During the first and subsequent exposures in the subway, Phyllis and the therapist used a number of cognitive and behavioral techniques. These included distraction, muscle and breathing relaxation, permission to leave the situation, coping statements to decatastrophize anxiety, and challenging automatic thoughts.

Stress management

Back in the office, Phyllis and the therapist engaged in stress management and began examining her cognitive distortions. Stress management included examination of the pros and cons of Phyllis's current job, acceptance of her anxiety variability, application of the double-standard technique to her intolerance of anxiety, and consideration of the occupational and training opportunities available to her.

Examining automatic thoughts and assumptions

Work with Phyllis's cognitive distortions began with identifying her negative automatic thoughts and maladaptive assumptions. Some of Phyllis's typical distorted automatic thoughts were as follows:

"I'll have a panic attack."
"I won't be able to get out."

"My heart will start racing."
"I won't be able to breathe."
"I'll have an asthmatic attack."
"I'll pass out."

And some of her maladaptive assumptions were as follows:

"Everyone thinks I have it together. If people find out I'm anxious, they'll think less of me."
"If I say something [about anxiety], I'll jinx it."
"What I don't know won't hurt me. You shouldn't talk about my agoraphobia. I'm too suggestible."
"If I think about anxiety, I'll have a panic attack."
"If it's possible it could happen, I should worry about it. If it's possible, it's probable. It's dangerous if my heart races."

A review of her automatic thoughts indicated considerable fortunetelling, catastrophic thinking, mind reading, and labeling. Her assumptions focused on the demand to eliminate all anxiety, her belief that her anxiety was dangerous and uncontrollable, and her belief in hypervigilance. As a consequence of these thoughts, Phyllis would escalate her catastrophizing and fortunetelling, and avoid any situations in which her anxiety might be present. Her fear of talking about anxiety was a substantial source of her ambivalence about being in therapy.

Sessions 5–8

Imaginal exposure

In-session imaginal exposure involved, first, asking Phyllis to imagine being on the subway and feeling anxious. She was asked to describe step by step exactly what she saw happening, to the conclusion of arriving home. This imaginal exposure scenario was

Rehearsing rational responses to automatic thoughts

repeated, this time with the therapist providing her with rational responses to her catastrophic thoughts. Imaginal exposure was then gone through a third time with the therapist playing devil's advocate and voicing Phyllis's catastrophic thoughts while Phyllis provided rational responses to them.

Another imaginal exposure exercise used was the following: Phyllis was asked to imagine herself on the subway alone in a crowded, hot car, feeling short of breath and dizzy. When her SUDs rating reached 8 during this imagery exercise, she was told to breathe slowly into her hands and to focus her breathing into her abdomen. Phyllis was told that she could have induced a panic attack by hyperventilating, but that this was unnecessary, since she could imagine a higher level of anxiety and practice rebreathing. In addition, Phyllis was instructed in other coping techniques to handle her hyperventilation, such as running in place, sitting down, or lying with her feet above her head in case of faintness. Finally, the therapist gave Phyllis the list of coping statements for patients (Form 3.6), as well as a "coping card" developed especially for her anxiety (Table 3.3).

Sessions 9–10

Increasing in vivo *exposure*

Phyllis began *in vivo* exposure on her own by taking a local subway that would stop every couple of minutes. She gradually increased her exposure to the express subway. Over subsequent weeks, she also began going out to restaurants and theaters more often. Before Phyllis began taking each step in the exposure hierarchy, the therapist would rehearse with her images of panic and anxiety in the feared situation, challenge her with her negative automatic thoughts (which she then had to refute), and provide her with behavioral techniques (e.g., rebreathing) to handle the physical manifestations of anxiety. Even the situation highest in her hierarchy (i.e., transatlantic travel) was similarly handled. As a result, she and her husband successfully flew to Europe and back.

Imaginal exposure, challenging negative thoughts, and using behavioral coping techniques

Sessions 11–12

Examining schemas and modifying them

Phyllis viewed herself through the schemas of control and rationality, and she viewed others as rejecting and evaluating. She compensated for her vulnerability to others' reactions by attempting

TABLE 3.3. "Coping Card" For Phyllis's Anxiety

1. Specifically, what am I predicting will happen?
2. How often do I predict incorrectly?
3. What is the worst outcome? The best outcome? The most likely outcome?
4. Aren't some anxiety and discomfort normal?
5. I've never stopped breathing. My heart has never stopped. I'm healthy.
6. Escape is not relevant, because there is no danger.
7. I have a lot of unrealistic, "magical" thoughts. These are just thoughts, not facts.
8. If I have a panic attack, I can think of it as a variation in arousal. It's not dangerous.
9. I've never had problems with hyperventilating. But if I did, I could breathe into my hands slowly. I could sit down. I could try to breathe into my stomach.

Examining schema compensation and avoidance

Submitting schemas to challenges

Examining origin of schemas

always to be strong, independent, logical, and in command of herself. She also avoided situations where she might be trapped (e.g., subways) or might be evaluated negatively for her anxiety.

Phyllis's all-or-nothing view of anxiety and control was addressed by using the cost–benefit technique, by examining evidence for and against the idea that she needed to have complete control, and by examining the origin of her schemas about emotionality. Phyllis recalled that her mother was a highly emotional (probably histrionic) individual who had caused her much embarrassment. As a result, Phyllis equated strong emotions with "weakness" and "irrationality," which she and the therapist contrasted with "being more fully alive" and "being a complete human being." Phyllis found the double-standard technique particularly useful when she applied it to friends who might be anxious.

Stress management for other areas of Phyllis's life

Phyllis had other sources of stress that she raised in therapy—specifically, her ambivalence and anger at feeling trapped in her job (a job she had chosen because of her comorbid social phobia). Cognitive therapy was helpful in challenging her self-critical thoughts about her position and in helping her examine her all-or-nothing thinking about anxiety and weakness.

Continued exposure

As therapy progressed, Phyllis began normalizing her life by using all forms of public transportation, as well as increasing the distances that she could walk comfortably in the city. She almost never used the rebreathing technique when she became anxious, but simply knowing that it might work helped her decatastrophize anxiety. Phyllis became quite adept at anticipating how she would handle future situations that might arouse anxiety.

Assertiveness

She also became more assertive at work (where she was "underemployed") and began considering the possibility of further professional training in graduate school. Her perfectionism about anxiety—that is, her early goal of trying to eliminate all anxiety—was challenged and modified by examining the value of accepting sensations and feelings; by examining whether they might be useful signs of other problems in her life (especially her resentment about feeling trapped in her job); and by decatastrophizing anxious arousal through recognizing that arousal seldom led to panic, that panic never led to losing total control, and that she was able to continue doing things even when she was anxious. Therapy was phased out by reducing sessions to biweekly and then once per month, with no relapse of symptoms. Reviewing her typical automatic thoughts and assumptions and providing her with an outline of the treatment plan helped her to phase out treatment comfortably.

DETAILED TREATMENT PLAN FOR PANIC DISORDER AND AGORAPHOBIA

Treatment Reports

Tables 3.4 and 3.5 are designed to help you in writing managed care treatment reports for patients with panic disorder alone or with panic disorder and agoraphobia. From Table 3.4, select the symptoms that are appropriate for your patient. (Zuckerman's [1995] *Clinician's Thesaurus* provides other applicable words and phrases.) Be sure also to specify the nature of the patient's impairments, including any dysfunction in academic, work, family, or social areas, with agoraphobia, this dysfunction is usually considerable. Table 3.5 lists sample treatment goals and matching interventions. Again, select those that are appropriate for the patient.

Session-by-Session Treatment Options

The clinician may choose to abbreviate therapy by emphasizing interventions focused on panic disorder and agoraphobia—such as muscle relaxation and breathing relaxation training, exposure to the fear hierarchy, cognitive restructuring (e.g., decatastrophizing anxiety), and in-session panic induction and exposure to panic symptoms. Clark and his colleagues at Oxford University report a high degree of success with an abbreviated treatment package. The treatment options outlined in Table 3.6 are for 12 sessions, but treatment may be lengthened or shortened where necessary. Once more, choose the options that are suitable for your patient.

TABLE 3.4. Sample Symptoms for Panic Disorder and Agoraphobia

Panic Disorder

Panic attacks (specify frequency)

Heart racing

Palpitations

Sweating

Shaking

Difficulty breathing

Chest pain

Tightness in chest

Nausea

Dizziness

Feeling faint

Derealization

Depersonalization

Numbness

Tingling

Chills

Hot flashes

Fear of losing control

Fear of dying

Fear of going crazy

Fear of having future panic attacks

Specify any change in behavior as a result of panic attacks

Agoraphobia

Specify situations feared—examples:
   Fear of being alone
   Fear of crowded places
   Fear of being in public
   Fear of bus, subway, car, train, plane
   Fear of having a panic attack

Unable to go places without a companion

Specify which feared situations are avoided

TABLE 3.5. Sample Treatment Goals and Interventions for Panic Disorder and Agoraphobia

Treatment goals	Interventions
Reducing physical symptoms of anxiety/panic	Muscle and breathing relaxation training
Acquiring breathing skills	Breathing relaxation and rebreathing training
Eliminating conditioned anxiety response to physical sensations	Exposure
Stating belief that physical anxiety symptoms are not harmful	Cognitive restructuring, behavioral experiments
Engaging in all previously avoided activities	Exposure
Eliminating safety behaviors	Exposure
Modifying schemas of vulnerability and need for control (or other schemas—specify)	Cognitive restructuring, developmental analysis
Reporting that fear of future panic attacks has been reduced to less than 1 on a scale of 0–10	Cognitive restructuring, skills review, and practice
Eliminating impairment (specify—depending on impairments, this may be several goals)	Cognitive restructuring, problem-solving training, or other skills training (specify)
No panic attacks for 1 month	All of the above
Eliminating all avoidance behavior	All of the above
SCL-90-R anxiety scores in normal range	All of the above
Acquiring relapse prevention skills	Reviewing and practicing techniques as necessary

TABLE 3.6. Session-by-Session Treatment Options for Panic Disorder and Agoraphobia

Session 1

Assessment

Inquire regarding all symptoms

Administer Initial Evaluation of Anxiety and Avoidance for Patients (Form 3.2)

Administer standard battery of intake measures (see Form 3.3), plus additional anxiety questionnaires as appropriate

Evaluate for comorbid conditions (e.g., major depression, other anxiety disorders)

Evaluate substance use; evaluate need for counseling or detoxification if patient has substance abuse or dependence

Evaluate need for medication

Homework

Assign Wilson's *Don't Panic* or Burns's *The Feeling Good Handbook*

Session 2

Socialization to Treatment

Inform patient of diagnosis

Develop list of treatment goals

Provide patient with information handouts on panic disorder and agoraphobia (Form 3.4) and on cognitive-behavioral therapy in general (Form B.1, Appendix B)

Cognitive-Behavioral Interventions

Train patient in muscle relaxation, breathing relaxation

Have patient begin constructing hierarchy of feared situations (Form 3.5)

Teach patient self-monitoring of anxiety/panic (Form 3.7)

Begin identifying automatic thoughts in feared situations (Form 3.8)

Medication

Consider medication (if patient is not already using it) and review side effects and efficacy

Homework

Have patient practice relaxation

Have patient begin self-monitoring of anxiety/panic

Session 3

Assessment

Evaluate anxiety (BAI) and depression (BDI)

Examine patient's hierarchy of feared situations (Form 3.5) and typical thoughts in those situations (Form 3.8)

Examine patient's self-monitoring of anxiety/panic (Form 3.7)

Evaluate patient's ability to induce relaxation in session

Evaluate homework

Cognitive-Behavioral Interventions

Continue training in muscle relaxation, breathing relaxation

Continue to elicit automatic thoughts associated with anxiety, and provide patient with challenges to thoughts (see Table B.3, Appendix B)

Medication
  Evaluate side effects
  Evaluate need to increase dosage
  If no improvement, either increase dosage, add another medication, or change class of
    medication (consider the need to taper or discontinue one class of medication when
    adding another class)

Homework
  Have patient practice relaxation and continue self-monitoring of automatic thoughts when
    anxious/panicking

Session 4

Assessment
  As in Session 3

Cognitive-Behavioral Interventions
  Focus on catastrophic thinking, fortunetelling, labeling, self-criticism
  Continue presenting challenges to automatic thoughts (see Table B.3)
  Identify and challenge underlying maladaptive assumptions
  Begin exposure by using imagery in session
  Plan and rehearse *in vivo* exposure outside of session

Medication
  As in Session 3

Homework
  Have patient practice relaxation
  Have patient record and challenge automatic thoughts

Sessions 5–8

Assessment
  As in Session 3

Cognitive-Behavioral Interventions
  Continue with imaginal exposure of panic
  Conduct actual in-session induction of panic symptoms—rebreathing or other techniques in
    session
  Focus on self-instruction to decatastrophize panic symptoms
  Have patient develop self-instructions for anxiety and stress
  Plan exposure to situations higher in hierarchy

Medication
  As in Session 3

Homework
  Have patient practice relaxation
  Assign *in vivo* exposure to situations higher in hierarchy—have patient write down
    predictions before exposure, cognitive challenges, and outcome; assign "worry time"

(cont.)

TABLE 3.6 *(cont.)*

Sessions 9–10

Assessment

As in Session 3

Examine increased exposure, decreased number of panic attacks

Cognitive-Behavioral Interventions

Review past negative predictions and outcomes

Review progress

Rewrite new, adaptive assumptions

Develop self-instructions for anxiety and stress

Plan phase-out of sessions for panic disorder/agoraphobia

Evaluate whether patient needs further work on panic disorder/agoraphobia or other problems

Evaluate situations that arouse anxiety or interpersonal conflict

Evaluate need for assertion training, relationship enhancement skills, mutual problem solving, ability to construct alternatives

Medication

As in Session 3

Homework

Have patient practice relaxation

Assign *in vivo* exposure to situations higher in hierarchy—have patient write down predictions before exposure, cognitive challenges, and outcome

Have patient monitor and challenge automatic thoughts related to current everyday conflicts

Sessions 11–12 (Scheduled Biweekly)

Assessment

As in Session 3

Readminister SCL-90-R, Fear Questionnaire

Cognitive-Behavioral Interventions

Review patient's ability to identify and challenge anxious thoughts

Review patient's interpretation of anxiety symptoms and ability to reduce anxiety through relaxation, rebreathing, reattribution, or self-instruction

Evaluate whether patient continues to expose self to anxiety-provoking situations

Homework

Assign continued exposure to anxiety-provoking situations

Have patient develop own homework

Have patient anticipate anxiety-provoking situations that might arise and list possible coping strategies (behavioral, interpersonal, and cognitive)

CHAPTER 4

Generalized Anxiety Disorder

DESCRIPTION AND DIAGNOSIS

Symptoms

The essential features of generalized anxiety disorder (abbreviated GAD in the text of this chapter) are apprehensive worry and physical symptoms such as restlessness, fatigue, problems with concentration, irritability, muscle tension, and/or insomnia (American Psychiatric Association, 1994). GAD is distinguished from other anxiety disorders in that the individual is worried about a variety of events; in other anxiety disorders, worry is confined to specific stimuli or issues. For example, in panic disorder the worry is focused on panic attacks, in social phobia the worry focuses on embarrassment in public, in obsessive–compulsive disorder the worry focuses on contamination or the fear of the consequences of not performing rituals, and in hypochondriasis the worry focuses on possible illness.

Prevalence and Life Course

Epidemiological studies indicate that the lifetime prevalence of GAD varies between 5.8% and 9%, with greater risk for women (the female-to-male ratio is 2.5:1), young adults, and blacks (Blazer, George, & Hughes, 1991; Breslau & Davis, 1985). Patients presenting with GAD often claim that the onset has been gradual and that they have been anxious since childhood; some studies indicate the average duration of this problem prior to treatment is 25 years (Butler, Fennell, Robson, & Geldeer, 1991; Rapee, 1989, 1991a, 1991b). Because of its chronicity, its self-perpetuating quality, and often its lack of response to treatment, some clinicians and researchers view GAD as a lifelong illness, similar to diabetes or essential hypertension.

Genetic/Biological Factors

Although some estimates indicate that GAD may have a moderate heritability of 30% (Kendler, Neale, Kessler, Heath, & Eaves, 1992), other findings suggest lack of specificity of transmission (Weissman & Merikangas, 1986). GAD is associated with other specific traits, such as nervousness, depression, low frustration tolerance, and inhibition (Angst & Vollrath, 1991).

Coexisting Conditions

Most patients with GAD present with a variety of other diagnoses, including social and specific phobia, major depression, irritable bowel syndrome, and personality disorders (see Borkovec & Roemer, 1996; Brown & Barlow, 1992; Brown, Moras, Zinberg, & Barlow, 1993; Sanderson & Wetzler, 1991). Ninety percent of individuals who develop GAD during their lifetimes also have another psychiatric condition, with 42% qualifying for a diagnosis of major depression or dysthymia (Sanderson, Di-Nardo, Rapee, & Barlow, 1990). The most common personality disorders associated with GAD are avoidant and dependent, with obsessive–compulsive personality disorder proving most common in one study (Nestadt et al., 1992). In another study, close to 50% of GAD patients qualified for a diagnosis of some personality disorder (Sanderson & Wetzler, 1991). Recent threatening events and recent life stresses are associated with GAD (Finlay-Jones & Brown, 1981; Blazer et al., 1991), although its chronicity suggests that the *perception* of stress and threat may partly result from GAD.

Differential Diagnosis

The nature of GAD is that the individual is worried about a number of things, not simply one or two. Consequently, GAD can be differentiated from specific phobia, in which patients fear a specific, well-defined stimulus (e.g., animals). It can also be distinguished from social phobia, in which patients are specifically worried about or avoid situations in which negative evaluation is expected. Furthermore, GAD can be distinguished from obsessive–compulsive disorder, panic disorder, other anxiety disorders, and disorders in other DSM-IV categories. (Figure 4.1 is a diagnostic flow chart that provides more details about differential diagnosis of GAD.) Note that when the diagnosis is anxiety disorder due to a general medical condition or substance-induced anxiety disorder, the substance use should be the top priority.

UNDERSTANDING GENERALIZED ANXIETY DISORDER IN COGNITIVE-BEHAVIORAL TERMS

Several cognitive-behavioral conceptualizations of GAD are of value to the clinician. In this section we first discuss behavioral models, emphasizing conditioned anxiety, and cognitive models, emphasizing information processing and appraisal of stress. We then discuss a number of models that combine cognitive and behavioral elements.

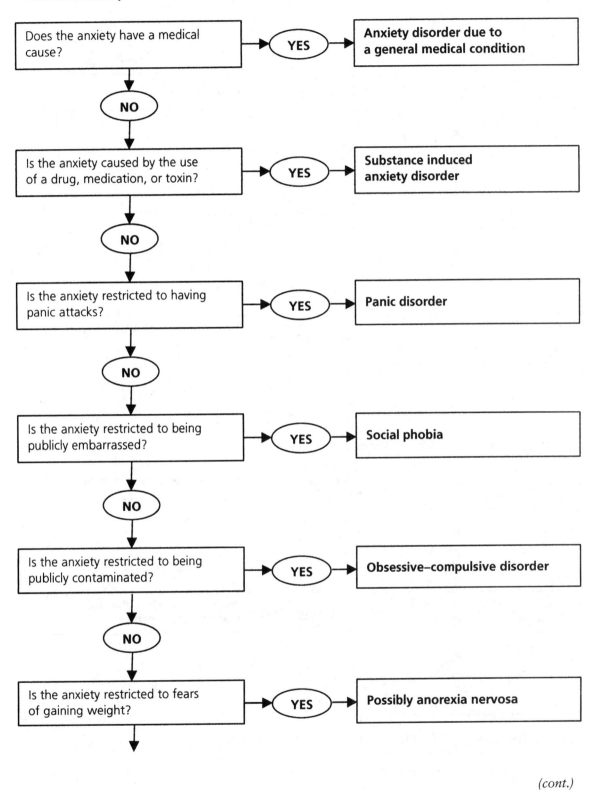

FIGURE 4.1. Diagnostic flow chart for generalized anxiety disorder.

(cont.)

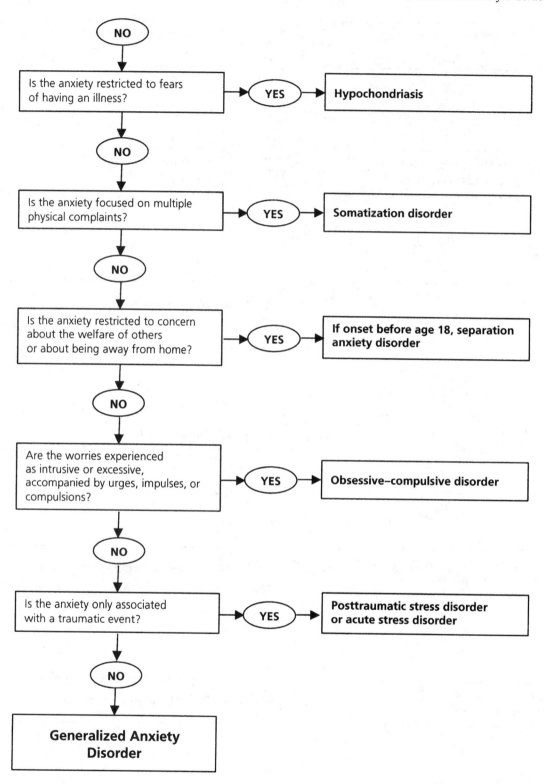

FIGURE 4.1 *(cont.)*

Behavioral Factors

Wolpe (1958) proposed that a neutral stimulus becomes conditioned to an unconditioned fear-arousing stimulus, leading to the acquisition of fear. His model of reciprocal inhibition proposes that fear may be "unlearned" by pairing the feared stimulus or response with a response that is incompatible with fear, such as relaxation, assertiveness, or sexual arousal. Other models of fear reduction include extinction, habituation, exposure, changes in expectancy, and self-efficacy. Although applying Wolpe's and other behavioral models of fear and anxiety to treatment may be somewhat more complex in GAD than in other anxiety disorders (because a patient with GAD worries about or fears many things, not just one or a few well-defined stimuli), the clinician treating a patient with GAD may use any number of behavioral techniques, depending on the patient's particular needs. These include the construction of fear hierarchies and planned exposure to various feared situations, images, or ideas; pairing of relaxation with exposure to these feared things, in some instances (i.e., self-directed desensitization); thought-stopping; modeling; vicarious reinforcement (and punishment); assertiveness training; self-efficacy training; and problem-solving training. Several of these techniques are discussed later in this chapter, and some are described in detail in Appendix A and in the CD-ROM accompanying this book.

Cognitive Factors

According to Beck et al. (1985), anxiety responses had adaptive value in the evolution of the human species. Anxiety responses, such as mobilization, inhibition, and demobilization, reflect active defense, avoidance of risky behavior, and collapse, respectively, which were protective responses in the face of various types of threats. Active defense, involving hypervigilance, sensitivity to sound, and increased heart rate, may assist the individual in either flight or fight. Inhibitory responses, such as blocking of thinking, clouding of consciousness, and muscle rigidity, prevent the individual from taking unnecessary risks (as evidenced in fear of heights or in social phobia). Demobilization is reflected in weakness, fatigue, lowered blood pressure, and lowered heart rate, leading to collapsing or freezing in place, which decrease the likelihood that the individual will be detected by predators (see Beck et al., 1985; Marks, 1987).

Responses to threat include fight, flight, freezing, fainting (collapse), retraction, dodging, clinging, calling for help, and other reflexes (eye blinking, gagging, coughing), with corresponding cognitive implications: "I have to get out of here," "I can't move," "What is happening to me?," or "Don't leave me." The cognitive model stresses the importance of various distortions in information processing in anxiety—specifically, hypervigilance, false alarms, loss of objectivity, generalization of danger to other stimuli, catastrophizing, excessive focus on negative outcomes, no tolerance for uncertainty, and "lack of habituation" (Beck et al., 1985). (Like Beck and colleagues, Lazarus emphasizes stress or threat appraisal; see Lazarus, 1991; Lazarus & Folkman, 1984.)

The cognitive model acknowledges that individuals may differ in being biologically predisposed toward the arousal of anxiety symptoms and the perception of threat. However, once the anxiety is aroused, it is increased or maintained by specific cognitive distortions. Some examples of the three types of these distortions in GAD are provided in Table 4.1.

Other Cognitive-Behavioral Models

Barlow's Model

The excellent work of Barlow has influenced the clinical treatment of anxiety disorders in general. GAD, with its focus on arousal, hypervigilance, and worry, is explained by reference to five factors operating in interaction with one another (Barlow, 1988): negative life events, biological vulnerability, diffuse stress response, psychological vulnerability (with accompanying sense of lack of control and predictability), and lack of coping skills or support that might mitigate lack of controllability. During the "anxious apprehension cycle," there may be accompanying "false alarms" that serve to exacerbate the sense of uncontrollability and vulnerability. With the focus on (sometimes) minor life events and the accompanying sense of loss of control over worry, the anxiety may gener-

---

TABLE 4.1. Examples of the Three Types of Cognitive Distortions in Generalized Anxiety Disorder

<u>Distorted automatic thoughts</u>

Catastrophizing: "Something terrible is going to happen," "I am going to fail."

Labeling: "I'm a failure," "My boss is a tyrant."

Dichotomous thinking: "I am always anxious," "I'm never good enough."

Overgeneralizing: "I can't handle my anxiety. I can't handle anything."

<u>Maladaptive assumptions</u>

"I must get rid of all anxiety—immediately and forever."

"Anxiety and worry are unhealthy."

"If people knew that I was anxious, they would reject me."

"Anxiety is a sign of weakness. I should never be weak."

"I shouldn't be anxious."

"I have to watch out for my anxiety so it doesn't catch me by surprise."

<u>Dysfunctional schemas</u>

Biological threat: "Anxiety means I'm sick."

Humiliation: "People will laugh at me."

Control: "I am either in complete control or I have no control."

Autonomy: "Anxiety means I'm weak and dependent. I can't survive on my own."

Abandonment: "I will be abandoned."

Note. Adapted from Leahy (1996). Copyright 1996 by Jason Aronson, Inc. Adapted by permission.

alize to a variety of innocuous situations and increase. The treatment recommended involves reducing autonomic arousal with relaxation techniques, improving coping skills, and cognitive restructuring.

Borkovec's Model

The model of worry advanced by Borkovec (Borkovec & Inz, 1990; Borkovec, Shadick, & Hopkins, 1991) stresses the role of attempts at suppression of negative images. The anxious individual, beset by concerns of negative and catastrophic outcomes, attempts to prevent these outcomes by anticipating escape or avoidance, which presumably will suppress the occurrence of the negative outcome image. For example, an anxious individual who begins to worry about going bankrupt examines all the evidence that he or she will not be able to pay her bills, attempting to figure out how these problems can occur and how they can be avoided or solved.

Wells and Butler's Model

Wells and Butler have advanced a metacognitive model of GAD, emphasizing the central role of *worrying* in this disorder. Wells and Butler (1997) indicate that GAD patients overestimate the likelihood of negative events, rate the cost of threatening events as very high, and interpret ambiguous events as more threatening than persons without GAD would interpret them. Wells (1994a, 1994b) and Wells and Butler (1997) propose that GAD patients have both positive and negative beliefs about worrying. That is they worry about worrying, but they also believe that giving up worrying may expose them to unforeseen threat or danger. Wells and Butler (1997, p. 167) indicate that these positive attitudes about worrying include the following beliefs: "Worrying helps me cope with future problems," "If I think of all the bad things that could happen, I'll be prepared to prevent them," and "I'll be tempting fate [if I don't worry]." Wells and Butler distinguish between Type 1 and Type 2 worry. Type 1 worry refers to concern or vigilance about external or internal (e.g., health) threats. Type 2 worry, or "metaworry," refers to negative appraisal of one's own cognitive processes—for example, "Worrying will make me crazy." According to this model, the anxious individual is locked in a conflict between the fear that worry is uncontrollable and the belief that worry protects him or her.

The therapeutic model derived from this theory involves identification of the patient's beliefs about the costs and benefits of worrying, the recognition of productive worrying, experiments in "letting go" of worry or postponing worry, challenging avoidance of activities or thoughts about which the patient worries, and constructing positive outcomes in imagery (Wells & Butler, 1997).

Outcome Studies for Cognitive-Behavioral Treatment

Given the apparent chronicity and poor spontaneous remission rates of GAD, it is promising that there are now treatments with some demonstrated efficacy. Borkovec and Whisman (1996) indicate that psychosocial treatments (especially cognitive-behavioral treatment) have proven to be more effective than nondirective treatment, a placebo or a benzodiazepine; that gains are maintained by cognitive-behavioral therapy or behavior therapy; that cognitive-behavioral therapy leads to a reduction of the use of benzodiazepines; that these gains are clinically significant; and that for some patients, gains actually improve even after therapy is discontinued. Schwiezer and Rickels (1996) indicate that 70% of GAD patients respond to benzodiazepines. Butler et al. (1991) found that cognitive-behavioral therapy was superior to behavior therapy in producing "good outcome" for patients 6 months after treatment ended (42% vs. 5%, respectively, although another study found statistically similar outcomes for cognitive-behavioral therapy and behavior therapy (58% and 38%, respectively) (Durham et al., 1994). When compared with psychoanalytic treatment, cognitive-behavioral therapy was far superior—a "good outcome" rate of 72% versus 31%, respectively (Durham, 1995).

ASSESSMENT AND TREATMENT

Rationale and Plan for Treatment

The patient presenting with GAD has symptoms that include physiological arousal (restlessness, muscle tension, sleep disturbance), as well as cognitive symptoms (worry, difficulty controlling worry, and inability to concentrate). The goals of treatment are to reduce to the overall level of autonomic arousal, to decrease the concern about worry, and to assist the patient in reducing worry to a reasonable level. Since the patient is worried about a variety of situations and themes, more "general" interventions are employed. That is, the therapist will use interventions such as progressive muscle relaxation, biofeedback, breathing relaxation, and behavioral treatment of insomnia in order to reduce overall levels of anxious arousal, and will employ a variety of cognitive interventions to address the worry. These cognitive interventions include assisting the patient in distinguishing between productive and unproductive worry, addressing the patient's concern that worrying too much may be harmful, assessing the patient's tendency to jump to conclusions and catastrophize, and helping him or her learn to distinguish between anxiety and actual facts. We have developed an extensive self-help form called Questions to Ask Yourself If You Are Worrying (see Form 4.5, below), which may be tailored to the needs of the individual patient. In addition, since a patient with GAD is worrying throughout the day, the clinician will assist the patient in limiting worry to "worry time" and will help the patient monitor the different themes of worry. Finally, the treatment approach will help the patient recognize that he or she may be quite able to cope with a variety of problems, should they arise.

The treatment of the patient with GAD often involves addressing more than one disorder, since 83–91% have a comorbid disorder (Barlow, DiNardo, Vermilyea, Vermilyea, & Blanchard, 1986; Sanderson et al., 1990). The treatment package for GAD is outlined in Table 4.2. In practice, the sequence of the elements listed in this table is variable, with the therapist often using several techniques simultaneously. Moreover, since GAD is so often comorbid with depression or other anxiety disorders, the clinician will usually need to employ more than one treatment package.

TABLE 4.2. General Plan of Treatment for Generalized Anxiety Disorder

Assessment
  Initial clinical evaluation of anxiety symptoms
  Tests and other evaluations
  Consideration of medication
Socialization to treatment
Relaxation training
Assessing and confronting avoidance: Exposure and other techniques
Desensitization: Pairing (or not pairing) exposure with relaxation
Monitoring worries and assigning "worry time"
Cognitive evaluation of the nature of worrying
Other techniques for countering worrying and rumination
Interpersonal interventions
Stress reduction and problem-solving training
Phasing out treatment

Assessment

Forms 4.1 and 4.2 provide guidance for therapists in the evaluation of GAD. Form 4.1 is a checklist to be completed by the patient that covers the DSM-IV symptoms of GAD, as well as some symptoms of other anxiety disorders. Form 4.2 provides space for recording the patient's scores on various assessment instruments, for noting other relevant aspects of the patient's history (substance use, previous anxiety episodes), and for recording treatment recommendations.

Initial Clinical Evaluation of Anxiety Symptoms

Form 4.1, the Leahy Anxiety Checklist for Patients, is a checklist that allows the patient to endorse the specific symptoms of anxiety he or she has been experiencing. The checklist covers not only the symptoms of GAD as specified by DSM-IV, but some symptoms (e.g., shortness of breath, dizziness, pounding heart) of other anxiety disorders (e.g., panic disorder); if these latter symptoms are endorsed, this gives the clinician a preliminary indication that comorbid anxiety disorders may be present and will need to be treated. Scores between 5 and 10 reflect mild anxiety, 11 and 15 moderate anxiety, and 16 or higher significant anxiety.

Tests and Other Evaluations

Evaluation of patients with GAD during the intake and at later points may involve a number of self-report or interview instruments, such as the BAI, BDI, GAF, SCID-II, and Locke–Wallace (see Chapters 2 and 3). The SCL-90-R (also mentioned in Chapters 2 and 3) has a scale (factor) evaluating anxiety that can be distinguished from phobia and obsessive–compulsive symptoms, although there is some overlap between the Obsessive–

FORM 4.1. Leahy Anxiety Checklist for Patients

Patient's Name: _____ Today's Date: _____

Place a number next to the answer that best describes how you have been feeling generally during the past month. Use the scale below:

   1 = Not at all   2 = Slightly true   3 = Somewhat true   4 = Very true

1. Feeling shaky   _____

2. Unable to relax   _____

3. Feeling restless   _____

4. Get tired easily   _____

5. Headaches   _____

6. Shortness of breath   _____

7. Dizzy or light-headed   _____

8. Need to urinate frequently   _____

9. Sweating (unrelated to heat)   _____

10. Heart pounding   _____

11. Heartburn or upset stomach   _____

12. Easily irritated   _____

13. Startled easily   _____

14. Difficulty sleeping   _____

15. Worried a lot   _____

16. Hard to control worries   _____

17. Difficulty concentrating   _____

FORM 4.2. Further Evaluation of Generalized Anxiety Disorder: Test Scores, Substance Use, History, Treatment Progress, and Recommendations

Patient's Name: _____ Today's Date: _____

Therapist's Name: _____ Sessions Completed: _____

Test data/scores

Beck Depression Inventory (BDI) _____   Beck Anxiety Inventory (BAI) _____

Global Assessment of Functioning (GAF) _____   Leahy Anxiety Checklist _____

Symptom Checklist 90—Revised (SCL-90-R) _____   Locke–Wallace Marital Adjustment Test _____

Structured Clinical Interview for DSM-III-R, Axis II (SCID-II) _____

Anxiety Disorders Interview Schedule—Revised (ADIS-R) _____

Other anxiety questionnaires (specify) _____

Substance use

Current use of psychiatric medications (include dosage) _____

_____

Who prescribes? _____

Use of alcohol/other drugs (kind, frequency, amount, consequences) _____

_____

History (intake only)

Previous episodes of anxiety (specify nature):

    Onset   Duration   Precipitating events   Treatment

Treatment progress (later evaluations only)

Situations still avoided: _____

_____

Situations approached that were previously avoided: _____

_____

Recommendations

Medication evaluation or reevaluation:

Increased intensity of services:

Behavioral interventions:

Cognitive interventions:

Interpersonal interventions:

Marital/couple therapy:

Other:

Compulsive and Anxiety scales. The ADIS-R (mentioned in Chapter 3), the Hamilton Anxiety Rating Scale (Hamilton, 1959), and the State–Trait Anxiety Inventory (Spielberger, Gorsuch, & Lushene, 1970) are additional anxiety questionnaires that may be used. Form 4.2 provides space for recording scores on these instruments. It also enables the therapist to record the patient's medication, alcohol, and other drug use; to record (at intake only) the history of any previous episodes of anxiety (the nature of these should be specified); and to indicate treatment recommendations.

Consideration of Medication

Treatment of GAD with medication may involve both acute and chronic (or maintenance) treatment. The three drug classes with proven efficacy for GAD are benzodiazepines, azapirones (especially buspirone), and antidepressants (especially imipramine and SSRIs). There is some evidence that patients presenting with somatic or adrenergic symptoms respond better to benzodiazepines; that patients with psychic symptoms such as worry, tension and irritability respond better to buspirone; and that patients with depressive symptoms and GAD respond better to imipramine (Schwiezer & Rickels, 1996). Although beta-blockers are sometimes used with patients with GAD, they have proven inferior to benzodiazepines, and consequently are not currently approved as treatments for GAD.

Socialization to Therapy

As we do with most patients, we recommend that patients with GAD read David Burns's *The Feeling Good Handbook* (Burns, 1980) and/or *Feeling Good: The New Mood Therapy* (Burns, 1989). In addition, specific focus on anxiety is provided by Reid Wilson's (1987) *Don't Panic*, an excellent description of the range of anxiety disorders and their treatment. The patient should be told that he or she has an anxiety disorder known as "generalized anxiety disorder" or "GAD." This means that the patient worries about a variety of things and may experience muscle tension, insomnia, physiological arousal, fatigue, and other symptoms. The patient may also experience depression or other anxiety disorders. We find it helpful to explain that everyone has worries some of the time, and that some worrying is productive (useful) while other worries are unproductive and cause unneeded anxiety. We indicate that medication may be included in the treatment plan, which will emphasize teaching the patient how to relax, improving his or her ability to handle stress, enhancing his or her ability to cope with interpersonal issues, evaluating how the patient is thinking about his or her worrying and other problems, and providing the patient with useful self-help techniques. Form 4.3 is an information handout about generalized anxiety disorder that can be given to patients. Our handout about cognitive-behavioral therapy in general (Form B.1 in Appendix B) can also be used.

Relaxation Training

The therapist may indicate to the patient that anxious thoughts and feelings are more likely to occur when the patient is physiologically aroused. Consequently, the patient can

What Is Generalized Anxiety Disorder?

All of us feel anxious at times. We may worry about things that *might* happen. We may have a restless night of sleep. But people with generalized anxiety disorder (or GAD) have physical symptoms that interfere with their normal lives. These problems may include restlessness, fatigue, problems with concentration, irritability, muscle tension, and/or insomnia. In addition, these individuals worry about a variety of events, such as health, financial problems, rejection, and performance, and they find it difficult to control their worry. Many people with GAD feel that their worry is "out of control" and that it will make them sick or make them go insane.

Who Has Generalized Anxiety Disorder?

About 7% of the population will suffer from GAD. Women are twice as likely as men to have this problem. This is a chronic condition, with many people saying that they have been "worriers" all their lives. Most people with GAD have a variety of other problems, including phobias, depression, irritable bowel syndrome, and relationship problems. Many people who have this problem find that they avoid others because of fear of rejection, or that they become overly dependent on others because of their lack of confidence.

What Are the Causes of Generalized Anxiety Disorder?

Only about 30% of the causes of GAD are inherited. There are certain traits that may make people more likely to develop this problem; these include general nervousness, depression, inability to tolerate frustration, and feeling inhibited. People with GAD also report more recent life stresses (such as conflicts with other people, changes in their work, and additional demands placed on them) than those without GAD do. People with GAD may not be as effective in solving problems in everyday life as they could be, or they may have personal conflicts in which they may not be as assertive or effective as they could be.

How Does Thinking Affect Generalized Anxiety Disorder?

People with GAD seem to be worried that bad things are going to happen most of the time. They predict that "terrible" things will happen, even when there is a very low probability of bad things happening. They think that the fact that they feel anxious means that something bad is going to happen—that is, they use their emotions as evidence that there is danger out there somewhere. Many people who worry believe that their excessive worry may keep them from being surprised, or that worrying may prepare them for the worst possible outcome. If you are a chronic worrier, you probably notice yourself saying, "Yes, but what if . . . ?" This "what-iffing" floods you with a range of possibly bad outcomes that you think you have to prepare yourself for. There seems to be no end to the things that you could worry about. In fact, even when things turn out to be OK, you may say to yourself, "Well, that's no guarantee that it couldn't happen in the future!"

In addition to worrying about things that might happen "outside of yourself," you may think that

(cont.)

"worrying will make me crazy" or "worrying will make me sick." If you have GAD, you may be locked in a conflict between the fear that worry is uncontrollable and the belief that worry protects you.

How Can Cognitive-Behavioral Therapy Help?

Cognitive-behavioral therapy for GAD can help you identify your beliefs about the costs and benefits of worrying, and show you how to recognize the difference between productive and unproductive worrying. Your therapist will help you carry out experiments in "letting go" of worry and postponing worry. In addition, you will learn how to overcome your avoidance of activities or thoughts about which you worry. Your therapist may also use interventions such as muscle relaxation, biofeedback, breathing exercises, time management techniques, and treatment of insomnia in order to reduce your overall levels of anxious arousal. Other interventions may include addressing your concern that worrying too much may be harmful, assessing your tendency to jump to conclusions that awful things will happen, and helping you learn to distinguish between anxiety and actual facts. Your therapist can teach you to use an extensive self-help form ("Questions to Ask Yourself If You Are Worrying") that can help you get a better perspective on worrying. Finally, since you are worrying throughout the day, your therapist will assist you in limiting worry to "worry time" and will help you keep track of the different themes of worry.

How Effective Is Cognitive-Behavioral Therapy for Generalized Anxiety Disorder?

Given the apparent long course of GAD, it is promising that new forms of treatment are proving to be effective. In some studies, cognitive-behavioral therapy has proven to be more effective than medications in the treatment of GAD. It leads to a reduction of the need to use medications, and in some cases patients continue to improve even more after therapy is completed. About 50% of patients with GAD show significant improvement.

Are Medications Useful?

Many patients with GAD also benefit from the use of medication, which can decrease the feeling of anxiety and apprehension. The value of medication is that it can make you feel less anxious very rapidly. Medication may be an essential part of your treatment, while you learn—in therapy—how to handle your problems more effectively.

What Is Expected of You as a Patient?

Because you may have been a worrier all your life, you may be pessimistic about the chances that anything will help you. It is true that you won't get better overnight, so you will have to work on your worries and anxiety on a regular basis. Your therapist will want you to come to sessions on a weekly basis, to keep track of your worries, to practice relaxation or breathing exercises at home, and to work on managing your schedule so that you are not overburdened. In addition, your therapist will help you identify your worries and help you view things in a more realistic perspective. To do this, you will be asked to write down the things that you are worried about, and to use self-help homework techniques to challenge your negative thinking. You may also be asked to work on solving problems more effectively and on learning how to interact with people more productively.

learn any number of relaxation techniques, such as progressive muscle relaxation, breathing relaxation, guided imagery, or meditation (see Appendix A and the CD-ROM for full discussions of the first two types). The patient can be encouraged to practice more than one relaxation technique. In addition, the use of stimulants (e.g., caffeinated beverages) should be discouraged, as should the excessive use of alcohol. Patients complaining about insomnia should be given the patient information handout on insomnia presented in Chapter 2 (Form 2.8); the use of the bed for sleep and sex only should be emphasized. Finally, overall relaxation is increased if the patient can engage regularly in aerobic exercise.

Assessing and Confronting Avoidance: Exposure and Other Techniques

A GAD patient may sometimes actually present with few anxious symptoms. On closer inquiry, the clinician may find that numerous situations are avoided and that the patient is underperforming at work or in personal relations because he or she fears an increase in anxiety. When this is the case, therapist and patient may construct a hierarchy of avoided situations, rate the SUDs for each situation, and identify the negative thoughts associated with these situations. (Forms 3.5 and 3.7 in Chapter 3 can be used for this purpose.) The therapist may then use behavioral rehearsal, cognitive rehearsal, and/or modeling of confronting avoidance. Or the therapist may guide the patient through imaginal exposure to the feared situations. Homework assignments may involve planned *in vivo* exposure to avoided situations. (See Appendix A and the CD-ROM for fuller discussions of exposure.)

Desensitization: Pairing (or Not Pairing) Exposure with Relaxation

The foregoing interventions (exposure, etc.) may be viewed as a form of desensitization. In addition, the patient may be trained in pairing his or her relaxation response with imaginal exposure to the feared stimulus, with the patient moving up the hierarchy from less to more feared thoughts or images. The patient may practice pairing relaxation with exposure in the actual situations. Alternatively, the patient may be instructed *not* to pair exposure to the stimulus with relaxation, so as to allow the patient the opportunity to learn that anxiety will decrease with increased length of exposure to the feared stimulus. One can view the difference between these two approaches as the difference between the "reciprocal inhibition" model advocated by Wolpe and the "cognitive disconfirmation" model advocated by Beck, Wells, and their associates.

Monitoring Worries and Assigning "Worry Time"

A distinguishing element for many patients with GAD is that their worries focus on more than one theme. A clinician and patient should assess various characteristics of worries: their content areas and situational elicitors, the specific predictions they entail, the level of anxiety these predictions generate, and the strength of the patient's confidence in these predictions. The Patient's Worry Log (Form 4.4) is useful in evaluating these specific

FORM 4.4. Patient's Worry Log

Content area for each worry	Factors in situation that bring out the worry	Prediction (Specify exactly what you think will happen and when it will happen)	Anxiety rating for each prediction (0–10)	Rating of confidence in accuracy of prediction (0–10)	Actual outcome (Exactly what happened?)	Anxiety rating at outcome (0–10)

worries and in helping the patient recognize his or her tendency to make "false predictions." As suggested by Borkovec and by Wells and Butler, worries are reinforced by the nonoccurrence of negative events and by the magical belief that worries are protective and preparatory.

In addition, "worry time" should be assigned to the patient. That is, the patient should be *required* to worry for a specific period of time (e.g., 20 minutes) at an assigned time and place. Other worries that occur during the day are to be delayed until worry time. This allows stimulus control of worries; it also helps the patient recognize that worries are about finite themes, and that worrying can be curtailed but not completely eliminated.

Cognitive Evaluation of the Nature of Worrying

Patients with GAD invest in worry as a hypervigilant strategy to avoid negative outcomes. They often think that worrying prepares them for the worst, helps them avoid negligence, and keeps them from regretting not having done something. With such a patient, the therapist can evaluate the costs and benefits of worrying, and can distinguish between "productive worry" (e.g., "Do I have enough gas in my car to make this trip?") and "unproductive worry" ("What if I were to get cancer?", "What if my business were to fail completely?"). In addition, the therapist should examine the patient's worrying about worrying, such as "I'm worrying so much I might go crazy" or "I should never worry" or "I have no control over my worrying."

The therapist can give the form called Questions to Ask Yourself If You Are Worrying (Form 4.5) to the patient. This allows the patient to evaluate specific predictions; the tendency to jump to conclusions; the difference between possibility and probability; the safety or protection factors available; the tendency to catastrophize outcomes; and other questions that may challenge the sense of negativity, imminence, and exaggerated outcome. (This form may be simplified, expanded, or modified by the therapist to fit the needs of the individual patient.) The therapist can also address the categories of distorted automatic thoughts evident in worries, such as labeling ("I'm incapable of handling stress"), catastrophizing ("I'm going to lose everything"), fortunetelling ("I'll get rejected"), dichotomous thinking ("Nothing is working out"), and discounting the positives ("I don't have anything going for me"). In addition, the therapist can focus on the patient's underlying maladaptive assumptions (his or her "rule book" about approval, perfectionism, certainty, and other "shoulds" and "musts"), as well as his or her dysfunctional schemas about self and others (involving such themes as rejection, defectiveness, demanding standards, or abandonment). Finally, the nature of the patient's rhetorical questions that reflect worrying, such as "What if it doesn't work out?" or "What's wrong with me?," can be examined and rephrased as "propositional statements" that can be tested, such as "Nothing will work out" or "Everything is wrong with me." Specific techniques for identifying and challenging the cognitive distortions involved in worries are outlined in Table B.3 of Appendix B, in the CD-ROM accompanying this book, in Leahy (1996), as well as in Judith S. Beck's (1995) *Cognitive Therapy: Basics and Beyond*.

FORM 4.5. Questions to Ask Yourself If You Are Worrying: A Self-Help Form for Patients

Specific worry: _____

Questions to ask yourself:	Your response:
Specifically, what are you predicting will happen?	
How likely (0–100%) is it that this will actually happen? How negative an outcome are you predicting (from 0% to 100%)?	Likelihood: How negative:
What is the worst outcome? The most likely outcome? The best outcome?	Worst: Most likely: Best:
Are you predicting catastrophes (awful things) that don't come true? What are some examples of the catastrophes that you are anticipating?	

What is the evidence (for and against) your worry that something really bad is going to happen?
    If you had to divide 100 points between the evidence for and against, how would you divide these points? (For example, would it be 50–50? 60–40?)
	Evidence for:
	
	Evidence against:
	
	Points: Evidence for = _____
	          Evidence against = _____

Are you using your emotions (your anxiety) to guide you? Are you saying to yourself, "I feel anxious, so something really bad is going to happen"?	
Is this a reasonable or logical way to make predictions? Why/why not?	
How many times have you been wrong in the past about your worries? What actually happened?	

(cont.)

Questions to ask yourself:	Your response:
What are the costs and benefits to you of worrying about this? If you had to divide 100 points between the costs and benefits, how would you divide these points? For example, would it be 50–50? 60–40?)	Costs: Benefits: Points: –___ (costs) ___ (benefits) Subtract costs from benefits: ___ – ___ = ___
What evidence do you have from the past that worrying has been helpful to you and hurtful to you?	
Are you able to give up any control in order to be worried less?	
Is there any way that worrying really gives you any control, or do you feel more out of control because you are worrying so much?	
If what you predict happens, what would that mean to you? What would happen next?	
How could you handle the kinds of problems that you are worrying about? What could you do?	
Has anything bad happened to you that you were not worried about? How were you able to handle that?	
Are you usually underestimating your ability to handle problems?	
Consider the thing you are worried about. How do you think you'll feel about this 2 days, 2 weeks, 2 months, and 2 years from now? Why would you feel differently?	
If someone else were facing the events that you are facing, would you encourage that person to worry as much as you? What advice would you give him or her?	

Other Techniques for Countering Worrying and Rumination

A variety of other techniques, both behavioral and cognitive, can be used as necessary to counter a patient's worrying and rumination. The patient can be trained in behavioral activation (reward planning and activity scheduling) as a means of both elevating mood and decreasing rumination time. Both Appendix A and Chapter 2 describe behavioral activation, and Chapter 2 provides forms for monitoring actual activities (Form 2.5) and for predicting the amount of pleasure and mastery that will result from planned activities (Form 2.6). Engaging in distraction can also be encouraged (this is also described in Appendix A). Finally, the patient can be helped to develop an "antirumination script," which might go something like this: "Instead of sitting here and fretting, I could be solving my problems, distracting myself, doing something productive, calling a friend, or challenging my negative thinking."

Interpersonal Interventions

Patients with GAD often have interpersonal problems that contribute to their worries and general discomfort. The clinician can assist such a patient in learning appropriate skills, such as assertiveness; rewarding and attending to others instead of complaining; mutual problem solving; active listening and other aspects of effective communication; acceptance of others; and negotiation and conflict resolution. Specific cognitive interventions may focus on various cognitive distortions (see above) as these are manifested in interpersonal relationships. The clinician may assist the patient in learning appropriate behavior through modeling and behavioral rehearsal and through constructing specific interpersonal goals, such as complimenting five people every day or calling up three people each week to pursue rewarding behaviors. Finally, many GAD patients experience conflict with their spouses or partners, partly because of their tendency to view neutral events as potentially negative or even dangerous. If necessary, a patient's spouse or partner may be included in the treatment; the emphasis in conjoint sessions should be on increasing positive reinforcement and positive tracking for both members of the couple, and on encouraging the anxious individual to avoid enunciating too many worrisome thoughts.

Stress Reduction and Problem-Solving Training

We indicate to patients the difference between a stressor (such as a demand by the boss) and the experience of stress (emotional discomfort) (see Lazarus & Folkman, 1984). The experience of stress or discomfort will result from increased arousal and the perception that one does not have the ability to handle the demands one is confronting. The therapist may utilize self-instructional training (Meichenbaum, 1977) and problem-solving training (Nezu & Nezu, 1989c), to reduce stress. In addition, time management (especially being careful not to plan too many things), introduction of "stress breaks," self-contingency contracting (e.g., establishing positive self-rewards), anger control (see Novaco, 1978), and other techniques are useful.

Troubleshooting Problems in Therapy

The majority of patients presenting with GAD have experienced significant anxiety for most of their lives. Consequently, they may be impatient, demanding, skeptical, hopeless, or minimally compliant with treatment. The following problems are often confronted in treatment.

Excessive Focus on Negative Feelings

Many anxious patients focus on how bad they feel—especially their physical sensations, their apprehension, and their general discomfort. The clinician can indicate to such a patient that the goal of therapy is to help the patient feel better, but that in order to accomplish this several goals must be addressed. The clinician can help the patient label feelings accurately (rating their intensity, tracking their variation, and gaining distance from them by "observing" their quality and variation across the day); can help the patient identify how feelings are related to situations and thoughts; can emphasize the difference between a feeling and a thought ("I *feel* anxious because I *think* I'll fail"); and can help the patient evaluate how feelings change as negative thoughts become less credible.

Difficulty in Identifying Automatic Thoughts

Because of the intensity of patients' feelings or because of their exclusive focus on their discomfort, many anxious patients claim that they cannot identify their thoughts. The therapist may ask such a patient to slow down the process through the use of guided imagery in the session, in which anxiety-provoking situations are described and the patient slowly goes through his or her feelings, images, and thoughts. If the patient describes visual images, these can then be used as primes for automatic thoughts, as in this example:

THERAPIST: You said that you had the image of your head exploding. Complete this sentence: "When I think of my head exploding, it makes me anxious because I think that what is happening is . . . "
PATIENT: I'm losing control. I'm going crazy.

Another technique that can be useful is to suggest automatic thoughts that the patient may or may not have had and ask, "Could this be what you were thinking?" (See J. S. Beck, 1995, for a description of these techniques.)

Demand for Immediate Results

Anxious patients often demand immediate, total relief from their negative feelings, hoping for a "magic bullet." This demand can be addressed in the following ways: clarifying that anxiety has been a lifelong problem that requires an investment of time and effort to treat; stressing that old habits of thinking, feeling, and behaving do not change overnight; examining the costs and benefits of demanding immediate results; examining what will happen if immediate results are not obtained and what will happen if results are obtained gradually; evaluating how the demand for immediate results (low frustration tolerance) actually results in greater vulnerability to anxiety; and indicating how these demands contribute to feelings of hopelessness.

Perfectionistic Beliefs in Anxiety Reduction

Similar to the demand for immediate results is the dichotomous belief about anxiety: "Either I am totally anxious, or I should have no anxiety." We tell patients that eliminating all anxiety is impossible, except for dead people! Reducing, moderating, coping with, and not catastrophizing anxiety are suggested as alternative appropriate goals. Furthermore, a patient can examine how small amounts of anxiety can be useful to motivate the self or to indicate that something may be problematic.

Demands for Certainty

Patients who ask rhetorical "What if . . . ?" questions may demand certainty about feared events or about the outcome of therapy. These demands for certainty in an uncertain world are modified in therapy to statements about probability: "What is the probability that you will fail? Be rejected? Have cancer?" Patients who dwell on "what if?" are asked to examine the costs and benefits of demanding certainty about every possible imagined event. The therapist may describe many situations—for example, driving a car, eating chicken in a restaurant, or walking across the street—that are possibly dangerous, but that are tolerated as acceptable risks. Magical, absolutistic beliefs about negligence and responsibility, which contribute to the demand for certainty (Salkovskis, 1996), are evaluated; the therapist indicates to the patient that responsibilities are not about all possible events, but about reasonable precautions taken by reasonable people.

Beliefs That Worries Are Realistic

Some patients believe that their worries are realistic. For example, a 45-year-old woman who was being treated for hypertension with medication thought that her blood pressure was still hypertensive because it was 135/80. She claimed that an ideal blood pressure was 120/70 (and that an ideal cholesterol reading was less than 140). These perfectionistic and incorrect beliefs that hypertension is defined by the absence of an ideal rating were directly addressed in treatment by providing the patient with corrective information. Other patients may claim that their worries are "realistic" because the things they worry about "could happen." This may be addressed by having such patients assign subjective probabilities to feared events and evaluating whether these are related to actual facts. For example, having heard of an airplane crash on the news, one patient estimated her chances of being in a similar crash at 10%. She was surprised to learn that the facts indicate that one can take a round trip on a commercial airliner every day for 45,000 years and expect one fatal accident. Confusing subjective feelings of anxiety with probabilities often contributes to extreme estimates of danger. Furthermore, a patient may be asked to estimate the sequence of probabilities of feared events: "I have a headache → I have something seriously wrong with me ($p = .10$) → It could go undiagnosed → ($p = .05$) → It could be a brain tumor → ($p = .001$) → I could die from it ($p = .10$)." Multiplying these sequential probabilities (each of which is exaggerated in its own right) yields the following: $.10 \times .05 \times .001 \times .10 = .0000005$. Thus, the chances of a headache's signaling a fatal brain tumor are rather remote.

Difficulty in Relaxing

Some patients describe difficulty in relaxing, even when given relaxation training. The therapist may increase a patient's ability to relax by including relaxation training in every session for several weeks to evaluate whether the patient is rushing through the exercises or not doing them properly. In addition, it is wise to train a patient in more than one exercise, to make sure that the patient does not have time pressures following the exercises, and to check whether he or she is practicing relaxation with distracting stimuli (such as music or TV). Some anxious patients fear that their relaxation will leave them vulnerable and unaware of danger, and these thoughts, when elicited, may be evaluated via the cognitive techniques described earlier. With patients with concomitant panic disorder, the decrease in tension may actually evoke a panic attack (see Chapter 3); the patients should be informed that this may happen in some cases, but that relaxation-induced panic usually subsides with continued practice of the exercises.

Refusal to Engage in Exposure

Some patients fear exposure so greatly that they refuse to confront feared situations. Interventions that may be helpful include using guided imagery in sessions before actual exposure is employed, extending the fear hierarchy downward to include even less anxiety-provoking events, modeling exposure, accompanying the patient in the feared situation, cognitive rehearsal of coping statements in the session, eliciting and challenging (through role plays and role reversals) the feared exposure, and using time projection ("How will you feel 30 minutes, 1 hour, 2 days after you have completed this task?").

Phasing Out Treatment

As in the case of panic disorder and agoraphobia, we caution against premature termination of treatment for GAD—especially since GAD in many cases has been chronic for years and is resistant to treatment. Accordingly, the treatment package described in this chapter calls for 20 sessions, although it may sometimes be possible to provide adequate treatment in fewer sessions. Phasing back to biweekly or monthly sessions after the patient shows some improvement helps the patient to begin functioning independently of therapy. During phase-out, as noted in connection with other disorders in other chapters, the patient is encouraged to self-assign homework; this can focus on various aspects of treatment that have been particularly challenging for the patient.

CASE EXAMPLE

Sessions 1–2

Assessment

Comorbid conditions

Jill was a 29-year-old manager, married with no children, who complained of having had anxiety and worries since she was a young adolescent. On intake, she indicated a moderate level of depression (her BDI score was 21); a high level of anxiety (her BAI score was 29); and elevations on the anxiety, obsessive–compulsive, and depression scales of the SCL-90-R. On the SCID-II and on interview, she gave indications of having obsessive–compulsive personality disorder. Her Locke–Wallace score (137) suggested a very high level of marital satisfaction, although later developments in the case called this into question (see below).

Caffeine and alcohol use; recent stressors

The patient indicated that she consumed no more than one cup of coffee per day and refrained from drinking alcohol. Recent stressors included her brother's recurring and spreading cancer, her own diagnosis and treatment for melanoma, a recent miscarriage, and pressures on her job. She had been married for 6 years and indicated that her husband had a history of alcohol abuse, but that his drinking was less in the last 2 years. In addition, she and her husband occupied the upper floor of a two-family house while her parents lived in the lower floor, and she indicated that she was often disturbed by her father's depression.

Socialization to treatment

In socializing Jill to treatment, the therapist gave her handouts on generalized anxiety and depression (Forms 4.3 and 2.4, respectively). The patient was provided with David Burns's *The Feeling Good Handbook* and was told that her diagnosis was GAD and major depression, with the focus on her anxiety and worries. She decided that she would work on her problems in therapy and declined medication as a treatment. Her short-term goals were to reduce her worries about work and to decrease her self-criticism. Both long-term and short-term goals focused on dealing with her feelings about her brother's illness and any fears of a recurrence of her own cancer. The therapist indicated that thoughts often create feelings, and that the overall goal of therapy would be to help her reduce her general level of anxiety through relaxation techniques and through identifying and modifying her habitual ways of thinking. A distinction was made between Jill's productive and unproductive worry, with the emphasis that her unproductive worry often focused on things that were beyond her control. In addition, her "worry about worry" was addressed by indicating that she not only worried about bad things' happening,

Monitoring worries

but also worried about her worrying's being out of control. Jill was asked to keep track of her worries with the Patient's Worry Log (Form 4.4).

Sessions 3–5

Progressive muscle relaxation

Stress management; "worry time"

Identifying and challenging distorted automatic thoughts

Jill was trained in progressive muscle relaxation and encouraged to examine how she could be assertive at work and set limits on her time schedule. Her Patient's Worry Log indicated that she was not worried about a recurrence of her melanoma, but that she feared that her brother's cancer was terminal. Her initial focus in therapy was on her worries and pressures at her job. She was instructed in the use of "worry time"—that is, limiting her worrying, as much as possible, to a specific time and place (usually a 30-minute period at home after work).

The pressures on Jill's job resulted in part from daily time pressures to complete tasks with inadequate technical and personnel support. However, they were also partly caused by her perfectionistic automatic thoughts, such as "It's not perfect. It's not the way it should be. I'll fail. I'm a failure. I can't get control over this." The therapist helped Jill categorize these thoughts (as fortunetelling, labeling, personalizing, catastrophizing, etc.) and had her rate (1) her confidence in their accuracy and (2) the intensity of the emotions associated with them (both on a scale of 0–100%). The therapist then employed various cognitive techniques to assist her in challenging the thoughts. These techniques included examining their costs and benefits, examining the evidence for and against them, vertical descent, decatastrophizing, the double-standard technique, and problem solving. In addition, Jill and the therapist examined her tendency to personalize the work problems. First, they evaluated sources of the problems other than herself (e.g., lack of support, technical limitations, unrealistic demands, prior workers' mistakes); Jill then divided up responsibility for the problems, using the "pie" technique. Finally, she rerated her original thoughts and emotions, and worked on developing new and more adaptive thoughts.

Identifying and challenging maladaptive assumptions about worrying and the utility of worrying

The therapist also examined Jill's underlying maladaptive assumptions about worrying (specifically, "Worrying will drive me crazy" and "I have to stop worrying completely") and about the utility of worrying ("I'll be prepared for the worst" and "I'll be motivated to do a better job"). Techniques that proved useful for challenging these assumptions were examining costs and benefits, evaluating the evidence for and against each assumption, rational role play, and the double-standard technique.

Sessions 6–8

Further monitoring of worries

Specific challenges to worries

Jill continued to track her worries with the Patient's Worry Log (Form 4.4), which indicated that she worried about things that were beyond her control (e.g., the amount of work assigned) and about incurring complaints from her boss (which seldom occurred). Jill was then given the Questions to Ask Yourself If You Are Worried form (Form 4.5) and instructed in its use; her filled-out version of this form for one worry is presented here as Table 4.3.

The continuing challenges to Jill's negative thoughts proved extremely helpful. She reported feeling much less depressed and anxious, and she indicated that she felt better able to "leave the work at work" when she went home. After eight sessions, there was a dramatic decrease in both her anxiety (BAI = 8) and her depression (BDI = 5). Therapy was phased back to once every 2 weeks and then once per month.

Sessions 9–15

Interpersonal interventions

During the course of Jill's treatment, her husband's drinking increased, resulting in an increase in marital conflict. She was encouraged to assert herself with him, and she was trained in active listening skills (especially rephrasing, empathy, and validation), as well as avoiding labeling and judging her husband when she was speaking. (It is interesting that her rating of the marriage before therapy was very favorable; note her high Locke–Wallace score as reported at the beginning of the case. Some patients enter treatment focused on specific worries or physical discomfort, but eventually acknowledge marital problems of considerable significance.) She was able to become appropriately assertive with her husband, which was moderately helpful in reducing the conflict and in encouraging him to decrease his drinking.

Identifying old and new schemas

Jill was also now able to summarize her old and new schemas about herself and others. Her old schemas were "I'm totally responsible" and "I'm inadequate." By contrast, her new, revised schemas were as follows: "I am only responsible for what is reasonable. I am human. I am competent, but not perfect. I don't have to please everyone. Others can take responsibility." She could now see how her worries at work were related to her schema about excessive personal responsibility, and she was able to attribute most of the problems at work to inadequate personnel. She modified her demands on time pressure and productivity, and began to accept a certain amount of "error" in the work environment.

TABLE 4.3. Questions to Ask Yourself If You Are Worrying: A Self-Help Form for Patients (Form 4.5), as Filled Out by Jill

Specific worry: *I've got too much work to do.*

Questions to ask yourself:	Your response:
Specifically, what are you predicting will happen?	*I'll fail to get the work done.*
How likely (0–100%) is it that this will actually happen? How negative an outcome are you predicting (from 0–100%)?	Likelihood: *90%* How negative: *85%*
What is the worst outcome? The most likely outcome? The best outcome?	Worst: *The boss will get so angry he'll fire me.* Most likely: *I'll get most of the work done and no one will say anything.* Best: *I'll get everything done.*
Are you predicting catastrophes (awful things) that don't come true? What are some examples of the catastrophes that you are anticipating?	*Yes. I won't get fired. I'm doing better than anyone else who's had this job.* *The computer will crash, my brother will die, I'll get fired, I'll never be able to have a kid, my marriage will break up.*

What is the evidence (for and against) your worry that something really bad is going to happen?
 	
    If you had to divide 100 points between the evidence for and against, how would you divide these points? (For example, would it be 50–50? 60–40?)
	Evidence for: *The work seldom gets completely done.*
	
	Evidence against: *This is part of the job. There's more work than there are resources to get it done. They need me and they won't fire me. They already know that the problem exists, and they decided it's cheaper to absorb the costs than pay to have everything overhauled.*
	Points: Evidence for = __5__
	            Evidence against = __95__

Are you using your emotions (your anxiety) to guide you? Are you saying to yourself, "I feel anxious, so something really bad is going to happen"? Is this a reasonable or logical way to make predictions? Why/why not?	*Yeah. I'm doing a lot of emotional reasoning. The fact is that nothing really terrible is happening at work.*
How many times have you been wrong in the past about your worries? What actually happened?	*I've always been wrong about my worries at work, because I'm able to get most of the work done and no one has ever thought of firing me.*

(cont.)

TABLE 4.3 *(cont.)*

What are the costs and benefits to you of worrying about this?	Costs: *Anxious, frustrated, self-critical, angry.* Benefits: *Maybe I'll try harder to get it done.* Points: – *80* (costs) *20* (benefits) Subtract costs from benefits: *20 – 80 = –60*
What evidence do you have from the past that worrying has been helpful to you and hurtful to you?	*Worrying about this hasn't helped me. It just makes my job more difficult.*
Are you able to give up any control in order to be worried less?	*I can try. I feel better when I accept what I can't control.*
Is there any way that worrying really gives you any control, or do you feel more out of control because you are worrying so much?	*No, it doesn't give me any control. It only makes me frustrated and then I try to do a perfect job—which is impossible.*
If what you predict happens, what would that mean to you? What would happen next?	*It means I'm incompetent. People will think I can't do my job.*
How could you handle the kinds of problems that you are worrying about? What could you do?	*I could be assertive and ask for support at work.*
Has anything bad happened to you that you were not worried about? How were you able to handle that?	*When I learned I had cancer I got treatment and I got better.*
Are you usually underestimating your ability to handle problems?	*Yes, I'm actually good at solving problems.*
Consider the thing you are worried about. How do you think you'll feel about this 2 days, 2 weeks, 2 months, and 2 years from now? Why would you feel differently?	*It always feels better later. Two days from now I'll really have forgotten about this.*
If someone else were facing the events that you are facing, would you encourage that person to worry as much as you? What advice would you give him or her?	*No—I wouldn't encourage them to worry. It's useless. I'd tell them, "You can only do so much. If they don't care enough to provide the support you need, it's their problem."*

Sessions 16–20

Life stressors

In the later months of her treatment, Jill got pregnant, and her brother's cancer became more ominous. She took a couple of months off from work to take care of him, and then he died. Her grief during this time was appropriate; she felt that she had done all that she could to support him during the difficult last months.

Goals to pursue after termination

Phasing out treatment

She summarized her need to continue to be assertive at work and at home, to accept limits on her responsibility and time, to continue using the forms she had been given to challenge her negative thoughts, and to recognize that others shared responsibility for their problems. The therapist played "devil's advocate" in role plays to help her continue recognizing that the problems at work, and in her family, were often out of her control and beyond her responsibility. Therapy was terminated by mutual consent, and Jill indicated that she would continue to use her self-help tools and assertion as needed.

DETAILED TREATMENT PLAN
FOR GENERALIZED ANXIETY DISORDER

Treatment Reports

Tables 4.4 and 4.5 are designed to help you in writing managed care treatment reports for patients with GAD. Table 4.4 shows sample specific symptoms; select the symptoms that are appropriate for your patient. (Zuckerman's [1995] *Clinician's Thesaurus* can be consulted for additional words and phrases.) Be sure also to specify the nature of the patient's impairments, including any dysfunction in academic, work, family, or social functioning. Table 4.5 lists sample goals and matching interventions. Again, select those that are appropriate for the patient.

Session-by-Session Treatment Options

Given the long-standing, chronic, and often treatment-resistant nature of GAD, we advocate that the treatment plan include at least 20 sessions of individual cognitive-behavioral treatment, with the opportunity for periodic follow-ups once regular treatment has been completed. Table 4.6 provides options for 20 treatment sessions for a patient with GAD. (As noted earlier, the sequence of interventions presented here may vary, depending on individual patients' needs.)

TABLE 4.4. Sample Symptoms for Generalized Anxiety Disorder

Anxious mood

Excessive worry

Irritable mood

Restlessness

Feeling on edge

Fatigue

Impaired concentration

Muscle tension

Insomnia

Specify length of time symptoms have been present

TABLE 4.5. Sample Treatment Goals and Interventions for Generalized Anxiety Disorder

Treatment goals	Interventions
Reducing physical symptoms of anxiety	Relaxation training
Reducing time spent worrying (<30 minutes/day)	Distraction, "worry time"
Reducing negative automatic thoughts	Cognitive restructuring
Eliminating avoidance (specify)	Exposure
Eliminating assumptions about dangerousness of anxiety, positive value of worry, or other assumptions (specify)	Cognitive restructuring, behavioral experiments
Modifying schemas of threat/vulnerability/need for control (or other schemas—specify)	Cognitive restructuring, developmental analysis
Eliminating impairment (specify—depending on impairments, this may be several goals)	Cognitive restructuring, problem-solving training, or other skills training (specify)
Eliminating all anxiety symptoms (SCL-90-R scores in normal range)	All of the above
Acquiring relapse prevention skills	Reviewing and practicing techniques as necessary

TABLE 4.6. Session-by-Session Treatment Options for Generalized Anxiety Disorder

Sessions 1–2

Assessment

Evaluate presenting problems

Evaluate specific anxiety symptoms with the Leahy Anxiety Checklist for Patients (Form 4.1)

Identify specific content of worries

Administer standard battery of intake measures (see Form 4.2), plus additional anxiety questionnaires as appropriate

Evaluate for comorbid conditions (e.g., major depression, other anxiety disorders)

Evaluate substance use (including use of caffeine or tobacco); evaluate need for counseling or detoxification if patient has substance abuse or dependence

Assess need for medication

Evaluate sleep disorders

Socialization to Treatment

Inform patient of diagnosis

Provide patient with information handouts on anxiety disorders (Form 4.3) and on cognitive-behavioral therapy in general (Form B.1, Appendix B)

Indicate how GAD involves motor tension and arousal

Indicate that worries are a central part of GAD, and that worries are reinforced by their nonoccurrence

Develop short-term and long-term goals

Cognitive Interventions

Normalize worrying—review productive versus nonproductive worrying

Determine whether patient "worries about worrying" (e.g., "Worrying means I'm going crazy or have no control over my thoughts and feelings.")

Introduce Patient's Worry Log (Form 4.4)

Homework

Have patient begin reading Burns's *The Feeling Good Handbook* or Wilson's *Don't Panic*

Assign use of Patient's Worry Log to monitor worries

Sessions 3–5

Assessment

Evaluate anxiety (BAI) and depression (BDI)

Continue to identify themes of patient's worries

Review Patient's Worry Log—frequency, duration, situations, precursors, and consequences of worries

Behavioral Interventions

Train patient in progressive muscle relaxation and/or breathing relaxation

Instruct patient in reward planning/activity scheduling

Describe and encourage "worry time"

Evaluate need for assertion training

Evaluate need for exposure to avoided situations; discuss exposure with patient

Encourage exercise

Treat insomnia, if necessary

(cont.)

TABLE 4.6 *(cont.)*

Cognitive Interventions

Introduce Questions to Ask Yourself If You Are Worrying form (Form 4.5)

Begin to identify and categorize automatic thoughts (with specific emphasis on fortunetelling, catastrophizing, discounting positives, etc.)

Begin challenging thoughts by evaluating costs and benefits of worrying, using other cognitive techniques (see Table B.3, Appendix B)

Medication

Evaluate side effects of medication

Evaluate need to increase dosage

If no improvement, either increase dosage, add another medication, or change class of medication (consider the need to taper or discontinue one class of medication when adding another class)

Homework

Assign breathing relaxation, progressive muscle relaxation

Have patient follow self-help tips for insomnia (Form 2.8)

Assign "worry time"

Have patient increase exercise

Have patient reward planning/activity scheduling

Have patient continue to monitor worries, test predictions, track negative thoughts, and categorize these thoughts

Assign continued reading

Sessions 5–8

Assessment

As in Session 3–5

Review homework

Behavioral Interventions

Train patient in generalizing relaxation to new situations

Have patient engage in self-directed desensitization (exposure with or without relaxation) to avoided situations, as appropriate

Encourage patient to decrease rumination time—develop an antirumination script

Examine situational/life sources of stress (e.g., financial, interpersonal, work, family, etc.)

Encourage patient to schedule stress breaks, self-reward for behavior

Introduce problem-solving skills

Cognitive Interventions

Identify patient's underlying maladaptive assumptions

Challenge assumptions via cost–benefit analysis, other cognitive techniques (see Table B.3)

Continue challenging automatic thoughts via cognitive techniques and use of Form 4.5

Introduce Daily Record of Dysfunctional Thoughts

Use vertical descent

What is the ultimate outcome or fear that the patient anticipates?

Distinguish between possible and probable outcomes

Examine worries for probability, plausibility

Introduce idea of "sequential probabilities" (i.e., multiplying the probabilities of negative events predicted)

Medication

As in Sessions 3–5

Homework

As in Sessions 3–5

Have patient schedule stress breaks, self-reward for behavior

Assign use of problem solving

Decrease rumination through distraction, reward planning/activity scheduling, rational responding

Sessions 9–15

Assessment

As in Sessions 6–8

Behavioral Interventions

Continue with self-directed desensitization

Continue with assertion training and introduce anger control training, as appropriate

Continue with problem-solving training

Begin self-efficacy training: Have patient list personal positives, take credit for positives, continue with self-reward

Cognitive Interventions

Continue evaluating and challenging automatic thoughts and assumptions

Identify, evaluate, and modify dysfunctional schemas

Examine how worries are related to schemas (about defectiveness, failure, biological vulnerability, control, abandonment, responsibility, etc.)

Continue to evaluate and modify maladaptive assumptions (about excessive responsibility, time pressure, what is "essential," and imminence of "disasters")

Medication

As in Sessions 3–5

Homework

As in Sessions 3–5 and 6–8

Have patient increase exposure to feared situations as appropriate

Assign assertion and anger control practice

Have patient increase self-reward

Have patient identify and challenge maladaptive assumptions and dysfunctional schemas

Sessions 16–20

Assessment

As in Sessions 6–8

(cont.)

TABLE 4.6 *(cont.)*

Behavioral Interventions
   Plan phase-out of treatment
   Have patient identify short-term and long-term goals for self-help
   Identify how behavioral techniques can be used in future

Cognitive Interventions
   Review what has been learned about automatic thoughts, assumptions, and schemas
   Use rational responding to play "devil's advocate" for patient

Homework
   Have patient self-assign homework focused on troubleshooting future problems

CHAPTER 5

Social Phobia

DESCRIPTION AND DIAGNOSIS

Symptoms

Social phobia is the fear of one or more social situations. Among the situations that commonly make people with social phobia anxious are public speaking, other types of public performance, social gatherings, meeting new people, eating in public, using public restrooms, disagreeing with others, and speaking to authority figures. Faced with such situations, these persons typically worry that they will do or say something that will lead to embarrassment or humiliation, or that their anxiety will be noticed by others who will then judge them negatively.

Some people with social phobia are afraid of only one or two social situations. This form of the disorder is commonly referred to as "discrete" or "performance" social phobia. DSM-IV (American Psychiatric Association, 1994) calls for patients who fear a number of social situations to be given the specifier "generalized" as part of the diagnosis. Many people who present complaining of discrete fears turn out to have some generalized fears as well. Approximately two-thirds of patients with social phobia who present at anxiety disorder clinics have the "generalized" form (Judd, 1994).

Those with social phobia either avoid the situations they fear or else endure them with considerable distress. They commonly report physical symptoms of anxiety when in social situations, including palpitations, trembling, sweating, tense muscles, stomach pain, dry throat, hot or cold flashes, and headaches. For some patients, the physical symptoms reach the level of a full-blown panic attack (Heckelman & Schneier, 1995; Judd, 1994).

Social phobia can result in serious impairment of academic, occupational, and social functioning. More than 50% of those with social phobia fail to complete high school. Seventy percent are in the lowest two quartiles of socioeconomic status, and over 20% are on welfare. Over half are single, divorced, or separated (Judd, 1994).

Social phobia is not believed to differ qualitatively from the symptoms of "shyness" that are reported by 20–40% of the population. Rather, social phobia is seen as a more extreme form of the same phenomenon, which is severe enough to lead to impairment in life functioning (Rapee, 1995).

Prevalence and Life Course

The National Comorbidity Survey found a lifetime prevalence rate for social phobia of 13.3% and a 12-month prevalence rate of 7.9%, making social phobia the third most common psychiatric disorder in the United States (Kessler et al., 1994). Other recent surveys have found similarly high prevalence rates (Chapman, Mannuzza, & Fyer, 1995). Epidemiological studies have consistently found a female-to-male ratio of approximately 2:1. However, in clinic samples the ratio is typically even or slightly higher for males. This may be due to the fact that traditional male roles demand greater assertion, both in dating and in careers; therefore, the symptoms of social phobia are likely to be more disturbing to males (Chapman et al., 1995).

The modal age of onset for social phobia is between 11 and 15 years. However, many patients report earlier onset, and social phobia can be diagnosed in children under age 10. The course of social phobia is typically chronic and unremitting. The mean age at presentation for treatment is 30, indicating that most patients have suffered for years before seeking help. The majority of those with social phobia never get treatment (Rapee, 1995).

Genetic/Biological Factors

Several lines of research point to a genetic role in social phobia. Two family studies (Fyer, Mannuzza, Chapman, Liebowitz, & Klein, 1993; Reich & Yates, 1988) found that the first-degree relatives of social phobia patients were almost three times as likely as the relatives of normal controls to meet criteria for social phobia. Plomin and Daniels (1986) found that adopted children who were shy were likely to have biological mothers who were socially anxious. Kendler et al. (1992) found a 24.4% concordance rate for monozygotic twins versus 15.3% for dizygotic twins, indicating that genetic factors contribute approximately 30% to the occurrence of social phobia.

Coexisting Conditions

Comorbidity is common with social phobia. In one community sample, 59% of social phobia patients reported lifetime occurrence of DSM-III-R simple phobia (DSM-IV specific phobia), 45% reported agoraphobia, 17% major depression, 12% dysthymia, 11% obsessive–compulsive disorder, and 5% panic disorder. In addition, 19% reported alcohol abuse and 13% reported other substance abuse. In 77% of these cases, social phobia preceded the development of the comorbid condition; in 85% of the cases involving alcohol abuse, it preceded the alcohol abuse (Schneier, Johnson, Hornig, Liebowitz, & Weissman, 1992). Patients with social phobia and an additional diagnosis have a suicide attempt rate of 15.7%, compared to 1.0% for patients with social phobia without a comorbid diagnosis and 0.9% for nonclinical populations (Judd, 1994).

The most common comorbid Axis II diagnoses found with social phobia are avoidant personality disorder and obsessive–compulsive personality disorder. In fact, 50–89% of patients with generalized social phobia and 21–23% of those with discrete social phobia meet criteria for avoidant personality disorder. No qualitative differences have been found between social phobia patients who have avoidant personality disorder and those who do not. It therefore appears that avoidant personality disorder represents a more severe form of social phobia (Heckelman & Schneier, 1995).

Differential Diagnosis

Social phobia may be difficult to differentiate from panic disorder and agoraphobia. Although some social phobia patients do have panic attacks, these are always triggered by social or performance situations. In addition, during panic attacks, they fear that others will notice and judge them for their anxiety symptoms, whereas panic disorder patients fear physical harm from the symptoms. If unexpected panic attacks occur in the absence of social cues, an additional diagnosis of panic disorder should be considered.

Social phobia patients may have substantial avoidance that restricts their functioning and can resemble agoraphobia. However, in social phobia the avoided situations always involve social interaction and the fear of judgment, whereas in agoraphobia patients fear situations in which they could have an unexpected panic attack and be unable to escape or get help. Therefore, patients with social phobia typically feel most comfortable when they are alone, while patients with agoraphobia are typically more comfortable when others are present.

Patients with generalized anxiety disorder may have excessive worries related to a number of issues, including social situations. If there is a specific fear of being embarrassed or humiliated, an additional diagnosis of social phobia should be given.

Social withdrawal and hypersensitivity to criticism may be present in major depression, especially when the specifier "with atypical features" applies. However, these symptoms are mood-dependent and remit when the depressive episode resolves. Social phobia should only be diagnosed if social fears and avoidance have occurred in the absence of a major depressive episode.

In schizophrenia and other psychotic disorders, and in schizoid and schizotypal personality disorders, avoidance of social contact is due to lack of interest in others and/or delusional fears of harm. In social phobia (and avoidant personality disorder), there is a desire for social interaction; however, this desire is inhibited by fears of humiliation or embarrassment (Donohue, Van Hasselt, & Hersen, 1994; Heckelman & Schneier, 1995).

A diagnostic flow chart for social phobia (Figure 5.1) illustrates the differential diagnosis of this disorder in more detail.

UNDERSTANDING SOCIAL PHOBIA IN COGNITIVE-BEHAVIORAL TERMS

Several different cognitive and behavioral models have been proposed to explain social phobia. Although the models overlap to some extent, each has led to a different set of treatment recommendations. The most recent research protocols have typically used a combination of these approaches. In this section we first outline the various theoretical models of social phobia and describe the treatment techniques based on each model or group of models. We then consider the outcome research.

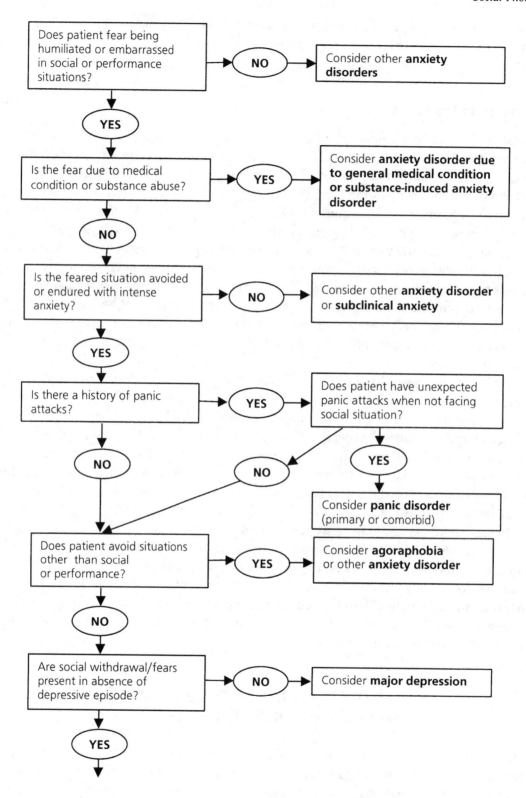

FIGURE 5.1. Diagnostic flow chart for social phobia.

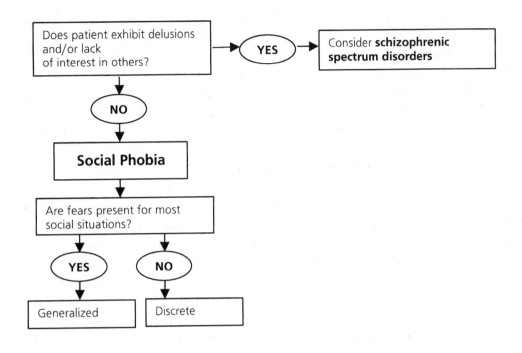

FIGURE 5.1. *(cont.)*

Behavioral Factors

Conditioning Models

As with other anxiety disorders, Mowrer's (1960) two-factor theory provides a model for understanding the role of conditioning in the acquisition and maintenance of social phobia. The experience of one or more traumatic or embarrassing social interactions may cause a person to acquire a conditioned response of anxiety, embarrassment, and/or humiliation. This conditioned response can then be evoked by similar social situations in the future. The range of social cues that elicit the fear response may expand over time through generalization. In addition, it is believed that social fears can be learned through vicarious observation of the fear responses of others. Ost and Hugdahl (1981) found that over 50% of patients with social phobia recalled a specific traumatic event that preceded their fears, while 13% recalled vicarious learning experiences.

The concept of "preparedness" (Seligman, 1971) has also been used to help explain the acquisition of social fears. Seligman suggests that species are genetically predisposed to acquire fears to stimuli that have posed survival threats in their evolutionary past. For example, humans more readily develop fears of the dark, snakes, and large animals (presumably realistic threats as they evolved) than of electrical appliances or automobiles. Such "prepared" fears are characterized by rapid acquisition, high resistance to extinction, and apparent irrationality (Mineka & Zimbarg, 1995). Applying this concept to social phobia, Baumeister and Tice (1990) point out that humans generally cannot survive in isolation. It would therefore be adaptive to have a mechanism for inhibiting behavior likely to lead to social exclusion. Such a mechanism would involve anxiety as a signal to terminate problematic behavior. Ohman and Dimberg (1978) have argued that social phobia is related to dominance hierarchies found in humans and other species. Behaviors typical of social phobia patients, such as gaze aversion and avoiding disagreement, may be seen as efforts to avoid attack by higher-status individuals. Research with nonhuman species supports the hypothesis that social fears may be "prepared" (Mineka & Zimbarg, 1995).

Regardless of how conditioned fears of social situations are acquired, avoidance serves to maintain them. When patients with social phobia avoid feared situations, they experience a decrease in anxiety, which reinforces the avoidance behavior. At the same time, such avoidance prevents these patients from experiencing social situations without negative consequences, and therefore from having their conditioned fears extinguished.

Conditioning-Based Treatments

Two behavioral techniques have been applied to social phobia based on conditioning models: (1) exposure and (2) applied relaxation. Exposure treatments seek to extinguish conditioned fear responses to social cues. This is accomplished by having patients expose themselves repeatedly to the feared cues until their anxiety decreases. As with other anxiety disorders, exposure may be imaginal (i.e., patients imagine themselves in a feared situation) or *in vivo* (i.e., patients engage in a feared social activity outside of the therapist's office). Exposure may also be accomplished through the use of role-play exercises, in which patients act out feared situations, either with the therapist or with other members of a treatment group.

Applied relaxation (Ost, 1987) aims to substitute a new conditioned response (relaxation) for the old conditioned response (fear). Patients are trained in a series of progressively shorter relaxation exercises, until they are able to relax quickly and automatically to a cue word. Patients are then taught to identify early warning signs of anxiety, such as physical symptoms, and to apply relaxation skills when the warning signs first appear. Finally, patients are assigned to practice applied relaxation in a variety of anxiety-provoking situations. Some variations of applied relaxation such as anxiety management training (Suinn & Richardson, 1971), include the use of positive coping statements and distraction techniques.

Skills Deficit Model

A second behavioral explanation offered for social phobia is that individuals who develop the disorder have deficits in their knowledge of social skills. However, there is controversy in the literature regarding whether social phobia patients actually lack social skills or are inhibited by anxiety from using skills they do have. Research on the subject has yielded mixed results (Rapee, 1995). Marks (1985) has argued that although many persons with social phobia do not in fact lack social skills, some, particularly those with more severe symptoms, do.

Social Skills Training

Social skills training has been developed as a treatment for social phobia based on the skills deficit model. The content varies from program to program (e.g., Stravynski, Marks, & Yule, 1982; Turner, Beidel, Cooley, Woody, & Messer, 1994), but generally includes such skills as introducing oneself, choosing appropriate topics of conversation, active listening, empathy, self-disclosure, initiating social activities, initiating and maintaining friendships, expressing disagreement, assertion, and (in some programs) public speaking. Therapists teach skills by providing specific instructions, modeling skills, having the patients role-play the skills, giving feedback (as other group members do), and assigning homework to practice the new skills in naturally occurring social situations.

Cognitive Factors

The Cognitive Model

A number of authors (e.g., Barlow, 1988; Butler, 1985; Butler & Wells, 1995; Clark & Wells, 1995; Heimberg & Barlow, 1991; Leary & Kowalski, 1995) have suggested that cognitive factors are central to social phobia. In fact, the DSM-IV criteria for social phobia imply cognition—that is, the belief that the person will be judged negatively by others.

Like those of patients with other anxiety disorders, the cognitive distortions of social phobia patients can be conceptualized on three levels: distorted automatic thoughts, underlying maladaptive assumptions, and dysfunctional schemas. Before, during, and after social or performance situations, these patients report conscious thoughts that they are failing to perform adequately, that their anxiety symptoms will be noticed, and that others are judging them. Underlying these automatic thoughts are assumptions that imply excessively high and perfectionistic standards for performance and/or an excessive need for approval. The self-schemas of social phobia patients often include beliefs that they are unacceptable, unattractive, or incompetent. Examples of cognitive distortions at all three levels are shown in Table 5.1.

There is considerable research support for the role of cognitive factors in social phobia. Those with social phobia have been found to report more negative and fewer positive thoughts during social interactions. They report more thoughts concerning the impressions they are making on others. They underestimate the quality of their social performance (relative to independent judges' estimates) and overestimate the degree to which their anxiety symptoms are visible. They make more negative interpretations of ambiguous feedback than normal controls do, make more catastrophic interpretations of mild negative feedback, and have better memory for negative social feedback. The percentage of time spent internally focused has been found to correlate with reported shyness. Finally, change in fear of negative evaluation has been found in several studies to be the best predictor of outcome in therapy for social phobia, regardless of the form of treatment (Clark & Wells, 1995; Leary & Kowalski, 1995; Rapee, 1995; Heimberg & Juster, 1995).

One important question for the cognitive model is how unrealistic negative beliefs are maintained in the face of contradictory evidence. Cognitive theorists have suggested

TABLE 5.1. Examples of the Three Types of Cognitive Distortions in Social Phobia

Distorted automatic thoughts

"I won't be able to think of anything to say."

"I'll say something stupid."

"I'll freeze."

"I'm boring."

"My face is hot. I'm blushing."

"My hands are shaking."

"I'm losing control."

"Everybody is looking at me."

"People can tell I'm nervous."

"I'm a loser."

"They think I'm stupid."

"They're better/smarter/funnier than me."

"They think I'm a fool."

"That was terrible."

"No one liked me."

"I blew it again."

Maladaptive assumptions

"If I'm quiet, people will think I'm boring."

"I have to have something intelligent or witty to say."

"If I'm not perfect, they'll reject me."

"If someone doesn't like me, it means there is something wrong with me."

"If they see I'm anxious, they'll think I'm incompetent."

"I have to make a good impression."

"I must get everyone's approval."

"I must not show any signs of weakness."

"If I disagree with someone, they'll get mad or think I'm stupid."

Dysfunctional schemas

"I'm odd."

"I'm different from everyone else."

"I'm weird."

"I'm a nerd."

"I'm stupid."

"I'm ugly."

"I'm weak."

"I don't have what it takes to be successful."

"I'm not likeable."

"I'm inadequate."

several factors that may play a role in the maintenance of dysfunctional beliefs in social phobia. These include the following:

1. **A shift in attention, when patients became anxious, from external cues to internal cues.** Faced with a social situation, patients often begin monitoring their own behavior for signs of social incompetence or visible anxiety. This prevents them from noticing positive feedback from others. Instead, they tend to use their internal feelings of anxiety as evidence that they are performing poorly, which only serves to increase their anxiety.

2. **Avoidance of social interactions.** This prevents testing and disconfirmation of negative beliefs.

3. **The use of "safety behaviors."** When patients with social phobia do participate in social interactions, they often engage in behaviors that are meant to protect them from possible embarrassment. These can include positive behaviors, such as holding a glass very tightly to prevent one's hand from shaking, or negative behaviors, such as avoiding asking questions in order not to look foolish. Like avoidance, these "safety behaviors" prevent the testing of negative beliefs.

4. **Self-fulfilling prophecies.** Patients often act in ways that make their negative beliefs come true. For example, a woman who does not speak in a group for fear of embarrassing herself may be perceived as cold, and therefore may be rejected, which may in turn confirm her fears that she is not socially acceptable.

5. **Schematic processing.** Social phobia patients often fail to notice or remember positive feedback from others, while easily recalling negative feedback. They also tend to interpret ambiguous feedback as negative.

Cognitive Treatments

In keeping with the cognitive model, cognitive restructuring has been proposed as a treatment for social phobia. The three types of cognitive restructuring that have been used most often in treatment studies are rational–emotive therapy (Ellis, 1962), cognitive therapy (Beck, 1976), and self-instructional training (Meichenbaum, 1977). Although the approaches differ somewhat in emphasis, all three involve teaching patients to identify negative beliefs and substitute more adaptive beliefs. The one study that compared these approaches in the treatment of social phobia (along with a fourth variation, interpersonal cognitive problem solving—Spivak, Platt, & Shure, 1976) found no difference in outcome among them (DiGiuseppe, McGowan, Simon, & Gardner, 1990). In the rest of this chapter, the generic term "cognitive therapy" is used to describe any approach that emphasizes changing maladaptive beliefs.

Outcome Studies

There have been a number of studies of treatment for social phobia. All forms of cognitive and behavioral therapy have been found to be superior to waiting-list conditions (Taylor, 1996). Of the individual treatment techniques, the strongest evidence exists for the effectiveness of exposure. Social skills training, applied relaxation, and cognitive restructuring have yielded mixed results when compared to other treatments (Donohue et al., 1994; Heimberg & Juster, 1995). No difference in effectiveness has been found between group and individual treatments. Two treatment packages that integrate cognitive and behavioral techniques have been tested for social phobia. Cognitive-behavioral group therapy (Heimberg, Dodge, Hope, Kennedy, & Zollo, 1990) emphasizes cognitive therapy and exposure, while social effectiveness therapy (Turner et al., 1994) combines social skills training and exposure. There is some evidence that combining exposure and cognitive restructuring may yield better outcome than either treatment alone (Heimberg & Juster, 1995; Taylor, 1996).

In general, patients have maintained their gains or improved further when followed for periods of up to 5 years after the end of therapy. The few studies that have shown a deterioration of gains have involved exposure-only treatments (Heimberg & Juster, 1995; Taylor, 1996). In spite of these positive findings, a substantial portion of patients have sought additional treatment after participating in research protocols; in some studies, more than 40% of patients have received additional treatment. Exposure-only treatments have yielded the highest percentage of additional-treatment seekers, whereas treatments combining exposure and cognitive restructuring have yielded the lowest. In general, the patients who sought further treatment had more severe symptoms at the start of treatment (Heimberg & Juster, 1995).

The amount of therapist contact provided in these outcome studies has ranged from 6 to 40 hours. There is some evidence that increasing the number of exposure sessions yields better outcome (Feske & Chambless, 1995). Two studies by Scholing and Emmelkamp (1993a, 1993b) found that 16 sessions of cognitive-behavioral treatment (after assessment) produced significantly better outcome than 8 sessions did.

Overall, the results of the outcome literature support the efficacy of cognitive, behavioral, and cognitive-behavioral treatments for social phobia. There is some evidence that treatments combining exposure and cognitive restructuring may yield better outcome, especially for maintaining gains and preventing the need for further treatment. Longer treatment (16 sessions or more) appears to provide better outcome than shorter treatment.

At the same time, it is apparent that current treatment packages for social phobia are not sufficient for the most severely impaired patients. Although existing research does not yet provide clear guidelines for helping these patients, several approaches would seem to be justified, including (1) combining cognitive-behavioral therapy and medication; (2) lengthening treatment, especially providing more exposure sessions; (3) adding treatment elements (i.e., cognitive therapy, social skills training, and applied relaxation) to exposure; and (4) focusing on underlying assumptions and schemas.

ASSESSMENT AND TREATMENT

Rationale and Plan for Treatment

In keeping with the findings of the outcome literature, the treatment package outlined in this chapter combines exposure and cognitive restructuring. Relaxation training and social skills training are included as options that can be used as needed.

Exposure is aimed at the symptoms of avoidance and the intense distress patients feel when they do face social situations. Exposure requires patients repeatedly to stay in contact with feared social cues until their anxiety diminishes. This process weakens the connection between the social cues and the fear reaction, and allows patients to learn that the embarrassment and humiliation they fear generally does not occur.

Cognitive restructuring directly targets the expectation of embarrassment and humiliation. This lessens anxiety and decreases avoidance.

Relaxation training provides patients with tools they can use to reduce the physical symptoms of anxiety. Social skills training teaches patients any social skills they may lack; this decreases expectations of social failure and increases the likelihood of positive feedback from others.

The treatment plan provides for 20 sessions of treatment, including assessment. Most of the sessions are 45 minutes in length, except for the first one or two exposure sessions, which are 90 minutes long. This amount of therapist contact is approximately in the middle of the range of contact provided in the research protocols. Patients with a single discrete social fear may require fewer sessions. Patients with severe generalized symptoms, especially those who also meet criteria for avoidant personality disorder, are likely to require longer-term treatment.

The treatment plan for social phobia is outlined in Table 5.2.

Assessment

The diagnosis of social phobia may be missed when patients initially present for treatment. It is not uncommon for patients to come to a first session describing other problems, such as depression, substance abuse, or panic attacks. Only on careful inquiry will it become apparent that social phobia has preceded and contributes to these conditions. Other patients will present with specific fears of performance situations. In such cases it is important to inquire about other, more generalized fears, as these are often present.

TABLE 5.2. General Plan of Treatment for Social Phobia

Assessment
    Initial clinical evaluation of anxiety and avoidance
    Tests and other evaluations
    Consideration of medication
    Socialization to treatment

Anxiety management training

Exposure

Cognitive restructuring

Coping with life problems

Phasing out treatment

Initial Clinical Evaluation of Anxiety and Avoidance

The initial assessment should include questions regarding all physical, cognitive, and behavioral symptoms of anxiety. The patient should be asked to list all of the situations he or she currently avoids or feels anxious about, and the degree of distress associated with each. In addition, the patient should be asked to list all safety behaviors. Forms 5.1 and 5.2 are provided here to assist patients in creating these lists. It may be helpful to ask patients to self-monitor and record any anxiety, avoidance, and safety behaviors for several weeks, as some of these behaviors may have become so automatic that they are not even recognized. (Note also that two forms in other chapters of this book—the Initial Evaluation of Anxiety and Avoidance for Patients [Form 3.2] and the Initial Fear Evaluation for Patients [Form 7.1]—may also be used in the initial evaluation of social phobia.)

The presence of any comorbid disorders should also be assessed. In addition, patients' interpersonal, educational, and occupational functioning should be assessed, as many individuals with social phobia have substantial deficits in these areas.

Tests and Other Evaluations

Self-report and interview instruments are also useful in assessing social phobia. The SCL-90-R (which is part of the standard intake battery described in previous chapters) includes an Interpersonal Sensitivity subscale, which provides a measure of social anxiety. The Social Phobia Questionnaire (SPQ) is a symptom checklist we developed for assessing patients. Patients' responses to individual items can help in making a diagnosis, and, when the scale is readministered later, can be used to evaluate therapeutic progress. A total score for the SPQ is derived by totalling the individual items. The SPQ is shown in Form 5.3. Other measures from the standard battery (the BAI, BDI, GAF, SCID-II, and Locke–Wallace), as well as other anxiety questionnaires (the ADIS-R, the Fear Questionnaire, the Hamilton Anxiety Rating Scale, etc.), may also be used as appropriate. Form 5.4 provides space for recording scores on the standard intake battery and additional anxiety questionnaires. It also enables the therapist to record the patient's medication, alcohol, and other drug use; to record (at intake only) the history of any previous episodes of anxiety (the nature of these should be specified); to note (on later evaluations) which situations are still avoided and which the patient can now approach; and to indicate treatment recommendations.

Consideration of Medication

Several different classes of medication have been studied for the treatment of social phobia (Lydiard & Falsetti, 1995; Potts & Davidson, 1995). Three controlled studies have found that the monoamine oxidase inhibitor (MAOI) phenelzine (Nardil) produced moderate to marked improvement in approximately two-thirds of treated patients. A second MAOI, tranylcypromine (Parnate), has been found effective in open trials.

The benzodiazapine clonazapam (Klonopin) has shown good response both in open trials and in one controlled study. Results have been more mixed for alprazolam

FORM 5.1. Social Anxiety Situations List for Patients

Patient's Name: _____ Week: _____

Instructions: Please list all social or performance situations that you avoid or that make you anxious. Note in the second column whether the situation is something you avoid. In the third column, note how much anxiety you feel (or would feel) when you are in the situation, from 0 (no anxiety) to 10 (maximum anxiety).

Social Situation	Avoided? (Yes/No)	Distress (0–10)

FORM 5.2. Safety Behaviors Inventory for Patients

Patient's Name: _____ Week: _____

Instructions: Please list any behaviors that you do or avoid doing in social situations in order to feel less anxious. Examples of behaviors you might do to feel less anxious are holding a glass tightly so no one sees your hand shaking or sitting in the back of a class so no one looks at you. Examples of behaviors you might avoid are introducing yourself to a stranger or disagreeing with someone. In the second column, please note how anxious you would feel if you changed the behavior, from 0 (no anxiety) to 10 (maximum anxiety).

Safety Behaviors	Distress (0–10)
Behaviors Done:	
_____	_____
_____	_____
_____	_____
_____	_____
_____	_____
_____	_____
Behaviors Avoided:	
_____	_____
_____	_____
_____	_____
_____	_____
_____	_____

FORM 5.3. Social Phobia Questionnaire (SPQ) for Patients

Listed below are social situations that commonly make people anxious. Please rate how anxious you usually feel in each situation. If the situation is one you avoid, rate how anxious you think you would feel if you were in the situation. Please add any additional social situations that cause you anxiety.

Situation	None (0)	A little (1)	Moderately (2)	A lot (3)
Speaking in front of other people	____	____	____	____
Going to parties	____	____	____	____
Meeting new people	____	____	____	____
Starting a conversation	____	____	____	____
Disagreeing with someone	____	____	____	____
Talking to a superior at work	____	____	____	____
Asking someone for a date	____	____	____	____
Going to business meetings	____	____	____	____
Looking someone in the eye	____	____	____	____
Eating or drinking in front of other people	____	____	____	____
Writing in front of other people	____	____	____	____
Asking for help or directions	____	____	____	____
Using public bathrooms when others are present	____	____	____	____
Other:				
_____	____	____	____	____
_____	____	____	____	____
_____	____	____	____	____

FORM 5.4. Further Evaluation of Social Phobia: Test Scores, Substance Use, History, Treatment Progress, and Recommendations

Patient's Name: _____ Today's Date: _____

Therapist's Name: _____ Sessions Completed: _____

Test data/scores

Beck Depression Inventory (BDI) _____   Beck Anxiety Inventory (BAI) _____

Global Assessment of Functioning (GAF) _____   Symptom Checklist 90—Revised (SCL-90-R) _____

Structured Clinical Interview for DSM-III-R, Axis II (SCID-II) _____

Locke–Wallace Marital Adjustment Test _____   Social Phobia Questionnaire _____

Anxiety Disorders Interview Schedule—Revised (ADIS-R) _____

Other anxiety questionnaires (specify) _____

Substance use

Current use of psychiatric medications (include dosage) _____

_____

Who prescribes? _____

Use of alcohol/other drugs (kind, frequency, amount, consequences) _____

_____

History (intake only)

Previous episodes of anxiety (specify nature):

    Onset   Duration   Precipitating events   Treatment

Treatment progress (later evaluations only)

Situations still avoided: _____

_____

Situations approached that were previously avoided: _____

_____

Recommendations

Medication evaluation or reevaluation:

Increased intensity of services:

Behavioral interventions:

Cognitive interventions:

Interpersonal interventions:

Marital/couple therapy:

Other:

(Xanax). Beta-blockers, such as propranolol (Inderal), are frequently used by musicians and other people with public performance fears. However, another beta-blocker, atenolol (Atenolol or Tenormin), has been found to produce only modest improvement in controlled studies, being less effective than phenelzine or exposure and not significantly better than placebo.

Recent studies have suggested that selective serotonin reuptake inhibitors (SSRIs) can be helpful in treating social phobia. Fluoxetine (Prozac), sertraline (Zoloft), paroxetine (Paxil), and fluvoxamine (Luvox) have all shown evidence of effectiveness. Interestingly, social phobia patients have not been found to have the same jitteriness when initiating treatment with fluoxetine that is often reported in panic disorder patients. Because MAOIs are often poorly tolerated by patients and benzodiazapines have the disadvantages of dependence and cross-reactivity with alcohol, some authors (e.g., Liebowitz & Marshall, 1995; Lydiard & Falsetti, 1995) have recommended that the SSRIs be used as first-line medications for social phobia.

Several medications commonly used for other anxiety disorders have been found not to be effective in most cases of social phobia, including the tricyclic antidepressants imipramine (Tofranil) and clomipramine (Anafranil), as well as buspirone (BuSpar) and bupropion (Wellbutrin).

One problem with all of these medications is relapse. Even the medications with the best research support, phenelzine and clonazapam, have shown substantial rates of relapse once they are discontinued.

Two studies comparing treatment with phenelzine to cognitive-behavioral group therapy (Heimberg et al., 1990) found that phenelzine produced more rapid response and produced slightly better outcome after 12 weeks of treatment, but that cognitive-behavioral group therapy was better at preventing relapse. Comparisons of cognitive-behavioral group therapy or exposure to atenolol and alprazolam have yielded superior results for the cognitive-behavioral therapies. No studies have yet examined the relative effectiveness of combining medication and psychotherapy (Heimberg & Juster, 1995).

Socialization to Treatment

Once a diagnosis is established, patients should be educated regarding social phobia, the rationale for treatment, and treatment options (including medication). Patients are often relieved to learn that their symptoms are common and that proven treatments are available. Form 5.5 is an educational handout about social phobia that can be given to patients.

Cognitive Restructuring

Cognitive restructuring targets patients' beliefs that they will be judged negatively by others. First, patients are taught to identify their distorted automatic thoughts by reviewing a recent social interaction and asking what emotions they were feeling and what thoughts were going through their minds at the time. Either the Patient's Daily Record of

FORM 5.5. Information for Patients about Social Phobia

What Is Social Phobia?

Social phobia is the fear of one or more social situations. Commonly feared situations include public speaking, meeting new people, being at parties, asking for dates, eating in public, using public restrooms, speaking to people in authority, and disagreeing with others.

People with social phobia are afraid they will act in ways that will make other people think badly of them. They often fear that others will see some sign of anxiety, such as blushing, trembling, or sweating. People with social phobia usually try to stay away from the situations that make them anxious. When they cannot, they tend to feel very anxious or embarrassed. Sometimes they may have panic attacks. Social phobia is a severe, disabling form of shyness and can cause problems in people's lives. Sometimes the problems are minor, such as not being able to speak up in class. Sometimes, however, the problems can be very serious. People with severe social phobia often have few friends, feel lonely, and have trouble reaching their goals in school or at work.

Who Gets Social Phobia?

Social phobia is very common. More than one out of eight people will suffer from social phobia at some point in their lives. Many more people have symptoms of shyness that are not severe enough to be called social phobia. Social phobia is twice as common for women as for men. However, men are more likely to try to find help for the problem. Social phobia usually starts when people are in their early teens, but it can begin much earlier. If people do not get help, the problem can last for years.

What Causes Social Phobia?

The exact causes of social phobia are not known. However, several things are believed to contribute to the problem:

- **Genetics.** People with social phobia often have relatives who are shy or have social phobia.
- **Prior experiences.** Many people with social phobia remember having been embarrassed or humiliated in the past. This leads them to be afraid that the same thing will happen again. Soon they start avoiding social situations. Over time, this tends to make them feel even more afraid.
- **Negative thinking.** People with social phobia often have negative automatic thoughts about what will happen in social situations. Common thoughts are "I won't be able to think of anything to say," "I'll make a fool of myself," and "People will see I'm anxious." They also tend to have standards that are hard to meet, such as "I should never be anxious," "You have to be beautiful and smart to be liked," or "I have to get everyone's approval." Often they have negative beliefs about themselves, such as "I'm boring," "I'm weird," or "I'm different from other people."
- **Lack of social skills.** Some people with social phobia never had the chance to learn social skills. This can cause them to have problems in social situations. Other people with this disorder have good social skills, but they get so anxious that they have a hard time using them.

(cont.)

How Does Cognitive-Behavioral Therapy for Social Phobia Work?

Cognitive-behavioral therapy helps you change the thoughts that cause your fear. Your therapist will teach you how to recognize your negative thoughts and to think more positively. He or she will also help you gradually face the situations you have been afraid of in the past. This allows you to discover that your fears usually do not come true, and you can become less fearful of these situations as a result. In addition, your therapist can teach you social skills and ways to relax, which can help you feel more confident.

A number of studies have shown that most people who get cognitive-behavioral therapy for social phobia feel less anxious. People usually continue to feel better even after therapy has stopped.

How Long Does Therapy Last?

For people with mild to moderate social phobia, 20 sessions is usually enough. People with fear of just one social situation, such as public speaking, may need fewer sessions. People with more serious symptoms may need more.

Can Medication Help?

Several different types of medication have been found to be helpful for social phobia. Your physician or a psychiatrist can recommend the one that would be best for you. One problem with medications for social phobia is that symptoms often return if the medication is stopped. For this reason, it is best that if you do take medication, you also get cognitive-behavioral therapy.

What Is Expected of You as a Patient?

Many people feel anxious at the beginning of therapy and wonder whether they can be helped. All you have to do is to be willing to give therapy a try. Your therapist will teach you things you can do to help yourself and ask you to practice them between sessions. Early exercises will be quite easy, but they will become more challenging as you feel more comfortable. The more you work on these exercises, the more likely it is that your social phobia will get better.

Dysfunctional Automatic Thoughts (Form 2.7 in Chapter 2) or the Patient's Event–Mood–Thought Record (Form B.4 in Appendix B) can be used for this purpose.

Patients are then taught to treat their negative thoughts as hypotheses to be tested rather than as reality. The skills of identifying the categories of distorted automatic thoughts being employed (see Form B.2 in Appendix B), gathering evidence, and developing rational responses to these thoughts are taught. Patients are then assigned to apply these skills to thoughts they have during naturally occurring social situations and during assigned exposure exercises.

A number of the cognitive techniques outlined in Table B.3 of Appendix B may be particularly helpful in challenging social phobia patients' automatic thoughts and helping them to develop rational responses. (Some of these techniques, as noted below, also allow patients to examine the maladaptive assumptions underlying their thoughts.) These include the following:

1. **Observing others' behavior.** Having patients observe the behaviors of other people can be an effective way of challenging negative thoughts. It can also help shift patients' focus from their own internal sensations of anxiety to external social cues, thereby reducing anxiety. For example, patients who fear that others will notice their anxiety can be asked to observe how many people are really looking at them at any given time. Usually the answer will be "Very few, if any." Patients who worry about being boring in conversations can be assigned to listen in on the conversation of others. Typically, they discover that most social conversation is rather mundane. Patients who assume that no one else feels anxious can be asked to look for signs of anxiety in others, either in social situations or on television. Again, they are likely to notice that others occasionally seem anxious and that generally nothing bad happens to them as a result.

2. **Testing predictions.** Before every social event (naturally occurring or assigned exposure), patients should be asked to write their predictions about what will happen—both how they think they will behave and how others will react. These should then be compared to what actually occurs. In most cases, patients begin to see that their predictions are inaccurate and negatively skewed.

3. **Double standard.** When patients fear that others will view them negatively if they make any mistakes or show any sign of anxiety (e.g., blushing, stammering), they can be asked what they would think if they saw someone else doing the same thing. Many patients judge others far less harshly than they expect to be judged themselves. The reasons for this discrepancy can then be explored. (Warning: Some patients are just as unforgiving of others as they are of themselves, and this exercise will not be helpful for them. In such cases, their assumptions about the need for—and possibility of—perfect behavior will need to be explored.)

4. **Surveying others.** Patients often assume that they are the only ones who feel anxious in performance or social situations. Patients can be assigned to ask people they know whether they ever feel anxious before giving a talk, going to a party full of strangers, or engaging in some other social interaction. Patients are often surprised to discover that others feel similar anxiety.

5. **How visible is anxiety?** Most people overestimate the degree to which their anxi-

ety is visible to others. This can be demonstrated in several ways: (a) Patients can be videotaped role-playing a social interaction or giving a speech. Before viewing the tape, they are asked to rate the degree of anxiety they felt from 0 to 10, to estimate how visible it was to others, and to specify what signs of anxiety they think were noticeable. Many patients are surprised, when they actually see themselves on tape, to discover that they do not look nearly as anxious as they feel. (b) Patients can be asked whether they remember any occasion when someone they know commented on being anxious when the patient had not been aware of it. Usually the answer is "yes." (c) Patients can ask others they observe in performance situations whether they felt anxious. Again, they will often be surprised to find that the answer was "yes," even though the patient did not observe any signs of anxiety.

6. **Behavioral experiments.** Patients who fear catastrophic negative reactions if they show any behavior they view as inept or as signalling anxiety (e.g., trembling, pausing too long in a conversation, etc.) can be asked to engage deliberately in the feared behavior and see what happens. Usually their fears are not confirmed.

7. **Vertical descent.** Some rejection is, of course, inevitable in social encounters. The technique called "vertical descent" can be used to uncover the assumptions that underlie patients' fear of rejection. These assumptions are typically that the negative judgment is accurate and that if the patients are rejected by one person, they will be rejected by all others. (These assumptions can be challenged by exploring alternative explanations and fighting overgeneralization; see below.) Patients can then be urged to ask the question, "So what?" For example, "Suppose you approach someone and he or she refuses to speak to you. Why would that bother you? What would happen next? And why would that bother you?" Generally, of course, patients conclude that what would "bother" them is not really that "bothersome."

8. **Alternative explanations.** Social phobia patients often take any rejection or unfriendly behavior as a sign that they are inadequate. It can be useful to have them consider alternative explanations. For example, could the person who was unfriendly have been having a bad day? Might this person have his or her own problems? Perhaps the person treats everyone this way? Would someone else simply consider the person rude?

9. **Fighting overgeneralization.** Patients with social phobia often overgeneralize the meaning of rejection. This is particularly a problem in dating situations, although it is also common for people with fears of making sales calls or looking for a job. Because they have been rejected by one person, they conclude that they are not good enough for anyone. Socratic questioning can be used to help patients understand that (a) attraction is a matter of taste, not absolute judgment; and (b) dating (or sales or interviewing) is a numbers game. Patients can be asked to assume a certain "hit ratio" (e.g., 1 "yes" for every 10 approaches) and urged to collect rejections. They can also be asked whether they would date (hire, buy from) anyone who approached them, and if not, whether the other person should conclude that no one would ever want him or her.

10. **"Feared fantasy" role play.** In this exercise, a therapist plays the role of a person who verbalizes all the terrible things a patient assumes others are thinking about him or her, and the patient must try to defend himself or herself. This serves several functions: (a) It allows patients to practice rational responses to their negative thoughts; (b) it pro-

vides a kind of exposure; and (c) patients are able to see that if anyone actually did judge them in such a manner, the patients would probably perceive that person as obnoxious and not worth trying to please.

As therapy progresses and patients become proficient at challenging their distorted automatic thoughts, the focus should shift to underlying maladaptive assumptions and to dysfunctional schemas about the self and others. These can be addressed by looking at the advantages and disadvantages of the assumptions and schemas, examining evidence across the patient's lives, examining whether patients' behavior leads to self-fulfilling prophecies that reinforce their schemas, and using developmental analysis to examine and challenge the origins of the schemas.

Exposure

The situations that a patient either avoids or finds anxiety-provoking have already been listed and rated for degree of distress during the assessment phase. These are now ranked from least to most anxiety-provoking, in order to create a hierarchy of feared situations for the patient to be exposed to. (Form 3.5 in Chapter 3, the Patient's Hierarchy of Feared Situations, can be used for this purpose.)

Three types of exposure may be used: imaginal, in-session role play, and *in vivo*. Whenever possible, *in vivo* exposure should be chosen, as this will ultimately be most effective. However, when an *in vivo* experience is not immediately available—for example, if someone has a fear of public speaking, but no immediate opportunity to give a presentation—imaginal exposure or role play can be helpful. In addition, if patients are very anxious about facing an actual situation, imaginal or role-play exposure may be used as a less anxiety-provoking item on the hierarchy, to be mastered before moving on to *in vivo* exposure. Alternatively, a therapist may accompany a patient on the first *in vivo* trial of a new exposure. In all cases, the patients should be assigned to repeat the exposure on their own (*in vivo*, if possible) as homework. Forms for recording exposure practice in sessions or as homework are provided in Appendix A (Form A.1 is for imaginal exposure practice and Form A.2 for *in vivo* practice).

Patients who normally engage in safety behaviors during social interactions should be instructed to drop such behaviors during *in vivo* exposure. This should include both omitting positive behaviors, such as frequent apologizing, and engaging in normally avoided behaviors, such as disagreeing with people or telling jokes. If patients fail to do this, exposure will not be complete, and some degree of anxiety and avoidance will remain.

For imaginal exposure, a therapist narrates a scenario in which a patient participates in an anxiety-provoking social situation. The patient is asked to imagine being in the situation and to describe how he or she would think, feel, and act. The process is audiotaped. The patient is then assigned to listen to the tape repeatedly, first in session and then as homework, until he or she is able to picture the situation without feeling anxious. In role-play exposure, the patient and therapist act out a social situation. Again, this is repeated until the patient's anxiety decreases.

It is important to include elements of the patient's catastrophic fears in both imaginal and role-play exposure. For example, a patient may be asked to imagine not only giving a musical performance, but making a mistake in a crucial passage; or the therapist may role-play a person who not only refuses an approach for conversation, but is rude or cruel. (More complete descriptions of exposure procedures can be found in Appendix A and in the CD-ROM that accompanies this book.)

Butler (1985) has pointed out that in therapy for social phobia, it may be difficult to stick to the ideal of prolonged exposure to clearly specified tasks that move precisely up a hierarchy of fears. Social situations are too variable, and many of them (e.g., asking for directions, introducing oneself) involve relatively brief encounters. These problems can be surmounted by having patients repeat brief situations numerous times and by emphasizing consistent practice (i.e., an hour a day of exposure to a variety of situations) rather than trying to follow a hierarchy exactly. Once patients master the idea of exposure, we have found it helpful simply to assign them to look for opportunities to make themselves anxious every day. These "opportunistic" exposures can be recorded for review in the next session.

Cognitive restructuring can be combined with exposure exercises. That is, patients may be asked to list their negative thoughts before starting an exposure and to develop rational responses. After the exposure, they report any new negative thoughts and come up with rational responses to those.

Social Skills Training

Therapists can assess the presence of social skills deficits by role-playing social situations with patients. When deficits are noted, a therapist should train a patient in the needed skills. These may range from basic skills (such as making eye contact, asking questions, and active listening) to complex ones (such as interviewing for a job or establishing and maintaining friendships). The therapist first models the skills and then has the patient practice them in role play with the therapist. Eventually the patient is assigned to apply the new skills during *in vivo* exposure.

Relaxation Training

Relaxation training can be helpful for patients whose performance in social situations is interfered with by physical symptoms of anxiety. Patients can be taught progressive muscle relaxation, breathing relaxation, or both (see Appendix A and the CD-ROM for detailed instructions). It is crucial in some cases to practice relaxation in exposure to anxiety-provoking situations.

In other cases, however, relaxation must be used with caution—especially with patients who fear that physical signs of anxiety, such as blushing or sweating, will be noticed by others. It is crucial that such patients do exposure exercises in which they do *not* attempt to control these symptoms, so that they realize other people are unlikely to notice or care. Otherwise, there is the danger that relaxation will become another safety behavior that maintains rather than breaks the cycle of anxiety.

Troubleshooting Problems in Therapy

Many of the potential problems with exposure-based treatments that will be described in connection with posttraumatic stress disorder in Chapter 6 can also be encountered in the therapy of social phobia. These include resistance to doing exposure, failure to become anxious, failure to habituate, and noncompliance with homework. Readers are referred to the "Troubleshooting . . . " section of Chapter 6 for a discussion of how to deal with these problems.

In addition to the standard problems with exposure, patients with social phobia frequently present unique problems related to their perception of therapy as yet another social situation in which they may be judged. These patients are often highly anxious during the initial evaluation. They may be reluctant to reveal personal information and may have difficulty communicating their concerns. In addition, they may feel "put on the spot" by repeated questions. As therapy progresses, they may be hypersensitive to perceived judgments by the therapist.

These behaviors provide both a problem and an opportunity. The first goal must be to help such patients feel comfortable. An approach that is gentle, tactful, empathic, and not too intrusive is important and takes precedence over acquiring all of the relevant details in the first meeting. Open-ended questions, statements, and empathic reflections may be more useful than direct questions. It can also be helpful to normalize patients' anxiety by informing them that it is common for people to feel anxious when they first come to therapy.

As therapy progresses, a therapist should be aware of any change in a patient's emotional state or behavior during sessions. The patient can be invited to collaborate with the therapist in looking at what led to such changes. This will often uncover beliefs that the therapist is making negative judgments about the patient. Evidence for these thoughts can then be explored. If, as is usually the case, the patient is wrong about the therapist's judgment, it can be helpful for the therapist to tell the patient what he or she was actually thinking. Such discussions are important for two reasons: (1) They provide further evidence to counter the patient's negative beliefs; and (2) they prevent the buildup of a negative perception by the patient of the therapist's feelings about him or her that could otherwise lead to premature termination.

Phasing Out Therapy

Before therapy can be terminated, several criteria should be met: (1) The patient should have experienced a significant decrease in subjective anxiety; (2) exposure to all items on the patient's hierarchy of feared situations should have been completed; (3) the patient should no longer manifest substantial avoidance behavior; and (4) the patient should be able to apply the skills of exposure and cognitive restructuring (as well as any other skills taught in therapy) independently.

In order to prepare the patient for termination, therapy should be tapered to every other week and finally to once a month. During this final stage, the patient should take increased responsibility for designing exposure homework. Before termination, the patient should review the techniques that he or she found particularly helpful. Situations that may prove difficult in the future should be discussed, along with ways of dealing with them. Whenever possible, the patient should have the option of recontacting the therapist should the need arise.

CASE EXAMPLE

The following case example illustrates the application of the treatment package to a case of discrete social phobia.

Sessions 1–2

Presenting problem

Sam was a 26-year-old single white male. He had recently moved to the area and taken a management-level job in a large corporation. This was his first management position, and he was proud to have gotten it while so young. In general, he felt confident about his abilities. However, one of his new responsibilities was making presentations to upper-level management. Sam had always feared public speaking and had avoided it whenever possible. A few weeks before intake, Sam was told that his first presentation would be in 3 months. Sam responded by becoming very anxious.

Specific symptoms

He reported that he was only sleeping 3–4 hours a night, had no appetite, and had lost 8 pounds. He also complained of stomach cramps. He felt depressed and was often tearful. During the day he felt "spaced out" and unmotivated to work. He reported that he had "totally lost all confidence" and felt worthless and guilty.

History

Sam denied any prior episodes of depression and said that he had never felt so anxious in his life. He did report that he had been shy as a child, but that he had been able to get over this on his own by challenging himself to try new situations.

Current fears

When the therapist asked what made Sam most anxious about the upcoming presentation, Sam said that he would be speaking before people he regarded as older authority figures. He feared that they would challenge him and he would not be able to answer their questions. He believed that he had to do the presentation "perfectly" and that he would be unable to meet this standard.

Assessment and diagnosis

Sam was administered the standard intake battery (see Form 5.4). His diagnosis was social phobia and major depression, single episode, mild. He was informed that public speaking was the most common social fear and that effective short-term treatment was available. He was given the information handouts on social phobia (Form 5.5) and on cognitive-behavioral therapy in general

Socialization to treatment

(Form B.1). He was also educated regarding the option of medication, but he indicated that he wanted to try to deal with the problem without drugs. Since Sam's symptoms had developed recently, the therapist agreed to proceed with therapy and suggested that medication could be considered if Sam's symptoms did not improve.

Relaxation training

Because of his high level of physical tension and difficulty sleeping, Sam was taught progressive muscle relaxation, breathing relaxation, and distraction in the second session. He was instructed to practice each of these techniques once a day. He was

Homework

also assigned to read the first four chapters of *Feeling Good* (Burns, 1980) and to write down his goals for therapy.

Sessions 3–4

Goals

Sam listed two goals: (1) no longer feeling anxious; and (2) feeling comfortable while doing presentations. He denied current fears of other social situations, avoidance of situations other than public speaking, or engaging in any safety behaviors. It was therefore agreed that treatment would focus on his fear of public speaking.

Developmental history

Sam reported that the relaxation exercises had helped him sleep better, but that he still felt stressed much of the time. In order to understand the possible origins of Sam's fears, the therapist inquired about his developmental history. Sam reported that when he was young his mother had pushed him into social situations, and that this had made him feel uncomfortable. He found he was better able to overcome his fears when he could set his own pace. One of the factors in the current situation that made him particularly anxious was that he felt he was being pushed to make the presentation, rather than being able to approach it in his own time.

Identifying automatic thoughts

Sam was next taught to identify his automatic thoughts. He was asked for an example of a recent time when he had been feeling anxious. He said he had been awake in the middle of the night several days earlier worrying about the presentation. When asked what had been going through his mind at the time, Sam reported the following thoughts:

> "I can't do this."
> "I'm going to screw it up."
> "Why would they want to listen to me?"
> "I'll lock up."
> "They'll question me and challenge me."
> "I won't have the answers."

"They won't believe me."
"I've been tossed to the lions."
"I should be able to deal with this."
"I have to do this perfectly right."

Homework
For homework at the end of the third session, Sam was assigned to write down his automatic thoughts whenever he felt anxious during the coming week.

Cognitive restructuring
The fourth session was spent teaching Sam the cognitive skills of examining evidence and rational responding. Table 5.3 shows some of the automatic thoughts Sam reported from the week and the rational responses he developed with the therapist's help. As homework, Sam was assigned to continue to write his negative thoughts, but now also to practice rational responding during the following week.

Sessions 5–6

In the next session, Sam reported that although he had been feeling somewhat better for most of the week, he had become very anxious again in the last 2 days and was worried that something was seriously wrong with him. The therapist explained the concept of schema activation, and suggested that the stress of having to make the presentation might have activated some old schemas related to his earlier shyness. The problem was exacerbated because Sam took his physical symptoms of anxiety as signs that he was losing control, which made him even more anxious. The therapist helped Sam develop rational responses to the negative thoughts he had written during the week. The results are shown in Table 5.4.

Further cognitive restructuring

TABLE 5.3. Sam's Automatic Thoughts and Rational Responses, Session 4

Automatic thoughts	Rational responses
I'm going to lock up and not be able to say anything.	I've never locked up before. I've never seen anyone else do it. I can still do things even when I'm nervous. I'll be able to practice beforehand, so I'll be less likely to freeze.
I'll be sweating. They'll see I'm sweating. They'll wonder, "What's wrong with this guy?"	Most people would understand being nervous about giving a presentation. Most people probably won't even notice. I might not even sweat.
They'll ask me questions and I won't know the answers.	I know the material better than they do. I probably will have answers. It's OK to say, "I don't know, I'll find out and get back to you."

TABLE 5.4. Sam's Automatic Thoughts and Rational Responses, Session 5

Automatic thoughts	Rational responses
I'm not going to be able to do this presentation. It's going to overwhelm me because I'm in this crazy state.	Eventually I'll get over this state and be able to deal with it. A little anxiety is normal. I can work while anxious
I'll sit at my desk and get worried and not be able to concentrate.	I did OK today. I usually do OK. When I get worried, I can do relaxation. Even if it happens a little, that won't keep me from completing the project.
I'll never get over it. I'll be this way for the rest of my life.	That's not likely to happen. It doesn't happen to other people. Anxiety doesn't last forever.

Planning exposure   In the same session, the rationale for exposure was discussed with Sam. It was agreed that since Sam did not have any immediate way to practice *in vivo* exposure to public speaking, imaginal exposure would be used. Sam was assigned to list situations related to the upcoming presentation and rate each for how anxious he thought they would make him, on a scale of 0–10 (the therapist explained that this is called a "subjective units of distress" or "SUDs" scale). The therapist also discussed ways Sam could do *in vivo* exposure before the actual presentation. He recommended that Sam try to find a public speaking club or class.

The sixth session was primarily devoted to exposure. Because Sam was not able to find a time when he could schedule a 90-minute session and his symptoms were relatively mild, the session was scheduled for 45 minutes. Sam reported that he had found a public speaking group and had signed up to join it. He also said that he had been feeling pretty good for most of the week, although he had felt some anxiety after talking to a friend who was job-hunting and had thought, "Any management job I get *Exposure hierarchy*   will be doing presentations. I'll never be able to do it." Sam's hierarchy of feared situations is shown in Table 5.5.

TABLE 5.5. Sam's Hierarchy of Feared Situations

Rank	Situation	Anxiety level (SUDs)
1	Night before—trying to sleep	3
2	Fielding questions afterward	3
3	Preparing presentation slides	5
4	Actually speaking	5
5	Waiting for my turn to speak	8

First imaginal exposure exercise

The therapist suggested starting with the situation of preparing slides, since the situations Sam had given a SUDs rating of 3 would probably not make him anxious enough for exposure to be effective. When asked about his fears concerning the slides, Sam said he was afraid he would become so anxious that he would be unable to work on them. The therapist then narrated and audiotaped a scenario in which this happened. Sam's SUDs rating reached 8 out of 10. When the scenario was played back for Sam in the session, his SUDs rating dropped slightly. Sam was assigned to listen to the tape daily as homework.

Sessions 7–9

In the next session, Sam reported that listening to the tape had been helpful. His SUDs rating for this situation had dropped to 2. He also said that he was not feeling as anxious in general and was coming to realize that the presentation was not such a big deal.

Second imaginal exposure exercise

A second imaginal exposure exercise was done during this session. Sam was asked to imagine first waiting to present and then speaking. The scenario the therapist asked him to imagine again included Sam's worst fears: He was so anxious he dropped his slides; he was asked questions he couldn't answer; he froze; he was laughed at; and he was eventually told to leave.

Further cognitive restructuring

In the same session, another set of Sam's negative thoughts was examined, including the ideas that he would never be comfortable doing presentations and that he had to be perfect. The therapist pointed out that Sam had once felt anxious meeting new people and had gotten over that fear by making himself face those situations, and that the same strategy would probably work for his public speaking fear. The therapist also discussed the impossibility of doing anything perfectly, and addressed the perfectionistic assumptions underlying this thought of Sam's.

Effects of exposure

In the following session, Sam reported feeling much better. He indicated that after listening to the tape of the second exposure session, he began to realize that his fears were exaggerated; he now felt he was able to "talk back" to them. He also reported that he had been attending the public speaking group, and that although he had not yet made his first speech, he felt that the group was helping as well. Sam indicated that he no longer felt the need for weekly therapy sessions.

Relapse prevention

Since Sam appeared to be moving toward termination, the therapist suggested working on relapse prevention. Sam was asked to make a list of the techniques that he had found helpful. His list was as follows:

1. Writing my negative thoughts and challenging them.
2. Listening to the exposure tapes.
3. Reading *Feeling Good*.
4. Having contact with what I'm afraid of.
5. Remembering there is nothing wrong with a little anxiety or with being imperfect.

Phasing out therapy

The therapist suggested meeting again in 2 weeks, and Sam agreed. However, Sam canceled the next appointment. When the therapist called to find out what had happened, Sam indicated that he was continuing to feel better and agreed to make an appointment 2 weeks later.

In his ninth appointment, Sam reported minimal anxiety. His first major presentation was in a couple of weeks, and he was looking forward to getting it over with. He had given his first talk *In vivo exposure* in the public speaking group. He had been nervous, but had done breathing relaxation, and the speech had gone well. Some of his *Further cognitive* fears about disagreeing with people (especially authority figures) *restructuring* were examined, and Sam was helped to develop rational responses to these fears. Sam and the therapist agreed to meet again in a month, after Sam's first presentation.

Sam called and canceled this last session. He indicated that the talk had gone well, that he was no longer feeling anxious or *Termination* depressed, and that he wished to terminate therapy.

DETAILED TREATMENT PLAN FOR SOCIAL PHOBIA

Tables 5.6 and 5.7 are designed to help you in writing managed care treatment reports for patients with social phobia. Table 5.6 shows sample specific symptoms; select the symptoms that are appropriate for your patient. (Zuckerman's [1995] *Clinician's Thesaurus* is a further source of appropriate words and phrases.) Be sure also to specify the nature of the patient's impairments, including any dysfunction in academic, work, family, or social functioning. Table 5.7 lists sample goals and matching interventions. Again, select those that are appropriate for the patient.

Session-by-Session Treatment Options

Table 5.8 shows the sequence of interventions for a standard 20-session course of treatment for social phobia. As noted above, patients with discrete fears may require fewer sessions, while patients with severe generalized symptoms may require more.

TABLE 5.6. Sample Symptoms for Social Phobia

Fear of social situations (specify)
Fear of negative judgment by others
Feelings of embarrassment or humiliation
Anxious mood
Specify physical symptoms of anxiety:
    Blushing
    Sweating
    Shaking
    Palpitations
    Difficulty breathing
    Chest pain
    Nausea
    Dizziness
    Feeling faint

    Numbness
    Tingling
    Chills
    Hot flashes
Specify cognitive symptoms:
    Mind going blank
    Difficulty speaking
    Loss of concentration
    Derealization
    Depersonalization
Specify behavioral symptoms:
    Panic attacks
    Avoidance (specify)

TABLE 5.7. Sample Treatment Goals and Interventions for Social Phobia

Treatment goals	Interventions
Reducing physical anxiety symptoms	Relaxation training
Reducing fear of scrutiny/evaluation	Cognitive restructuring
Eliminating safety behaviors	Self-monitoring, exposure
Acquiring social skills	Social skills training (modeling, role play, *in vivo* practice)
Reducing anxiety in specific social situations to 2 or less on a scale of 0–10	Cognitive restructuring, exposure
Eliminating avoidance of social situations (specify)	Exposure
Modifying assumption of need for approval (or other assumptions—specify)	Cognitive restructuring
Modifying schema of inadequacy (or other schemas—specify)	Cognitive restructuring, developemental analysis
Eliminating impairment (specify—depending on impairments, this may be several goals)	Cognitive restructuring, problem-solving training, or other skills training (specify)
Eliminating all anxiety symptoms (SCL-90-R and/or SPQ scores in normal range)	All of the above
Acquiring relapse prevention skills	Reviewing and practicing techniques as necessary

TABLE 5.8. Session-by-Session Treatment Options for Social Phobia

Sessions 1–2

Assessment

Ascertain presenting problems
Inquire regarding all symptoms
Assess avoidance and safety behaviors (have patient fill out Forms 5.1 and 5.2)
Assess impairment in social, educational, and occupational functioning
Administer SPQ (Form 5.3)
Administer standard battery of intake measures (see Form 5.4), plus additional anxiety
    questionnaires as appropriate
Evaluate for comorbid conditions (e.g., major depression, other anxiety disorders)
Evaluate substance use; evaluate need for counseling or detoxification if patient has
    substance abuse or dependence
Assess need for medication

Socialization to Treatment

Inform patient of diagnosis
Indicate that disorder is common and brief treatment is available
Educate patient regarding option of medication
Discuss any fears/reservations patient has regarding treatment
Provide patient with information handouts on social phobia (Form 5.5) and on cognitive-
    behavioral therapy in general (Form B.1, Appendix B)
Begin developing short-term and long-term goals for therapy

Homework

Have patient begin reading Burns's *Feeling Good* or *The Feeling Good Handbook*, or
    Wilson's *Don't Panic*
Have patient begin using Forms 5.1 and 5.2 to self-monitor avoided situations and safety
    behaviors
Have patient write out goals for therapy

Sessions 3–4

Assessment

Evaluate homework
Evaluate anxiety (BAI) and depression (BDI)

Cognitive Interventions

Teach identification of automatic thoughts, using recent social situation

Behavioral Interventions

Assess need for relaxation training
If indicated, begin teaching progressive muscle relaxation and breathing relaxation

Homework

Have patient continue to self-monitor avoided situations, safety behaviors
Have patient begin recording automatic thoughts (on Form 2.7 or on Form B.4, Appendix
    B)
Have patient begin practicing relaxation at home (if indicated)

Assessment
As in Sessions 3–4

Sessions 5–6

Cognitive Interventions
Teach categorization of automatic thoughts, examination of evidence, and rational responding

Behavioral Interventions
Help patient create hierarchy for exposure; plan first exposures
Assess social skills deficits and discuss rationale for training (if indicated)
Continue teaching relaxation techniques (if indicated)

Homework
As in Sessions 3–4

Sessions 7–13

Note: The first session involving exposure should be 90 minutes; subsequent sessions may be 45 minutes, if patient is able to habituate in that time

Assessment
As in Sessions 3–4

Cognitive Interventions
Obtain automatic thoughts before, during, and after exposure, and have patient practice rational responding
Note changes in patient mood during sessions, obtain automatic thoughts, and dispute
Introduce concepts of maladaptive assumptions, dysfunctional schemas

Behavioral Interventions
Begin exposure: imaginal, role-play, and/or therapist-guided *in vivo* exposure
As each item is mastered, have patient move up exposure hierarchy
If exposure is primarily self-directed *in vivo*, use sessions to discuss prior exposures and plan new ones
Continue with social skills training (if indicated) via modeling, role play
Teach release-only relaxation, cue-controlled relaxation (if indicated)
Have patient apply relaxation during in-session exposures (if indicated)

Homework
As in Sessions 3–4
Have patient listen to tapes of imaginal exposure
Self directed *in vivo* exposure, self-directed application of cognitive skills during exposure
Have patient practice social skills, relaxation in exposure situations (if indicated)

Sessions 14–16 (Scheduled Biweekly)

Assessment
As in Sessions 3–4

(cont.)

TABLE 5.8 *(cont.)*

Cognitive Interventions
    Continue identifying and challenging automatic thoughts, underlying assumptions, and schemas

Behavioral Interventions
    Have patient complete exposure hierarchy
    Continue work on relaxation, social skills (if indicated)

Homework
    As in Sessions 7–13

Sessions 17–20 (Scheduled Biweekly or Monthly)

Assessment
    As in Sessions 3–4

Cognitive Interventions
    Continue to focus on assumptions and schemas
    Review techniques patient has found useful
    Discuss possible future problems and ways of coping with them

Behavioral Interventions
    Have patient design own exposures
    Review techniques patient has found useful
    Discuss possible future problems and ways of coping with them

Homework
    Have patient seek opportunities to be anxious and use these for further exposure
    Encourage continued practice of all cognitive skills
    Encourage continued practice of social skills and relaxation (if indicated)

CHAPTER 6

Posttraumatic Stress Disorder

DESCRIPTION AND DIAGNOSIS

Symptoms

Posttraumatic stress disorder (abbreviated PTSD in the text of this chapter) is the only diagnosis in the DSM-IV (American Psychiatric Association, 1994) that specifies an etiology. By definition, PTSD is a reaction to an extreme traumatic event. In order to qualify as "extreme," the event must involve death, threat of death, serious physical injury, or threat to physical integrity. Typical experiences that can lead to PTSD include combat, sexual or physical assault, serious accident, human-made or natural disasters, incarceration or torture, and being diagnosed with a life-threatening illness.

PTSD has three cardinal sets of symptoms: (1) reexperiencing of the trauma (including memories, nightmares, and/or flashbacks); (2) avoidance of internal and external cues associated with the trauma (which can include feelings of numbness or detachment); and (3) increased arousal (including insomnia, irritability, impaired concentration, and hypervigilance).

Prevalence and Life Course

Lifetime prevalence estimates for PTSD in community samples range from 1% to 14% (American Psychiatric Association, 1994). In populations that have been exposed to traumatic events, the prevalence is much higher. For example, a prevalence rate of 30% was found for Vietnam veterans in one study (Foy, 1992), while prevalence rates between 31% and 57% have been found for rape victims (Foa & Riggs, 1994).

PTSD can occur at any age. Symptoms generally appear shortly after the trauma; however, in some cases symptoms will not develop until months or even years after the event. In approximately half of cases, the symptoms spontaneously remit after 3 months (American Psychiatric Association, 1994). However, in other cases symptoms can persist, often for many years, and can cause long-term impairment in life functioning.

It is not clear why some people who are exposed to trauma develop PTSD and some do not. Some characteristics of the trauma are known to predict the likelihood and severity of symptoms. Direct exposure to the event, greater severity, longer duration, and perceived threat of death are all associated with increased risk. Premorbid factors that predict development of PTSD include a family history of mental disorder, previous psychiatric illness, personality traits of high neuroticism and poor self-confidence, early separation from parents, poverty, limited education, parental abuse, misconduct in childhood, and a prior history of trauma. Good social supports after the event can moderate the risk (Davidson, 1995).

Genetic/Biological Factors

Little has been written about the role of genetic and biological factors in PTSD, probably because environmental events play a central role in the disorder. Foy (1992) has suggested that biological factors may play a mediating role in determining who develops the disorder after a traumatic event and who does not. However, he does not specify the nature of the biological factors or the mechanism involved.

Coexisting Conditions

It has been estimated that between 60% and 100% of PTSD sufferers meet criteria for at least one other Axis I disorder (Litz, Penk, Gerardi, & Keane, 1992). The most common comorbid disorders are major depression and substance abuse. Other anxiety disorders are also common, including panic disorder, agoraphobia, obsessive–compulsive disorder, and social phobia (American Psychiatric Association, 1994). Psychotic disorders are less common, but can cooccur with PTSD. Axis II disorders are common, including borderline, antisocial, paranoid, obsessive–compulsive, and schizoid personality disorders.

A number of features are commonly associated with PTSD, including intense feelings of guilt, shame, disgust and/or despair; excessive anger and hostility; impaired interpersonal relationships; marital/couple distress and sexual difficulties; poor work performance; impaired affect regulation; impulsive and self-destructive behavior; and somatic complaints, such as headaches, joint pain, colitis, and respiratory problems.

Differential Diagnosis

PTSD is differentiated from adjustment disorder by the severity of the traumatic event; in order for a diagnosis of PTSD to be given, the event must be extreme. Acute stress disorder is given as a diagnosis if the symptom picture resembles PTSD but the event occurred less than 4 weeks ago. If intrusive thoughts are present, they must be related to a trauma; otherwise, a diagnosis of obsessive–compulsive disorder should be considered. Similarly, intense flashbacks may at times resemble the hallucinations associated with psychotic disorders. However, as long as they are associated with a trauma, PTSD is the more likely diagnosis.

An important differential diagnosis to be made with PTSD involves malingering. This must be ruled out any time there is the possibility of gain from the disorder (e.g., a damage award or veterans' benefits). In such cases, verification of the trauma should be obtained, most commonly from police or military records. More extensive assessment, including use of the Minnesota Multiphasic Personality Inventory (MMPI), may be appropriate. The clinical presentation may also hold some clues. If the patient tells the trauma story with eagerness or ease (as opposed to the avoidance more commonly seen), or if the trauma appears vague and nonspecific, the clinician should be alert to the possibility of malingering.

Figure 6.1 is a diagnostic flow chart that depicts the differential diagnosis of PTSD in greater detail.

UNDERSTANDING POSTTRAUMATIC STRESS DISORDER IN COGNITIVE-BEHAVIORAL TERMS

Behavioral Factors

The behavioral conceptualization of PTSD is based on Mowrer's (1960) two-factor theory of anxiety. According to this model, anxiety and other emotions experienced during a traumatic event become linked in the patient's mind to sights, sounds, and other sensations that occur during the event. This process is a form of classical conditioning. These sights, sounds, and other sensations thus become cues that evoke anxiety when they are experienced again later.

The range of cues that can elicit anxiety increases over time, due to two processes: (1) generalization, whereby cues that are similar to the original cue begin to evoke anxiety; and (2) higher-order conditioning, whereby a cue that was originally neutral begins to evoke anxiety because it has become associated with anxiety triggered by other cues. For example, a woman who was raped while walking home alone at night may begin to fear not only being out at night (the original cue), but also any dark place (generalization). She may also come to fear her therapist's office, where she has been discussing the rape (higher-order conditioning). It should be noted that anxiety-arousing cues can be external (places, sights, sounds) or internal (thoughts, memories, or emotional states).

The second part of the two-factor theory involves avoidance. Because cues that remind the person of the event evoke anxiety, he or she tries to avoid them. When a cue is avoided, the person's anxiety decreases. The reduction in anxiety serves as a reward that increases the likelihood of the person's avoiding the cue in the future. This is a form of operant conditioning. Thus avoidance becomes used increasingly often as a coping strategy. Because the cues that are avoided can be internal, such as thoughts or emotions, avoidance may lead to emotional numbing. Often alcohol or drugs are used as a way to avoid internal cues, and this leads to substance abuse or dependence.

Cognitive Factors

The behavioral model provides explanations for both the reexperiencing and avoidance symptoms of PTSD. However, it has been criticized as failing to account adequately for the repeated alternation between reexperiencing and avoidance/numbing that is com-

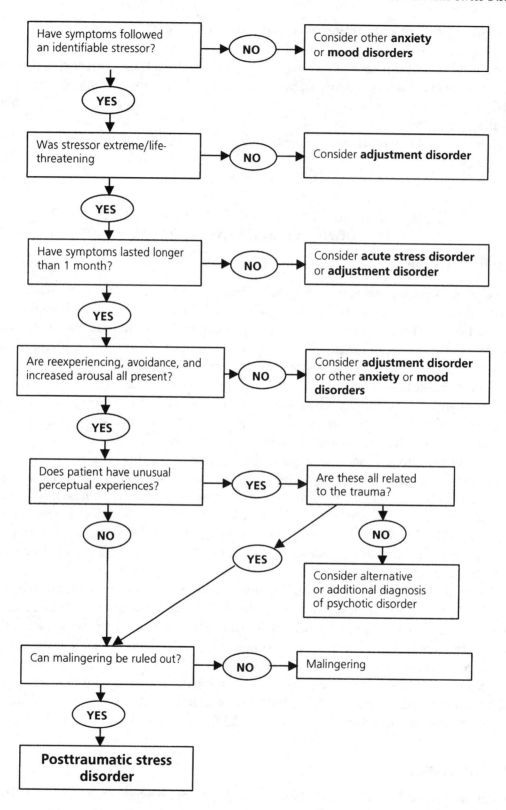

FIGURE 6.1. Diagnostic flow chart for posttraumatic stress disorder.

monly seen in the disorder, or for the persistent hyperarousal. It also fails to account for the altered sense of meaning that many PTSD patients report (Foa & Riggs, 1994).

Foa and her colleagues (Foa & Riggs, 1994; Foa, Rothbaum, & Molnar, 1995; Foa, Steketee, & Rothbaum, 1989) have proposed a cognitive model of PTSD that incorporates elements of the behavioral model. They propose that when a person experiences a trauma, a "fear structure" is formed in memory, consisting of three elements: (1) stimuli (the sights, sounds, and other sensations associated with the event); (2) responses (physiological and emotional reactions to the event); and (3) the meanings associated with the stimuli and responses. This fear structure forms a program for escaping from danger. Like the behavioral model, Foa's model proposes that cues associated with the trauma activate the fear structure—causing reexperiencing of the memories and responses, and leading to attempts to avoid such cues.

However, Foa's model also emphasizes the importance of the meaning element of the fear structure. Traumatic events often violate several commonly held assumptions and schemas: (1) "The world is safe," (2) "Events are predictable and controllable," (3) "Extreme negative events will not happen to me," and (4) "I can cope with whatever events arise." In keeping with Piagetian theory, Foa proposes that when an event is experienced that contradicts such basic schemas, there is a natural push to make sense of the experience. If the meanings associated with the trauma (e.g., "Dangerous events can happen without warning," "They can happen to me," and "I may be unable to cope") cannot be assimilated into existing schemas, there will be a need to revise the schemas—a process referred to as "accommodation."

What makes this cognitive processing of the trauma difficult for people with PTSD is the fact that activating the meaning element of the fear structure also activates the response element, leading the person to reexperience the intense emotional responses associated with the trauma. Since the emotions feel overwhelming, the person then tries to stop thinking about the memories. This avoidance blocks the process of assimilation and accommodation. A pattern then develops of alternating between attempts to assimilate (which lead to reexperiencing), and attempts to avoid the memories and negative emotions. According to Foa's model, the tension between the need to find meaning and the need for avoidance leaves the person in a persistent state of hyperarousal.

Examples of the distorted automatic thoughts, maladaptive assumptions, and dysfunctional schemas found in patients with PTSD are provided in Table 6.1.

Outcome Studies for Cognitive-Behavioral Treatments

Most of the cognitive-behavioral treatments developed for PTSD have been based on some form of exposure. Early studies typically utilized systematic desensitization, in which the patient is repeatedly exposed to brief presentations of trauma cues in imagination while undergoing relaxation. More recent studies have used prolonged exposure, in which the patient is exposed to cues (either in imagination or *in vivo*) for extended periods without using relaxation, until the anxiety response diminishes. Prolonged exposure is now believed to be more effective than systematic desensitization (Foa et al., 1995). A variant of exposure, eye movement desensitization and reprocessing (EMDR), has been introduced by Shapiro

TABLE 6.1. Examples of the Three Types of Cognitive Distortions in Posttraumatic Stress Disorder

Distorted automatic thoughts

"What happened is my fault."
"I should have been able to prevent it."
"I should have been able to handle the situation."
"I should be over this by now."
"I am weak."
"I can't stand these feelings."
"Something terrible could happen at any minute."
"I'm in danger now."
"I can't let my guard down."
"I can't handle this situation."
"I'm helpless."
"You can't trust anyone."
"No one cares."
"No one will be there to help me if I need it."

Maladaptive assumptions

"Because I could not control what happened, there is no point in trying to control anything."
"Because I could be in danger at any time, I must maintain control at all times."
"I must always be on the alert."
"I'll be overwhelmed if I think about what happened."
"It is better to avoid any potentially dangerous situation than endure risk."
"All risk is bad."
"I wouldn't be able to stand another loss."

Dysfunctional schemas

"The world is inherently unpredictable and dangerous."
"Bad things can happen at any time."
"You can't trust anyone."
"I am powerless to prevent catastrophe."
"I am a bad person."
"Life is meaningless."
"The future is bleak."

(1989). Controversy exists regarding the mechanisms responsible for the effectiveness of EMDR and whether they differ substantially from those at work in standard imaginal exposure (Acierno, Hersen, Van Hasselt, Tremont, & Meuser, 1994).

In addition to exposure, two other cognitive-behavioral techniques have been studied for PTSD: cognitive restructuring and anxiety management training. Cognitive restructuring uses standard cognitive techniques to address the meaning element of the fear structure. Anxiety management training uses a variety of techniques, including progressive muscle relaxation, visualization, biofeedback, assertion training, thought stopping, and distraction, to help patients manage their emotional and physiological responses.

van Etten and Taylor (1998) performed a meta-analytic review of 39 studies of PTSD treatment. They found that behavior therapy (generally including some form of exposure, and sometimes including cognitive restructuring and/or anxiety management training) and EMDR were equally effective, and that both were more effective than control conditions. Both behavior therapy and EMDR produced larger effect sizes than other forms of psychotherapy. The effectiveness of behavior therapy and EMDR was comparable to the effectiveness of SSRIs, and superior to that of other forms of medication. Patient gains were found to be well maintained at follow-up periods averaging 15 weeks after the end of treatment.

Foa and her colleagues have recently attempted to determine the relative contribution of various techniques in cognitive-behavioral treatment of PTSD. In a series of studies (Foa, Rothbaum, Riggs, & Murdock, 1991; Foa et al., 1995), they compared stress inoculation training, which includes anxiety management and cognitive restructuring; prolonged exposure; supportive counseling; a waiting-list condition; and the combination of stress inoculation training and prolonged exposure. Both cognitive-behavioral treatments were found to be superior to counseling or the waiting-list condition. Those patients who received the combination of stress inoculation training and prolonged exposure had the best outcome at follow-up.

Overall, these results support the effectiveness of cognitive-behavioral approaches for treating PTSD. It appears that a treatment combining anxiety management, cognitive restructuring, and exposure is likely to yield the best results.

ASSESSMENT AND TREATMENT

Rationale and Plan for Treatment

In keeping with the findings of the outcome literature, the treatment package described in this chapter combines anxiety management training, prolonged exposure, and cognitive restructuring to address the symptoms of PTSD.

Anxiety management training is used to reduce symptoms of hyperarousal and the emotional distress associated with reexperiencing. Exposure targets the symptoms of reexperiencing and avoidance. Repeated exposure to memories of the event weakens the association between the memories and the emotional reactions they evoke, so that patients are able to think about what happened to them without feeling distress. Exposure to previously avoided situations breaks the pattern of avoidance and reduces emotional responses to environmental cues. Cognitive restructuring is used to eliminate the pattern of alternating between thinking about and avoiding thinking about the trauma. It does this by altering maladaptive meanings associated with the event and helping patients either assimilate the experience into existing assumptions or modify those assumptions to accommodate the knowledge of what has happened.

Most studies of cognitive-behavioral treatment for PTSD have involved between 10 and 15 sessions lasting from 60 to 120 minutes each, scheduled once to twice a week (Marmar, Foy, Kagan, & Pynoos, 1994). Although this intensity will be required for some patients, it is not practical in many clinical settings, where 45-minute sessions have become the rule. We have attempted to address this in designing the treatment package by having a substantial portion of the imaginal exposure take place as homework. Still, it is advisable to leave 90 minutes for at least the first, and possibly the first several, exposure sessions. Using this approach, we have found that 12 to 20 sessions, the majority of which last 45 minutes, are often sufficient for patients who have had a single trauma. Patients who have severe or chronic PTSD, who have a history of multiple traumas, or who show substantial disturbance in life functioning will frequently require longer treatment.

The treatment plan for PTSD is outlined in Table 6.2.

Assessment

While some patients with PTSD will present for treatment describing their symptoms as a response to a specific traumatic event, many others will present complaining of anxiety, depression, substance abuse, or problems of living without revealing a history of trauma. This may be because they do not make the link between their symptoms and the event, or because they are reluctant to discuss the trauma.

Initial Clinical Evaluation of Trauma and Related Symptoms

Given the high prevalence of PTSD in clinical populations, all patients, regardless of their presenting problems, should be screened for a history of trauma. Questions that can be included in standard intake interviews include the following:

What is the most upsetting thing that ever happened to you?
Have you ever felt your life was in danger?
Have you ever been attacked or assaulted?
Have you ever been physically or sexually abused?

Even when patients reveal a recent trauma, clinicians should always inquire about any history of prior trauma.

TABLE 6.2. General Plan of Treatment for Posttraumatic Stress Disorder

Assessment
    Initial clinical evaluation of trauma and related symptoms
    Tests and other evaluations
    Consideration of medication
Socialization to treatment
Anxiety management training
Exposure
    Imaginal exposure to trauma memory and to related cues
    In vivo exposure to avoided situations
Cognitive restructuring
Coping with life problems
Phasing out treatment

Once a patient has disclosed a traumatic event, he or she should first be asked to describe the event in an open-ended manner. Even this process may be therapeutic, as it may be the first opportunity the patient has had to tell a neutral and sympathetic party about what happened.

After the patient has told his or her story, the clinician should inquire about any details of the event and its aftermath that have been omitted, including (1) physiological and emotional reactions at the time of the event; (2) choice points and actions taken before, during, and after the event; (3) meanings attached to the event, the patient's reactions, and his or her behaviors; (4) responses of others to the patient during and after the event; (5) cues that trigger memories; (6) the specific nature of reexperiencing symptoms; (7) all avoidance, including situations avoided, attempts to avoid memories/thoughts/emotions, and psychic numbing; (8) symptoms of physiological arousal (insomnia, startle responses, etc.); and (9) any difficulties in interpersonal, academic, or work functioning that have developed since the trauma. The patient's current social supports should also be assessed. The patient should be asked to list all cues that trigger memories on the Patient's Trauma Trigger Record (Form 6.1). This can be used either to list cues that have triggered memories in the past, or as a log to record any triggers and intrusive memories experienced between sessions.

Patients who have been diagnosed with PTSD should also be evaluated for comorbid conditions, including depression and other anxiety disorders. If the patient is so depressed that he or she is suicidal or cannot actively participate in therapy, the depression must be treated before treatment for PTSD is undertaken.

Any legal or financial issues related to the PTSD should be explored, and malingering should be ruled out. Inquiry should be made regarding the patient's premorbid level of functioning, including strengths and weaknesses, as well as developmental history. If the trauma included head injury, possible cognitive deficits need to be assessed.

Tests and Other Evaluations

Self-report questionnaires can be useful for assessing patients with PTSD. The Posttraumatic Stress Questionnaire (PTSQ) for Patients, which we have developed, allows patients to rate the degree to which they are bothered by common PTSD symptoms. This scale is shown in Form 6.2. Noting the degree of distress for each symptom can help in making a diagnosis. Totalling the items of the PTSQ yields a total score, which can be used to evaluate progress when the scale is readministered during therapy.

Another self-report measure is the Crime-Related Post-Traumatic Stress Disorder Scale (CR-PTSD), developed by Saunders, Arata, and Kilpatrick (1990) and based on 28 items selected from the SCL-90-R (Derogatis, 1977). The 28 items are as follows: 3, 12, 13, 14, 17, 18, 23, 24, 28, 38, 39, 41, 44, 45, 51, 54, 56, 59, 66, 68, 70, 79, 80, 81, 82, 84, 86, and 89. The authors recommend that the entire SCL-90-R be administered, rather than just these 28 items. The CR-PTSD score is then calculated by averaging the scores for each of the 28 items. A cutoff score of 0.89 was found to maximize correct classification. Because this scale was validated on samples of female sexual assault victims, it may not be as successful in classifying victims of other types of traumas.

FORM 6.1. Patient's Trauma Trigger Record

Patient's Name: _____ Week: _____

Instructions: Please list any sensations, places, or situations that evoke traumatic memories, or that you avoid out of fear they might evoke memories. In the second column, write the memory or sensation that you get when you are in contact with the trigger. In the third column, note whether the trigger is something you avoid. Finally, note how much distress you feel (or would feel) when you encounter the trigger, from 0 (no distress) to 10 (maximum distress).

Trigger	Memory or Sensation	Avoided? (Yes/No)	Distress (0–10)

FORM 6.2. Posttraumatic Stress Questionnaire (PTSQ) for Patients

Patient's Name: _____ Today's Date: _____

Listed below are symptoms people often have after experiencing a traumatic event or events. Please check how much you have been bothered by each symptom in the past month.

Symptom	None (0)	A little (1)	Moder- ately (2)	A lot (3)
Upsetting memories about what happened.	___	___	___	___
Nightmares about the event(s).	___	___	___	___
Feeling like you are living the event(s) all over again (flashbacks).	___	___	___	___
Anxiety or distress when you see or hear things that remind you of the event(s).	___	___	___	___
Avoiding things that remind you of the event(s).	___	___	___	___
Lack of interest in work and/or leisure activities.	___	___	___	___
Difficulty feeling close to other people.	___	___	___	___
Feeling emotionally numb.	___	___	___	___
Feeling unable to imagine the future.	___	___	___	___
Difficulty sleeping.	___	___	___	___
Feeling irritable or angry.	___	___	___	___
Finding it hard to concentrate.	___	___	___	___
Feeling on edge or unable to relax.	___	___	___	___

In addition to the PTSQ and SCL-90-R patients should be given other measures from the standard intake battery described in earlier chapters (the BAI, BDI, GAF, SCID-II, and Locke–Wallace) and perhaps other anxiety questionnaires (the ADIS-R, the Fear Questionnaire, etc.), as appropriate. Form 6.3 provides space for recording scores on the standard intake battery and other questionnaires. It also enables the therapist to record a patient's medication, alcohol, and other drug use (it should be emphasized that any substance abuse or dependence must be treated before treatment of PTSD can be undertaken); to record (at intake only) the history of any previous traumatic episodes or other anxiety episodes; to note (on later evaluations) which situations are now avoided and which the patient can now approach; and to indicate treatment recommendations.

Consideration of Medication

Medication is considered an adjunctive rather than a primary treatment for PTSD. It is generally recognized that some form of psychotherapy is necessary in treating the disorder (Marmar et al., 1994; Peterson, Prout, & Schwarz, 1991). However, in cases of severe or chronic PTSD, medication may provide enough symptom relief to allow patients to participate in therapy. In addition, medication can be helpful in treating comorbid conditions and related features of the disorder, such as depression, substance abuse, rage, and impulsivity (Friedman & Southwick, 1995).

There have been case reports involving almost every class of psychotropic drugs in the treatment of PTSD, including antidepressants, benzodiazepines, mood stabilizers, and neuroleptics. van Etten and Taylor (1998), in their meta-analysis of controlled studies, found that the SSRIs were more effective than other forms of medication. The mood stabilizer carbamazepine was found to be as effective as the SSRIs in one study. Benzodiazepines were not found to be very effective, which is notable because these medications have been widely prescribed for PTSD in the past. No data are available for the effectiveness of medication after discontinuation.

Socialization to Treatment

Once a diagnosis is established, the patients should be educated regarding PTSD, the rationale for treatment, and treatment options (including medication). This often has a therapeutic effect, as it may be the first time many patients have had a way to understand their symptoms and may allay fears that they are "going crazy." Discussing the rationale for treatment and getting a patient's specific consent before proceeding will also help build and maintain motivation for the treatment phase. Form 6.4 is an educational handout about PTSD that can be given to patients. The handout about cognitive-behavioral therapy in general (Form B.1 in Appendix B) can also be used.

Anxiety Management Training

The goal of anxiety management training is to provide patients with ways to cope with their heightened arousal and other emotional and physiological reactions to reex-

FORM 6.3. Further Evaluation of Posttraumatic Stress Disorder: Test Scores, Substance Use, History, Treatment Progress, and Recommendations

Patient's Name: _____ Today's Date: _____

Therapist's Name: _____ Sessions Completed: _____

Test data/scores

Beck Depression Inventory (BDI) _____

Beck Anxiety Inventory (BAI) _____

Global Assessment of Functioning (GAF) _____

Crime-Related Post-Traumatic Stress Disorder Scale (CR-PTSD) _____

Other Symptom Checklist 90—Revised (SCL-90-R) scales _____

Structured Clinical Interview for DSM-III-R, Axis II (SCID-II) _____

Locke–Wallace Marital Adjustment Test _____

Anxiety Disorders Interview Schedule—Revised (ADIS-R) _____

Other anxiety questionnaires (specify): _____

_____

Substance use

Current use of psychiatric medications (include dosage) _____

_____

Who prescribes? _____

_____

Use of alcohol/other drugs (kind, frequency, amount, consequences) _____

_____

History (intake only)

Previous traumatic episodes (specify nature):

    Onset   Duration   Precipitating events   Treatment

Previous episodes of other anxiety (specify nature):

    Onset   Duration   Precipitating events   Treatment

(cont.)

Treatment progress (later evaluations only)

Situations still avoided: _____

_____

_____

Situations approached that were previously avoided: _____

_____

_____

Recommendations

Medication evaluation or reevaluation:

Increased intensity of services:

Behavioral interventions:

Cognitive interventions:

Interpersonal interventions:

Marital/couple therapy:

Other:

_____

FORM 6.4. Information for Patients about Posttraumatic Stress Disorder

What Is Posttraumatic Stress Disorder?

Posttraumatic stress disorder (or PTSD) is a common reaction to very stressful or traumatic events. Many different kinds of events can lead to PTSD, including being in a car accident; being raped or being the victim of another crime; being physically or sexually abused; living through a disaster such as a flood or a bombing; or seeing someone else die.

People with PTSD have three main types of problems or symptoms:

1. **Reliving the trauma**. This can include memories that seem out of control, nightmares, and flashbacks that make people feel as if they are living the event all over again. Memories often come back when something people see or hear reminds them of the event.

2. **Avoiding**. Because it is upsetting to remember what happened, people with PTSD try not to think about it. They also stay away from people, places, or things that bring back memories. Often they feel numb or detached from other people. Some turn to alcohol or drugs to dull the pain.

3. **Signs of physical stress**. These can include trouble sleeping, feeling irritable or angry all the time, trouble concentrating, and feeling tense or on guard.

What Causes Posttraumatic Stress Disorder?

When people live through a trauma, the memories of what happened get connected in their minds with what they saw, heard, smelled, or felt at the time. Later a similar sight, sound, smell, or other feeling can bring the memories and emotions flooding back.

A second reason why the memories come back is that people have a need to make sense of what happened. Traumatic events often make people question things they once believed—for example, that the world is basically safe or that bad things won't happen to them. To understand the trauma, they have to think about it. But thinking about it brings the memories and feelings back. So they try not to think about it. Instead of finding understanding and peace, people often end up going back and forth between remembering and trying to forget.

How Does Posttraumatic Stress Disorder Develop?

Most people begin to have symptoms of PTSD shortly after the trauma. For about half of these people, the symptoms get better on their own within 3 months. For others, the symptoms can last for years. Some people don't start to have symptoms until many years after the event.

How Does Cognitive-Behavioral Therapy for Posttraumatic Stress Disorder Help?

There are three steps in cognitive-behavioral therapy for PTSD. First, your therapist will teach you ways to cope with the feelings and tension that come with the memories. These include ways to relax your body and to take your mind off the pain.

(cont.)

Second, your therapist will help you face the memories. He or she will guide you in retelling the story of what happened. The more you do this, the less upsetting the memories will become, and the more you will be able to find a sense of peace.

Finally, your therapist will teach you ways to change negative thinking and handle problems in your life.

A number of studies have found that cognitive-behavioral therapy helps people with PTSD feel better. These studies have included combat veterans as well as victims of rape, assault, and other traumas.

How Long Does Therapy Last?

How long treatment for PTSD lasts depends on how many traumas you suffered and how severe they were, how bad your symptoms are now, and how many other problems you are having in your life. For people who have been through a single traumatic event, 12 to 20 sessions are usually enough. Most of these sessions will be 45 to 50 minutes long, but a few may be as long as 90 minutes.

Can Medications Help?

Drugs by themselves are usually not enough for treating PTSD. However, they can be helpful for some people when combined with therapy. Your physician or a psychiatrist can suggest which medication might be best for you.

What Is Expected of You as a Patient?

It is best not to start treatment for PTSD if you are currently abusing drugs or alcohol or have a major crisis in your life. Your therapist can help you deal with these problems first, and then can help you begin working on your PTSD symptoms. Other than that, all you need to do is to be willing to try therapy and to spend some time each week practicing the things you learn.

periencing the trauma. This provides a degree of immediate relief for their distress, increases their sense of self-efficacy, and helps them tolerate the arousal necessary for exposure and the emotional processing of the trauma. Although a number of techniques are useful, we most commonly use the following: (1) breathing relaxation, (2) progressive muscle relaxation, (3) visualization, (4) thought stopping, and (5) distraction. The procedures for these techniques are described in detail in Appendix A and in the CD-ROM that accompanies this book. Each patient is taught all of the anxiety management techniques and is asked to practice them as homework before exposure is initiated.

Exposure

There are three primary targets for exposure: (1) the memory of the trauma; (2) other internal and external cues that trigger anxiety and reexperiencing; and (3) situations that are avoided. Of these, exposure to the memory of the trauma is the most important. Note, however, that before exposure work begins, any therapy-interfering behaviors need to be addressed. See the "Coping with Life Problems" section later in this chapter.

Imaginal Exposure to the Trauma Memory and to Related Cues

Exposure to the trauma memory is initiated in the therapist's office. The first exposure session should be scheduled for 90 minutes in order to allow enough time for habituation to occur. The patient is asked to relax in a comfortable position with eyes closed and to tell the story of the trauma while attempting to visualize it in his or her mind. This procedure is tape-recorded. The therapist functions as a guide and asks questions, which serve two main functions: (1) to focus the patient on details (such as specific sights, sounds, smells, and other sensory experiences, as well as emotions and internal physical sensations) in order to help fully activate the memory; and (2) to ensure that all significant details of the story are included and nothing is avoided. Periodically during the retelling of the story, the patient is asked to rate the distress he or she is feeling on a scale from 0 to 10. The therapist explains that these are called "subjective units of distress" or "SUDs" ratings.

The second step in the exposure session is to have the patient listen to the tape recording of the story, again closing his or her eyes and attempting to "relive" the experience. During this process, the patient again gives SUDs ratings. The patient listens to the tape repeatedly until the SUDs ratings begin to decrease. Ideally, exposure should continue until the SUDs ratings have decreased by at least half. When the trauma is complex or involves multiple events, it may be necessary to break the story into segments, and to devote several sessions to the telling of the whole story.

It is crucial that exposure not be terminated until the patient has experienced some decrease in anxiety. This is important for two reasons. First, terminating exposure while the patient is highly distressed will only serve to strengthen the association between the memory and the emotional distress. Second, the first time a patient experiences a reduction in distress during exposure is usually a very powerful experience. It contradicts the patient's belief that focusing on memories will make him or her feel even more anxious, and it provides motivation to continue exposure work.

Once the patient has habituated to the tape of the trauma story in the therapist's office, he or she is assigned to continue listening to the tape as homework. The patient is instructed to set aside at least 45 minutes each day for this purpose, and to listen to the tape repeatedly until the SUDs score for that day is reduced by half. The results of practice sessions (either in the office or as homework) should be recorded on the Patient's Imaginal Exposure Practice Record (Form A.1 in Appendix A).

After the initial session, if the patient is able to do the exposure homework successfully, it may be possible to shorten the exposure sessions to 45 minutes and have most of the work of habituation done through listening to the tape as homework. In addition to retelling the story, exposure to trauma memories may be accomplished by having the patient write about the trauma or draw or paint images from the trauma.

Patients who have anxiety reactions to specific cues can be exposed to these during sessions. For example, a patient who has been in an automobile accident and has developed a startle reaction to loud noises can be repeatedly presented with loud noises in the therapist's office, until he or she habituates to them and the anxiety decreases.

In Vivo *Exposure to Avoided Situations*

Once the patient has completed exposure work to the trauma memory, *in vivo* exposure should be undertaken for any avoided situations. For example, a patient who has avoided driving on limited-access highways since experiencing an automobile accident can be assigned to begin driving again. *In vivo* exposure can generally be done as homework without the therapist present. However, in cases where the patient is extremely anxious, it may be necessary to have another person (such as a supportive family member) present during early exposure trials. When the PTSD has been chronic, the patient may have developed extensive avoidance. In such cases it will be helpful to develop a hierarchy of feared situations, ranked from least to most anxiety-producing and to have the patient work slowly up the hierarchy. A more complete description of exposure procedures can be found in Appendix A; *in vivo* exposure practice should be recorded on Form A.2 in Appendix A.

Cognitive Restructuring

Cognitive restructuring in PTSD targets the patient's distorted automatic thoughts, maladaptive assumptions, and dysfunctional schemas associated with the trauma. The most common categories of distorted automatic thoughts in PTSD are overgeneralization, all-or-nothing thinking, and personalization. These reflect underlying assumptions about how things "must" or "should" be, and even deeeper-seated schemas about the nature of the self and others. In other words, faced with a traumatic event that contradicts commonly held assumptions about the safety of the world, the predictability and controllability of events, and the ability of the self to cope, people who develop PTSD tend to go to the opposite extreme—seeing everything and everyone as dangerous, unpredictable, and malevolent, and themselves as weak and incompetent. It should be noted that people who have had multiple prior traumas may have already developed extremely negative assumptions and schemas. In such cases, the most recent trauma may have served to strengthen existing negative assumptions and schemas, rather than to contradict positive ones.

The goal of cognitive restructuring for PTSD is to return the patient to a more balanced view, in which the world is seen as safe within limits, events are seen as generally predictable and controllable, and the self is seen as competent to cope with most situations, while at the same time there is acknowledgment of the existential reality that sudden, unpredictable, and extreme negative events, including death, can and do happen. Table 6.3 lists some techniques that may be helpful in addressing typical cognitive distortions in PTSD. (Many of these techniques are among the cognitive techniques listed in Table B.3 of Appendix B, but some are behavioral in nature.)

It should be noted that exposure alone will often lead to cognitive change. This is because exposure reduces the anxiety and avoidance associated with the trauma memories and allows the natural process of assimilation and accommodation to take place.

Coping with Life Problems

People who present with PTSD often have problems of living that are related to the trauma. Depending on the severity of the trauma, the chronicity of the PTSD, and personality factors, these problems can range from relatively mild to complex and highly disruptive. In addition, the type of life problems faced varies with the type of traumatic event. The issues faced by a woman who has been raped are likely to be different from those faced by a male combat veteran.

In general, any problem that has the potential to interfere with therapy needs to be addressed before exposure work can begin. For instance, substance abuse or dependence must be treated first, and the patient must have established a period of sobriety before undergoing treatment for PTSD symptoms. In addition, the patient must have a stable living situation and be in good physical health. For some patients, this means that substantial therapeutic work must be done before beginning PTSD treatment.

For many patients, however, this phase of therapy can be done after exposure has been completed. The full range of cognitive-behavioral techniques can be brought to bear on these life problems, including cognitive restructuring, exposure, and skills training. It may be helpful to include a patient's spouse or significant other in some sessions. Interventions that help the patient locate and/or utilize social supports may be particularly important. In some cases, the therapist may need to act as an advocate on the patient's behalf.

Troubleshooting Problems in Therapy

Several problems commonly arise when exposure-based treatment for PTSD is employed. These are described below, with recommendations for how to deal with each one.

TABLE 6.3. Examples of Techniques for Addressing Trauma-Related Cognitive Distortions

Target belief	Techniques
"The world is dangerous."	1. Calculating probabilities of specific events. 2. Listing advantages/disadvantages of world view. 3. Doing a cost–benefit analysis of specific vigilance and avoidance behaviors. 4. Identifying reasonable precautions.
"Events are unpredictable and uncontrollable."	1. Listing advantages/disadvantages of belief. 2. Listing all areas of life in which patient has some control, and rating degree of control for each. 3. Doing a cost–benefit analysis of specific efforts at prediction/control. 4. Keeping a daily log of behaviors that produce predicted outcomes. 5. Engaging in behaviors with high probability of predictable outcome. 6. Accepting that some events are unpredictable.
"What happened was my fault."	1. Examining knowledge and choices available to patient at the time. Were any better choices actually available? Could patient reasonably have predicted outcomes? 2. Using double-standard technique: "Would you blame a friend in a similar situation?" 3. Constructing a "pie chart" assigning responsibility for event to all relevant parties. 4. Examining societal biases (e.g., men are sent to war, then blamed for killing; women are urged to look "sexy," then blamed for being raped). 5. Practicing self-forgiveness—all humans make mistakes.
"I am incompetent."	1. Examining evidence for competence in daily life. 2. Examining unreasonable expectation of competence in extreme and unusual circumstances. 3. Keeping a daily log of competent coping. 4. Using graded task assignment (see Appendix A).
"Other people cannot be trusted."	1. Listing known persons who are trustworthy, and listing specific ways in which each can be trusted. 2. Rating people on a continuum of trustworthiness. 3. Examining patient's history of relationship choices. Are better alternatives available? 4. Carrying out behavioral experiments that involve trusting others in small ways. 5. Keeping a daily log of people who honor commitments.
"Life is meaningless."	1. Listing activities that formerly were rewarding (see Appendix A). 2. Scheduling pleasurable/rewarding activities (see Appendix A). 3. Recognizing feelings of loss as a way of confirming meaning. 4. Examining which goals and activities no longer seem meaningful and which now appear more important. 5. Working toward an acceptance of death. 6. Finding meaning in each day.

Resistance to Doing Exposure Work

The patient's beliefs about doing exposure should be elicited. Usually they involve fear that the anxiety will be overwhelming and unbearable, that it will go on forever, and/or that exposure will not work. The patient's understanding of the rationale for exposure should be reviewed. The patient can be asked this question: "If you were to tell the story 10 times in a row, how upset do you think you would feel by the tenth telling? How upset by the 100th? How upset by the 1,000th?" Most patients are able to see that eventually they would become "bored" and their anxiety would decrease. Patients can also be told of the experience of others who have been through exposure. Finally, a therapist and patient can contract to start the exposure work with some portion of the story or other cue that evokes less than maximum anxiety, so that the patient can experience habituation.

Failure to Become Anxious during Exposure

The most common causes for failure to become anxious during exposure are as follows: (1) The patient is distracting himself or herself from the anxiety-provoking cues; and (2) the cues being used in the exposure are not the ones that actually trigger anxiety.

The patient should first be asked about anything he or she is doing to attempt to reduce anxiety during exposure. The need to experience anxiety temporarily in order to get better should be emphasized, and the patient should be asked to focus his or her full attention on the exposure task. If the patient continues to experience minimal anxiety, other cues should be tried.

Becoming Overwhelmed with Anxiety during Exposure

As patients tell the trauma story, they usually move from cues that evoke mild to moderate anxiety to cues that evoke maximal anxiety. If a patient begins to feel overwhelmed during the exposure session, it is advisable to return to an earlier part of the story and allow the patient to habituate to that part before continuing with the most difficult cues. In general, if the patient's SUDs rating reaches 7 or 8, it is a good idea to allow some habituation to take place before proceeding. It may be necessary in some cases to have the patient employ anxiety management skills (e.g., distraction or relaxation) before resuming exposure. It is not advisable to terminate exposure while the patient is in a high state of anxiety, as this will strengthen rather than weaken the connection between the cues and the patient's emotional reaction. In such a case, it may be necessary to meet more than once a week during the initial phase of exposure, in order to help the patient cope with the strong emotions elicited.

Failure to Habituate

The most common reason for failure to habituate is that exposure has not continued long enough. Some patients will require an hour or more before habituating. Patients who complain of failure to habituate during homework are usually making their exposure sessions too short. An alternative explanation is that the patients are distracting themselves during exposure, thereby preventing habituation.

Noncompliance with Homework

Patients who do not complete homework assignments should be asked what kept them from doing the homework. Simple explanations, such as lack of time, should be explored first. In such a case, a therapist can work with a patient in the session to schedule time for exposure homework during the following week. If this fails, motivational factors should be explored. Further in-session exposure may be needed in order for the patient to experience sufficient habituation to feel motivated to continue on his or her own. Advantages and disadvantages of doing exposure homework can be reviewed. Finally, the possibility of resistance from one or more members of the patient's social support system, or of secondary gains from the patient's symptoms, should be considered.

CASE EXAMPLE

The following example is based on a composite of cases.

Sessions 1–2

Presenting problem   Ralph was a 25-year-old single white male. He lived with his divorced mother and worked as a salesman. When asked what brought him in for treatment, he replied, "Death."

Trauma history   Ralph reported that 3 years earlier he had been in an automobile accident in which his girlfriend of 5 years, Sara, was killed. They had spent the day at the beach and waited until late evening to drive home in order to avoid traffic. Although they'd both had three or four beers during the day, Ralph denied that either of them had been drunk. Because Ralph was feeling sleepy, Sara had volunteered to drive. Ralph had no memory of what happened next, except that he knew from later reports that their car left the road and struck a tree. Sara was thrown from the car and killed instantly. Ralph sustained a broken leg. Ralph's only memories of the accident were of looking up and seeing Sara's body, and of himself being carried on a stretcher to the ambulance. Ralph was kept overnight in the hospital and released the next day. While he was in the hospital, he was informed of Sara's death. Ralph attended Sara's funeral and recalled being shocked at the sight of her body in the casket.

Symptoms and impairment   After the accident, Ralph became depressed and started drinking daily. He had previously been considered a good worker, but his work attendance and performance became erratic, and he was fired from two jobs. He also withdrew from friends and did not date. This pattern continued for 2 years. Eight months prior to intake, Ralph was threatened with being fired again and decided to seek help. He underwent a brief hospital detoxification and began attending Alcoholics Anonymous (AA) meetings. He also resumed going to church. He stayed sober until shortly before the intake and maintained stable employment during that time. However, he continued to be socially isolated.

A few weeks before the initial session, Ralph learned that a cousin, Kate, to whom he had been close as a child, was in the hospital with AIDS complications. Ralph reacted by becoming depressed and resuming his drinking. He went on a 4-day "bender," missing several days of work. It was this event that prompted him to seek treatment.

Current symptoms   When asked how the accident affected him now, Ralph reported that he had nightmares about it and that he still thought about Sara "constantly." He did not want to date, because "It's not worth the trouble to get involved and have to go through hell like that again." He also reported that he was unable to go to hospitals to visit sick relatives or friends, and that he avoided funerals. He reported difficulty sleeping, was often irritable, and frequently got into conflicts at work. Ralph reported automatic *Automatic* thoughts such as the following: "If I get close to someone else, *thoughts* they'll die on me," "If I have to say goodbye to people, I will have a nervous breakdown," "Everything is a waste," and "Why is the world so cruel?" Ralph also felt responsible for Sara's death because he had asked her to drive that night.

Socialization The therapist told Ralph that his symptoms were common for *to treatment* someone who had been in an accident and had seen someone die. Ralph was given assessment forms to complete—the Patient's Trauma Trigger Record (Form 6.1), the PTSQ (Form 6.2), and the standard intake battery (see Form 6.3)—as well as information *Assessment and* handouts about PTSD (Form 6.4) and cognitive-behavioral ther-*homework* apy (Form B.1). He was assigned to write his goals for therapy as homework.

Session 3

Goals   Ralph brought in the following goals: (1) being able to go to hos-
Assessment results   pitals and funerals, and (2) staying sober. Ralph's assessment forms, combined with the clinical interview, indicated that he met *Comorbid* criteria for major depression and alcohol dependence in addition *conditions* to PTSD. He denied any thoughts of killing himself, but did say,

"I'll be glad when I'm dead." The therapist explained that treatment could not proceed if Ralph resumed drinking. He agreed to remain abstinent and to attend AA meetings. At Ralph's request, the therapist called his boss to confirm that Ralph was undergoing treatment, which was a condition of his return to work.

Coping with life problems

When asked about his family history, Ralph reported that his parents had separated when he was 8. His father had moved to another state and had since been largely uninvolved in Ralph's life. Ralph's mother had not remarried. She worked two jobs to support Ralph and his younger brother as they were growing up, and consequently she was often emotionally unavailable. Although Ralph was a poor student, he completed high school. He reported no prior history of trauma. He reported a history of heavy weekend drinking in high school, but denied having had any serious problems with alcohol prior to the accident.

Developmental history

The therapist and Ralph then further discussed the cognitive-behavioral model of PTSD and the nature of the treatment. Ralph agreed to proceed. He reported that just talking about the accident felt good, because he had never talked to anyone about it before. For homework, Ralph was asked to list any cues that triggered memories of the accident. He quickly replied, "Just hospitals, funerals, and driving." He was asked to notice anything else that triggered memories in the coming week and write it down, again using the Patient's Trauma Trigger Record (Form 6.1).

Further socialization to treatment

Homework

Sessions 4–6

The main tasks in the fourth through sixth sessions were anxiety management training and preparing Ralph for exposure. First, however, Ralph was asked what activities he found relaxing or pleasurable. He listed taking walks, working in his mother's garden, and calling old friends. He was assigned as homework to engage in these activities. When Ralph was asked what might keep him from reaching out to friends, he reported these automatic thoughts: "I am going to say something stupid," and "Everyone is too busy." These thoughts were used to teach Ralph rational responding.

Reward planning/ activity scheduling

Rational responding to automatic thoughts

Next Ralph was taught several anxiety management skills, including breathing relaxation, progressive muscle relaxation, thought stopping, and distraction. He was assigned to practice these between sessions.

Anxiety management training

In the sixth session, Ralph's guilt about the accident was discussed. Using Socratic dialogue, the therapist helped Ralph see

Cognitive restructuring

that the choice to have Sara drive was a rational one at the time. Because of his fatigue, it might not have been safe for him to drive. Sara had said she felt "OK" to drive. In fact, each of them had often driven while the other one slept. Finally, since the cause of the accident had never been determined, there was no way to know whether Ralph could have prevented it had he been driving.

By the end of the sixth session, Ralph reported feeling somewhat better. He found the progressive muscle relaxation particularly helpful, and his sleep had improved. He was more active and felt less depressed.

Planning exposure   Ralph had not been able to add any triggers to his original list of funerals, hospitals, and driving. Because he expressed anxiety about exposure, the therapist agreed to begin with something other than the actual memory of the accident. Ralph's cousin Kate was out of the hospital and reportedly doing better, so it was decided to start with an imaginary scenario in which he visited Kate in the hospital. The next meeting, which would be the first exposure session, was scheduled for 90 minutes.

Session 7

Imaginal exposure   After briefly explaining the exposure procedure, the therapist narrated an imaginary scenario for Ralph that included his arriving at the hospital, seeing other patients, seeing Kate, and then learning she had only a few weeks to live. Periodically throughout the scenario, Ralph was asked to describe what he was seeing, hearing, and feeling. All of this was tape-recorded.

During the initial exposure, Ralph's SUDs rating rose to 8. However, after he listened twice to the scenario played back on tape, his SUDs level dropped to 5. Ralph was pleased with this reduction in distress. He was assigned to listen to the tape daily as homework.

Homework

Sessions 8–11

Further imaginal exposure   In the eighth session, Ralph reported that he had listened to the exposure tape several times and that his SUDs ratings had continued to decrease. Another imaginal exposure scenario was done, this time of Ralph's attending a funeral. Ralph's SUDs rating peaked at 7 and decreased minimally after he listened to the tape one time. Although the session was only scheduled for 45 minutes, Ralph was offered the option of continuing in order to have time to habituate. He declined and said he would rather work on the tape at home.

Imaginal exposure to the accident

The ninth session was scheduled for 90 minutes, in order to do exposure to the memory of the accident and Sara's funeral. Ralph told the story in detail, with prompting by the therapist, and then listened to the tape several times. His maximum SUDs ratings declined from 8 to 4. At the end of the session, he commented:

Cognitive effects of exposure

> "It doesn't feel as depressing. I still love her and would like to have her back. But I don't feel angry or too much alone. . . . I feel kind of rested. Like I've been carrying a lot of weight alone and I just put it down."

Ralph then expressed some fears about letting go of Sara, including that if he got married to someone else he wouldn't get to see her in heaven. He finally concluded, "I would like to put her down for a while. I don't want to lose her either. I guess I already did."

Further exposure to the accident

The 10th session was again scheduled for 45 minutes. Ralph said that he had listened to the memory tape only twice. After he listened to the tape once more in the session, he reported that he had begun to recall some additional details about the accident. He continued to express ambivalence about letting go of Sara emotionally, but indicated that he was beginning to imagine what it would be like to date again. He was assigned to listen to the tape daily.

Coping with life problems

Homework

In the next session, Ralph reported that listening to the tape of the accident was "like a rerun now. Like I went to a movie and someone died. I feel sad, but not really upset." He reported a dream in which he met an attractive girl and started going out with her. He said he had been thinking more about dating someone else, and was starting to accept the idea. He also reported spending more time with friends. When the therapist commented that it sounded as though he was handling the pain of his loss, Ralph replied, "Everyone else does it. I know I can, too." Ralph also reported that Kate was back in the hospital. He was assigned as homework to go visit her.

Homework

Sessions 12–13

Coping with life problems

In the 12th session, Ralph reported that he had not been able to see Kate because her condition had worsened and she was no longer allowed to have visitors. He reported that he thought he would be able to handle going to her funeral. He commented, "I can't believe I wasted all this time and missed seeing her. Now I'll be in a hurry to do everything so I can catch up." He also reported that he met a woman while bicycling with friends. He had asked her out, but she already had a boyfriend.

Phasing out treatment

Ralph said that he was feeling much better and wanted to meet with the therapist less often. His negative automatic thoughts and other cognitive distortions associated with the accident had, in large part, spontaneously changed during exposure. Ralph was making progress in resuming his social life and had continued to be abstinent from alcohol. The therapist recommended meeting in 2 weeks.

Coping with life problems

In the next session, Ralph reported that Kate had died and that he had attended her funeral with no difficulty. He had been glad to see many family members there whom he had not seen in some time. He had also gone bicycling again with the woman he met several weeks earlier. In the session he talked about future plans, including traveling, buying a house, and eventually getting married. Since he was continuing to do well, Ralph and the therapist agreed to wait a month before meeting again.

Session 14

Phasing out treatment

In the final session, Ralph reported that he was feeling good and had no desire to drink. He had continued to attend AA meetings and church. He also said that he hardly ever thought about Sara. Although he was not yet dating anyone, he was socially active and meeting women he found attractive. He felt he had met his goals for therapy. The therapist had Ralph review which techniques he had found helpful and what he would do if he found himself under stress in the future. The therapist reminded Ralph that he could always contact him if he had further problems, and therapy was terminated.

DETAILED TREATMENT PLAN FOR POSTTRAUMATIC STRESS DISORDER

Treatment Reports

Tables 6.4 and 6.5 are designed to help you in writing managed care treatment reports for patients with PTSD. Table 6.4 shows sample specific symptoms; select the symptoms that are appropriate for your patient. (See Zuckerman's [1995] *Clinician's Thesaurus* for other suitable words and phrases.) Be sure also to specify the nature of the patient's impairments, including any dysfunction in academic, work, family, or social functioning. Table 6.5 lists sample goals and matching interventions. Again, select those that are appropriate for the patient.

TABLE 6.4. Sample Symptoms for Posttraumatic Stress Disorder

Specify traumatic event(s)
Intrusive memories
Nightmares
Flashbacks
Intense distress when exposed to memories or cues
Avoidance (specify what is avoided)
Inability to recall parts of the trauma
Withdrawal from usual activities (specify)
Detachment
Emotional numbness
Restricted affect
Inability to imagine the future
Insomnia
Irritability
Anger outbursts
Impaired concentration
Hypervigilance
Startle response

TABLE 6.5. Sample Treatment Goals and Interventions for Posttraumatic Stress Disorder

Treatment goals	Interventions
Reducing symptoms of hyperarousal	Anxiety management training
Reducing distress associated with memories to 2 or less on a scale of 0-10	Imaginal exposure
Eliminating avoidance of memories	*In vivo* exposure
Engaging in previously avoided activities (specify)	*In vivo* exposure
Eliminating anger outbursts	Anger management training
Increasing range of affect	Exposure to emotional cues
Increasing social contacts to three times a week	Activity scheduling, support groups
Eliminating feelings of guilt	Cognitive restructuring
Stating reduced belief (10%) in schemas of danger, lack of predictability/control (or other schemas—specify)	Cognitive restructuring, developmental analysis
Eliminating intrusive memories (and/or flashbacks/nightmares)	Imaginal exposure
Eliminating impairment (specify—depending on impairments, this may be several goals)	Cognitive restructuring, problem-solving training, or other skills training (specify)
Finding sources of meaning in life	Life review, activity scheduling/reward planning
Eliminating all anxiety symptoms (SCL-90-R and/or PTSQ scores in normal range)	All of the above
Acquiring relapse prevention skills	Reviewing and practicing techniques as necessary

Phasing Out Treatment

Four criteria should be met before a patient is considered ready to terminate treatment: (1) Symptoms have remitted sufficiently that the patient no longer meets criteria for PTSD; (2) the patient can discuss the trauma without feeling overwhelmed by emotion; (3) avoidance no longer interferes with the patient's daily functioning; and (4) significant cognitive distortions have been modified.

As with all disorders, we recommend emphasizing relapse prevention in the final phase of treatment for PTSD. The patient is asked to review the techniques he or she has found most helpful. The possibility that the patient may have a recurrence of symptoms when subject to life stress is discussed, and the patient is asked to envision which techniques he or she would use under those circumstances. In order to build patients' confidence in their ability to manage their symptoms, patients are encouraged to assign their own homework in later sessions, and the last several sessions are spaced 2 weeks to a month apart.

Session-by-Session Treatment Options

Table 6.6 shows the sequence of interventions for a 16-session course of treatment for PTSD. We have found this format to be useful in working with patients whose symptoms are responses to a single, discrete traumatic event. Patients who have suffered multiple traumas, who have serious impairment in life functioning, and/or who present with significant Axis II psychopathology may require more sessions, although the components of the treatment remain the same. This package can also be used as part of more complex treatment when PTSD is one, but not the only, presenting problem.

TABLE 6.6. Session-by-Session Treatment Options for Posttraumatic Stress Disorder

Sessions 1–2

Assessment

Ascertain presenting problems

Inquire about history of trauma, including possible multiple traumas

Inquire about triggers (Form 6.1) and about reexperiencing, avoidance, and hyperarousal symptoms (the PTSQ—Form 6.2)

Administer standard battery of intake measures (see Form 6.3), plus additional anxiety questionnaire as appropriate

Evaluate for comorbid conditions (e.g., major depression, other anxiety disorders)

Assess need for medication

Rule out contraindications for PTSD treatment (e.g., current substance abuse/dependence, current suicidal threat, unstable life circumstances)

Rule out malingering (use MMPI if necessary)

Assess premorbid functioning (including strengths, weaknesses, prior treatment, etc.)

Obtain developmental history

Assess social supports

Socialization to Treatment

Inform patient of diagnosis

Indicate that the symptoms are a common and understandable response to a traumatic event

Inform patient that short-term treatment is available with high probability of a significant reduction in distress

Provide patient with information handouts on PTSD (Form 6.4) and in cognitive-behavioral therapy in general (Form B.1, Appendix B)

Discuss option of medication

Explore and discuss any fears/reservations patient has regarding treatment

Homework

Have patient begin using Form 6.1 to monitor trauma triggers

Have patient begin listing avoided situations

Have patient write out goals for therapy

Session 3

Assessment

Evaluate homework

Evaluate anxiety (BAI and PTSQ) and depression (BDI)

Assess automatic thoughts, assumptions, and schemas related to the trauma

Socialization to Treatment

Continue discussing conceptualization of PTSD, treatment, and rationale

Discuss advantages/disadvantages of proceeding with treatment

Obtain patient's consent to proceed

Coping with Life Problems

Discuss any current life problems that might interfere with treatment

Intervene on patient's behalf if necessary

Homework

Have patient continue monitoring triggers, avoided situations

Sessions 4–6

Assessment

Evaluate homework

Evaluate anxiety (BAI and PTSQ) and depression (BDI)

Assess patient's current coping skills

Behavioral Interventions

Teach anxiety management techniques (breathing relaxation, progressive muscle relaxation, visualization, thought stopping, and distraction)

Have patient write out list of possible coping strategies (including patient's own preferred methods) to use when distressed

Cognitive Interventions

Teach patient to identify and write automatic thoughts

Teach patient rational responding

Homework

As in Session 3

Assign practice of at least one anxiety management technique daily

Have patient write automatic thoughts and rational responses

Session 7

Note: Be sure to allow a minimum of 90 minutes for this session

Assessment

Evaluate homework

Evaluate anxiety (BAI and PTSQ) and depression (BDI)

Behavioral Interventions

Create first imaginal exposure tape

Have patient listen to tape in session until habituation occurs

Homework

Have patient continue practicing anxiety management techniques

Have patient listen to exposure tape daily; this should continue until some habituation has occurred

Sessions 8–11

Assessment

As in Session 7

Note: Depending on how quickly patient habituates and the extent to which patient is able to do self-directed exposure homework, some of these sessions may need to be 90 minutes long

Behavioral Interventions

Review progress of anxiety management practice and deal with any problems encountered

Continue imaginal exposure to trauma memory until entire event is covered and patient can discuss it without significant anxiety

Expose patient in session to cues that trigger trauma memories

Plan self-directed *in vivo* exposure to avoided situations

(cont.)

TABLE 6.6 *(cont.)*

Cognitive Interventions
   Note cognitive distortions (at all three levels) revealed during exposure
   If cognitive distortions do not spontaneously change with continued exposure, use various techniques to challenge them (see Table B.3, Appendix B)

Homework
   Have patient continue practicing anxiety management techniques
   Have patient continue listening to exposure tape
   Have patient continue writing automatic thoughts and rational responses
   Assign self-directed *in vivo* exposure to avoided situations

Sessions 12–13
Assessment
   As in Session 7

Behavioral Interventions
   Encourage continued practice of anxiety management techniques
   Continue any exposure items not completed

Cognitive Interventions
   Identify any problematic cognitions remaining and challenge these

Coping with Life Problems
   Identify any remaining life problems and teach patient appropriate coping skills

Homework
   As in Sessions 8–11
   Have patient practice coping strategies for life problems

Sessions 14–16 (Scheduled Biweekly or Monthly)
Assessment
   As in Session 7

Behavioral Interventions
   Encourage continued practice of anxiety management techniques
   Continue exposure to any cues that remain problematic
   Review techniques patient has found useful
   Discuss possible sources of stress in future, predict possibility of temporary renewal of symptoms, and discuss ways of coping with them

Cognitive Interventions
   Address any remaining cognitive distortions
   Review techniques patient has found useful
   Discuss possible sources of stress in future, predict possibility of temporary renewal of symptoms, and discuss ways of coping with them

Coping with Life Problems
   Discuss ways of coping with any remaining life problems

Homework

Have patient self-assign homework

Encourage continued practice of anxiety management techniques

Encourage self-assigned exposure to avoided situations

Encourage continued practice of cognitive techniques

Encourage continued practice of life-problem-related skills

Have patient write list of favorite techniques to be used after termination

CHAPTER 7

Specific Phobia

DESCRIPTION AND DIAGNOSIS

Symptoms

DSM-IV (American Psychiatric Association, 1994) distinguishes several types of specific phobia—namely, "animal type," "natural environment type," "blood–injection–injury type," "situational type," and "other type." The distinguishing features of specific phobia are (1) that the person has intense fear when in or anticipating the presence of the stimulus; (2) that being exposed to the stimulus results in an anxiety reaction (which may become a full-fledged panic attack); and (3) that the person either avoids the stimulus or tolerates it with great discomfort. The individual is afraid of the stimulus itself, rather than concerned that others will see his or her anxiety (as in social phobia) or that the anxiety will lead to loss of control, insanity, or death (as in panic disorder).

Prevalence and Life Course

Phobias are common in the general population, with 60% of adults reporting some fears and 11.25% of the adult population qualifying for a diagnosis of specific phobia during their lifetime (Eaton et al., 1991). Some phobias are more likely to occur initially during childhood (e.g., fears of animals, being left alone, the dark, or ghosts) and may pass with increasing age. Females are more likely than males to exhibit specific phobia; they constitute from 55% to 90% of those with this diagnosis, depending on the content of the phobia. Types of phobia appear to run in families. If a phobia persists from childhood into adulthood, there is a very high probability that it will persist throughout life (Chapman, 1997).

Genetic/Biological Factors

Although many psychologists and their clients may believe that all fears are established through learning, surveys indicate that only a very small percentage of patients with specific phobia can trace the onset of their fears to specific frightening events reflecting either classical conditioning or imitation (Menzies & Clarke, 1994, 1995). As also discussed in connection with panic disorder and agoraphobia in Chapter 3, most fears—such as fears of snakes, insects, water, animals, lightning, blood/injury, and heights—have biological value in primitive environments. The excellent review provided by Marks (1987) illustrates that many phobias (e.g., fears of heights, open spaces, strangers, and other species) are manifested across a variety of species. The Darwinian explanation suggests that the cross-species manifestation of fear, its early onset (e.g., the visual cliff for infants, or the fear of crossing a transparent surface at a height), its universality across all human cultures, and the nonrandom nature of fears (i.e., the fact that certain stimuli are more likely to be feared than others) all suggest a strong evolutionary basis for fear. Furthermore, there is a reasonable heritability for most phobias, suggesting that genetic factors may be more important than direct experience. Genetic/biological models have a variety of expressions, including arguments for innate releasing mechanisms or innate patterns of behavior (Eibl-Eibesfeldt, 1972; Lorenz, 1966; Tinbergen, 1951); arguments favoring strong genetic predisposition (Marks, 1987); models proposing "preparedness" for classical conditioning to single trial learning (Seligman, 1971); and strict "learning theory" positions, such as Watson and Rayner's (1920) arguing for the primacy of experience. Although one can take a genetic/biological view of fear acquisition, this does not preclude the use of exposure as an intervention.

Coexisting Conditions

Although specific phobia is widespread, most individuals who present with such a phobia plus another anxiety disorder are usually treated for the other anxiety disorder rather than the specific phobia. Indeed, because of the overlapping criteria in evaluating specific phobia, the phobic patient may often be diagnosed as having agoraphobia, social phobia, or obsessive–compulsive disorder. In some cases, the phobia is so pronounced as to cause occupational problems (e.g., inability to travel or take elevators) and/or marital/couple distress.

Differential Diagnosis

Specific phobia must be distinguished from other disorders in which there is significant distress or avoidance related to anxiety. Panic disorder with agoraphobia is characterized by pervasive anxiety not specifically elicited by a single stimulus, as is found in specific phobia. The patient with panic disorder has many more panic attacks in a variety of situations, is apprehensive about having panic attacks, and fears that the panic attack may result in loss of control. In social phobia, the fear is less about the specific stimulus than about the risk of negative social evaluation. Posttraumatic stress disorder is elicited by life-threatening events, unlike specific phobia, and includes recurrent flashbacks and other symptoms not seen in specific phobia. With obsessive–compulsive disorder, the fear is of the content of the situation (e.g., contamination), not of the stimulus per se. (Figure 7.1 is a flow chart that provides further guidance in the differential diagnosis of specific phobia.)

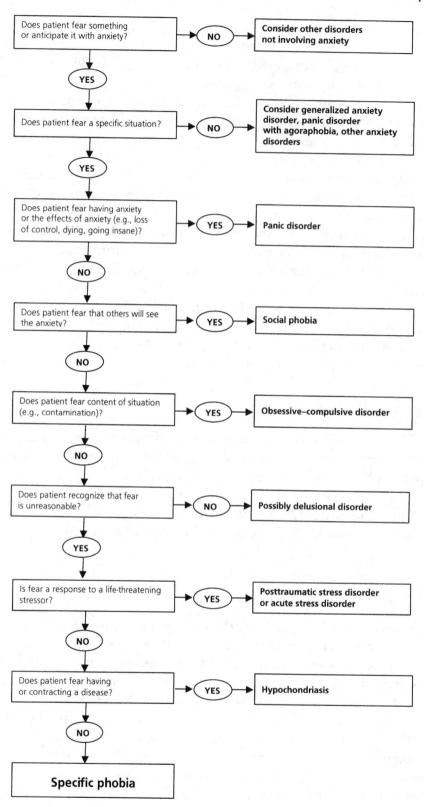

FIGURE 7.1. Diagnostic flow chart for specific phobia.

UNDERSTANDING SPECIFIC PHOBIA
IN COGNITIVE-BEHAVIORAL TERMS

In addition to discussing behavioral and cognitive factors per se in specific phobia, we also briefly mention ethological models and interpersonal factors and consequences in this section.

Behavioral Factors

The behavioral models of specific phobia describe two stages in the learning and maintenance of such a phobia. The first stage, *acquisition*, is based on contiguity or associationist learning—that is, classical conditioning. According to this model, the individual experiences a negative consequence in the presence of a previously neutral stimulus. Other learning models of acquisition of fear stress the effect of modeling and imitation (Bandura, 1969; Rachman, 1978). However, once the fear is established, it is maintained through the second stage—avoidance. Avoidance is presumed to reflect operant conditioning; that is, avoidance of or escape from the feared stimulus is negatively reinforced by the reduction of fear (Mowrer, 1947, 1960). This two-factor model accounts for the fact that a fear may be acquired (through classical conditioning) and maintained over a long period of time through the negative reinforcement of avoidance and escape, resulting in the "conservation of fear" (Mowrer, 1939, 1947).

According to an alternative model of fear maintenance, avoidance does not provide disconfirming information that would lead to the recognition that the initial pairing of the phobic stimulus and the negative consequence no longer holds (Arntz, Hildebrand, & van den Hout, 1994; Arntz, Rauner, & van den Hout, 1995). Treatment recommendations address the second phase—that is, maintenance of fear through avoidance and escape. The patient with specific phobia must experience prolonged exposure to the feared stimulus in order to learn that the stimulus is no longer dangerous.

Cognitive Factors

The cognitive model of phobia proposes that early developmental experiences may give rise to specific threat schemas that result in selective attention, evaluation, memories of, and strategies for dealing with feared stimuli. However, unlike more generalized "personal schemas" that refer to issues such as autonomy, abandonment, or demanding standards, these specific phobia threat schemas are centered on the content of the biological threat (e.g., water, heights). The cognitive model for phobia is less focused on automatic thoughts and assumptions and more focussed on information-processing biases. Since there is individual variation in the effects of biological disposition and traumatic experience in giving rise to phobias, the cognitive model attempts to explain these differences as a consequence of the *meanings* attached to the specific phobic stimulus and to the experience of anxiety (see Beck et al., 1985).

Ethological Factors

A third model of fear is based on ethological or evolutionary theory (see above). According to this model, individuals are innately predisposed to fear some stimuli rather than others, because these stimuli represent danger in a primitive environment. Thus surveys of fears in the general population indicate that the most common fears are fears of snakes, rats, insects, water, darkness, animals, strangers, heights, lightning, and close spaces—rather than fears of stimuli in the recent industrialized world, such as electricity. A variation of the ethological model has been proposed by Seligman (1971), who has suggested that individuals are *prepared* to acquire fears of certain stimuli more easily than fears of others, because of the adaptive value of these fears. This ethological/conditioning model helps account for both individual differences in fears and the nonrandom distribution of fears (i.e., the selectively higher frequency of certain fears).

Interpersonal Factors and Consequences

Many people in the nonclinical population will have at least one strong fear or diagnosable phobia. Perhaps because of its relative frequency, there is less of a stigma attached to specific phobia than to other disorders, such as social phobia or depression. In many cases, patients believe that their phobias are not entirely irrational and may defend them by referring to the protective nature of the fears. However, some fears (e.g., fears of airplanes) may have significant interpersonal consequences when they prevent partners from sharing in valued activities. A clinician working with a patient who has a specific phobia may need to counsel both partners to assure them that phobias are seldom voluntary "choices" made by one partner to "punish" the other, and that cajoling of the partner with the phobia only serves to exacerbate the fear.

Outcome Studies of Cognitive-Behavioral Treatments

Outcome studies are quite favorable for cognitive-behavioral treatments of specific phobia, with clinically significant improvement after rapid treatment for 74–94% of patients, depending on the class of specific phobia (Ost, 1997). Greater efficacy is obtained when behavioral treatment involves massed versus spaced exposure and *in vivo* versus imaginal exposure.

ASSESSMENT AND TREATMENT

Rationale and Plan for Treatment

The treatment of specific phobia directly links assessment to treatment. During the ongoing assessment, the clinician evaluates the content of specific fears, establishes a hierarchy of fears, evaluates the patient for safety behaviors, and determines the impact of the phobia on general functioning. Socialization stresses educating the patient about the "evolutionary adaptiveness" of phobias (in order to "depathologize" phobia for the patient) and instructing the patient on how avoidance maintains fears and how exposure is helpful in overcoming fear. Cognitive interventions stress the importance of selective exposure to information, filtering, memory biases, exaggeration of threat and probability, and the tendency to "forget" events that disconfirm danger.

The general plan of treatment for specific phobia is outlined in Table 7.1.

Assessment

Initial Clinical Evaluation of Fears and Phobias

During the intake, the therapist should inquire of all patients whether there are any situations or things that they avoid or tolerate only with anxiety and discomfort. Since many patients with specific phobia have arranged their lives around their phobia, they may not initiate a discussion of their phobia unless it presents new and difficult problems (e.g., threat to employment, marital/couple conflict). The phobia has thus become "normalized" for some people.

The Initial Fear Evaluation for Patients (Form 7.1) is a useful form for an initial evaluation of specific phobia, as well as of panic disorder with agoraphobia and social phobia. (Form 3.2 in Chapter 3, and Forms 5.1 and 5.2 in Chapter 5, can be used when more focused evaluation of the latter two disorders is desired.) The clinician should then continue the inquiry to determine the specific content area of the phobia—that is, whether the phobia is the animal type, natural environment type, blood–injection–injury type, situational type (e.g., fear of elevators, flying, closed spaces, etc.), or other type. In making the differential diagnosis, the clinician should determine whether the patient fears a specific situation (specific phobia), fears that others will see the anxiety (social phobia), or fears that an anxiety attack will lead to loss of control or threat to health (panic disorder).

TABLE 7.1. General Plan of Treatment for Specific Phobia

Assessment
> Initial clinical evaluation of fears and phobias
> Tests and other evaluations
> Consideration of medication

Socialization to treatment

Exposure
> Construction of a fear hierarchy
> Exposure (imaginal or *in vivo*) to hierarchy
> Eliminating safety behaviors

Relaxation training (if indicated)

Cognitive interventions

Establishing generalization

Phasing out treatment

FORM 7.1. Initial Fear Evaluation for Patients

Patient's Name: _____ Today's Date: _____

Therapist's Name: _____

Choose a number from the scale below to show how much you fear each of the situations listed below, and write that number next to each fear.

0	25	50	75	100
None	Somewhat	Moderate	Very	Extreme

1. Flying	11. Meeting strangers	21. Traveling in a bus, train, or subway
2. Elevators	12. Speaking in public	22. Walking alone
3. Heights	13. Using a public bathroom	23. Being alone at home
4. Insects	14. Eating in public	24. Dirt or soiled things
5. Snakes	15. People seeing I'm nervous	25. Lightning or thunder
6. Animals	16. Crowded stores	26. Darkness or night
7. Blood or injections	17. Malls	27. Standing in line waiting
8. Rats and mice	18. Restaurants, churches, movies	28. Exercise
9. Water	19. Closed spaces	29. Increasing my heart rate
10. Hospitals	20. Open spaces	30. People criticizing me

Tests and Other Evaluations

The evaluation of patients with specific phobia during the intake and at later points may also involve the standard intake battery of assessment instruments described in earlier chapters (the BAI, BDI, GAF, SCL-90-R, SCID-II, and Locke–Wallace; the SCL-90-R has a scale assessing phobias in general, but not the specific content of phobias). Other anxiety questionnaires mentioned in earlier chapters (the ADIS-R, the Fear Questionnaire, the Hamilton Anxiety Rating Scale, etc.) can also be administered as appropriate. Form 7.2 provides space for recording scores on these instruments. It also enables the therapist to record the patient's medication, alcohol, and other drug use; to record (at intake only) the history of any previous episodes of anxiety (the nature of these should be specified); to note (on later evaluations) in which a feared stimulus is still avoided and in which it can now be approached; and to note treatment recommendations.

Consideration of Medication

Medication should be avoided, if possible, since (1) there is no evidence of its efficacy in the treatment of phobia and (2) tranquilizing the patient may interfere with appropriate exposure to feared stimuli. However, if the patient has comorbid depression or another anxiety disorder, then appropriate medication for *those* disorders can be considered and prescribed.

Socialization to Treatment

During the socialization phase of therapy, we provide patients with an information handout on specific phobia (Form 7.3), as well as the handout on cognitive-behavioral therapy in general (Form B.1 in Appendix B). We also describe the behavioral, cognitive, and ethological models of fears and phobias. It is our experience that patients find the ethological/evolutionary model remarkably relieving, since it normalizes their fears as in fact *adaptive*, but in a different, prehistoric environment. Many patients immediately understand that their fears of heights, closed spaces, animals, and so on, may be reflective of fears that their ancestors had, which allowed them to survive in environments where these things were dangerous. We like to tell patients that their fears indicate that they have "the right response at the wrong time," and that the reason why their fears are so convincing to them is that these fears worked for thousands of years to protect human beings.

Next, we explain to patients that once the fear was learned, they also learned that their anxiety could be reduced if they avoided the things making them anxious. This is why fears persist when patients do not come into contact with the feared stimulus. It is like drinking two Scotches each time a person feels anxious: The person will immediately reduce his or her anxiety, but will also acquire an alcohol problem. Avoidance and escape persist because, like alcohol, they work immediately to reduce anxiety. We indicate that avoidance leads patients to believe that they cannot face the feared stimulus, and thus have begun to feel less effective in general. Treatment is aimed at helping patients learn

FORM 7.2. Further Evaluation of Specific Phobia: Test Scores, Substance Use, History, Treatment Progress, and Recommendations

Patient's Name: _____ Today's Date: _____

Therapist's Name: _____ Sessions Completed: _____

Test data/scores

Beck Depression Inventory (BDI) _____   Beck Anxiety Inventory (BAI) _____

Global Assessment of Functioning (GAF) _____   Locke–Wallace Marital Adjustment Test _____

Symptom Checklist 90–Revised (SCL-90-R) _____

Structured Clinical Interview for DSM-III-R, Axis II (SCID-II) _____

Anxiety Disorders Interview Schedule–Revised (ADIS-R) _____

Other anxiety questionnaires (specify) _____

Substance use

Current use of psychiatric medications (include dosage) _____

_____

Who prescribes? _____

Use of alcohol/other drugs (kind, frequency, amount, consequences) _____

_____

History (intake only)

Previous episodes of anxiety (specify nature):

    Onset   Duration   Precipitating events   Treatment

Treatment progress (later evaluations only)

Situations in which stimulus is still avoided: _____

_____

Situations in which stimulus is approached but was previously avoided: _____

_____

Recommendations

Medication evaluation or reevaluation:

Increased intensity of services:

Behavioral interventions:

Cognitive interventions:

Interpersonal interventions:

Marital/couple therapy:

Other:

FORM 7.3. Information for Patients about Specific Phobia

What Is Specific Phobia?

Specific phobia is a fear of a particular object, animal, or situation. The fear is great enough that you wish to avoid the situation or experience it only with considerable anxiety. Fears and phobias are very common. In a recent national survey, 60% of the people interviewed reported that they feared some situation or thing. The most common fears were fears of bugs, mice, snakes, bats, heights, water, public transportation, storms, closed spaces, tunnels, and bridges. Many people reported that they feared several things and that they consciously avoided them. In fact, over 11% of the people indicated that their fears qualified as specific phobias. That is, their fears were persistent and associated with intense anxiety; they avoided or wanted to avoid certain situations; they realized that their fears were excessive or unreasonable; and their fears resulted in distress and difficulty in their normal lives.

What Are the Causes of Specific Phobia?

There are several causes of specific phobia. Psychologists make a distinction between how you learned to fear something and why you still fear that thing even years later.

Some theories suggest that people tend to develop phobias about objects, animals, or situations that were dangerous in prehistoric times. For example, bugs, mice, snakes, many other animals, heights, strangers, bridges, and water were all potentially dangerous for early humans. In a wild environment, these fears were very adaptive and useful. People with these fears were better prepared to avoid contamination, poisonous bites, falling off cliffs or bridges, being murdered by strangers, or drowning. But in today's technological world, these fears are no longer as accurate as they once were.

A second origin of phobias is through learning—either connecting a bad experience with the thing you are afraid of (for example, perhaps you were bitten by a dog and developed a fear of dogs) or observing someone who is afraid and learning from their fear (for example, perhaps other family members had a fear of flying and you learned that fear from them). A third reason for phobias may be distortions in thinking. For example, a phobia may be based on incorrect information, on a tendency to predict the worst, on a tendency not to use evidence that challenges the phobia, or on a belief that you cannot tolerate anxiety.

Once you learn a fear or phobia, there are a number of ways in which it is maintained. The most important reason is that you avoid the situation you fear. If you fear flying, you feel less anxious every time that you decide to avoid getting onto a plane. Each time you avoid flying, you teach yourself that "the way to reduce my fear is to avoid"—that is, you learn to avoid. This is like taking a drink every time that you are anxious—you learn to drink more because it temporarily reduces your anxiety. But by avoiding the thing you fear, you never learn that you can overcome your fear. Another way you may maintain your fear is by engaging in "safety behaviors." These are things you do or say that you think will protect you. For example, in an elevator you may hold onto its side, or in an airplane you may hold onto your seat. Or you may repeat prayers or otherwise seek reassurance when you are in a feared situation. You can come to believe that these safety behaviors are necessary for you to overcome your fear.

(cont.)

How Can Cognitive-Behavioral Therapy Help?

Your fear and anxiety will begin to fade when you learn, from experience, that your phobia is unfounded. Cognitive-behavioral therapy for specific phobia is about helping you face what you fear rather than avoiding it. In order to overcome your fear, your therapist will have you make a list of the objects or situations that you fear, describe how intense your fear is, and indicate what your beliefs are about each object or situation (for example, do you think that you will be contaminated, die, be attacked, or go insane?). You will be taught how to relax when you are feeling tense. Your therapist may ask you to form images in your mind about a feared situation and hold these images in mind until you feel less anxious. You may observe your therapist doing the things that you fear, and later you may imitate him or her. Your exposure to the things that you fear will be gradual: Your therapist will explain everything before you do it; you are free to refuse to do anything; there will be no surprises sprung on you; and you will determine the pace at which you make progress. Most patients using these techniques find that they feel much less tense, become able to do things that they feared, and feel more effective in their lives. Many patients are able to improve rapidly with a few prolonged sessions (for example, 2- to 3-hour sessions) that allow intense exposure to the feared objects or situations. Depending on the fear, between 74% and 94% of patients improve when they use these techniques. Although some patients may use antidepressants or antianxiety medications for these fears, the treatments that we have described do not require these medications.

What Is Expected of You as a Patient?

Overcoming fears may require you to gradually put yourself into situations that make you anxious. You should let your therapist know which situations or things make you most anxious, what kinds of thoughts you have about those things, and whether you are willing to experience some anxiety in order to overcome your fears. Your therapist will help guide you through gradual exposure to these situations. You will have to carry out some self-help homework between therapy sessions, with which you will practice many of the same things that you are learning in the sessions with your therapist.

they can effectively deal with the things or situations they fear. The patient may be referred to Wilson's book *Don't Panic* for its general description of anxiety, fear, and the techniques that are useful in overcoming these problems.

Exposure

Behavioral interventions for specific phobia stress *exposure* to the feared stimulus. (See Appendix A and the CD-ROM accompanying this book for a full discussion of exposure.) Exposure may be imaginal or *in vivo*, graded or intense (flooding), massed or spaced, and therapist-directed or self-directed (see Craske & Rowe, 1997).

Construction of a Fear Hierarchy

Once a patient has been diagnosed with specific phobia and educated about its nature, he or she should be told about exposure as a form of treatment for this disorder. If the patient expresses willingness to proceed with exposure treatment, the therapist and patient construct a fear hierarchy for the phobia (or the most important phobia, if the patient has more than one). That is, various situations in which the patient might encounter the feared stimulus are described. The patient is then instructed to rank these in order from least to most feared, and to assign each situation a "subjective units of distress" or "SUDs" rating on a scale from 0 (no discomfort) to 10 (overwhelming anxiety or fear). The patient can use Form 7.4 to assist him or her in constructing the hierarchy. The clinician should also ask the patient whether the fear is greater when exits from the situation are blocked or when he or she is accompanied by someone. In addition, both imaginal and *in vivo* situations should be described; that is, the patient should be asked to give SUDs ratings for situations that he or she would only imagine versus situations that he or she would actually encounter (*in vivo*).

Exposure to the Fear Hierarchy

The therapist may employ imaginal rather than *in vivo* (real-life) exposure, with the images depicting increasing intensity of threat. However, the clinician should keep in mind that *in vivo* exposure is more effective than imaginal exposure. The *in vivo* exposure can occur either during the session (if this is practicable) or outside of the session. Wherever it occurs, it involves direct experience of the phobic stimulus. For example, for fear of spiders the patient may be asked initially to observe a spider, then to observe the spider on the therapist's hand, and then to allow a spider to crawl on his or her own hand.

During exposure to the feared stimulus, the patient can practice progressive muscle relaxation or breathing relaxation (see the discussion of relaxation training, below). Whether or not relaxation is incorporated into the exposure exercise, exposure continues until there is sufficient reduction of the SUDs rating. Then the therapist moves up the hierarchy to the next, more feared stimulus. Failure to continue the exposure long enough to allow habituation (i.e., decrease in fear level) may lead to an increased sensitization to the feared stimulus, making the fear worse in some cases. Consequently, it is essential

FORM 7.4. Patient's Fear Hierarchy for Specific Phobia

Patient's Name: _____ Today's Date: _____

Instructions: We are interested in the degree to which you fear a specific thing. For example, if you had a fear of flying, you might have a greater degree of fear if you were in an airplane during a storm, and a lot less fear if you were just sitting in your house and thinking about an airplane. We want you to decide what fear you want treatment for (for example, a fear of flying, elevators, heights, water, animals, blood, injection, snakes, etc.). Now we want you to imagine a number of different ways that you could come into contact with that feared situation or thing. Rank these in order from least to most frightening, and then write these in the boxes under "Situation." For example, if you had fear of flying, rank how frightening you would find these different situations: driving to the airport, getting onto the plane, engines starting up, planes taking off, flying, and landing. In the last column, note how afraid each situation would make you, from 0 (no fear) to 10 (maximum fear). Also, sometimes people feel more or less anxious if someone is accompanying them. You may also note this in constructing your list or "hierarchy" of feared situations—for example, are you more or less anxious if someone is with you on the plane?

Rank	Situation	Avoided? (Yes/No)	Fear Level (0–10)

that the therapist encourage staying with the feared stimulus long enough that the fear may diminish significantly. In the absence of enough habituation, the therapist may return to a less frightening stimulus in the hierarchy, engage in exposure, note habituation, and either return to the more frightening stimulus or end the session with the success of habituating to the less frightening stimulus. Failure to habituate may be due to the presence of "safety behaviors" (see below) that mask the exposure stimulus, too short a period of exposure, the need to identify a stimulus of intermediate fear potential, or dysfunctional thoughts that are associated with the particular stimulus.

One way of making sure that habituation occurs is to conduct "massed" exposure (i.e., exposure in a session lasting two or three times the length of a normal session). This "rapid treatment" of specific phobia often yields dramatic and immediate results, especially when the patient is encouraged to practice self-directed exposure outside of sessions (Ost, 1997). Another way is to conduct "flooding" (i.e., repeated imaginal or *in vivo* exposure to the stimulus in situations high on the patient's fear hierarchy). However, massed exposure is sometimes not practical within a clinical context, and flooding should only be undertaken with caution and after careful preparation of the patient. The more usual procedures in cases of specific phobia are to space exposure over several sessions with exposure practice between sessions, and to proceed in a graded manner up a patient's fear hierarchy as described above.

Homework assignments include continued, self-directed exposure to feared stimuli between sessions, in order to increase habituation and establish generalization of the effect. The patient can use Form 7.5 to record his or her exposure practice both within and between sessions. (Forms A.1 and A.2 in Appendix A can also be used for imaginal and *in vivo* exposure practice, respectively.) The patient is encouraged to schedule daily exposure to feared stimuli. Exposure to a specific stimulus is continued until the fear is reduced (this may vary—we recommend reducing fear to a SUDs level of 2.5 or to one-half of the initial SUDs level, whichever is less). Once the fear is reduced, the patient moves up to the next stimulus in the hierarchy and engages in exposure to that stimulus. Throughout the exposure experience, the patient should be directly praised by the therapist for tolerating the feared stimulus, and should also be encouraged to employ self-reward by praising himself or herself.

Eliminating Safety Behaviors

Many patients with specific phobia utilize "safety behaviors" (i.e., avoidant behaviors, which may often be covert) during the exposure to the stimulus. Since safety behaviors inhibit direct exposure (thereby interfering with habituation), they must be eliminated if possible. Examples of safety behaviors are holding onto a piece of furniture or a wall to prevent fainting, clenching muscles to establish readiness of response, scanning the environment for visual or auditory signs of danger, repeating prayers or self-reassurance statements, exhibiting anxious tics, holding one's breath, or trying to form images that distract one from the situation. In addition, some patients self-medicate with alcohol or anxiolytics, and then attribute their ability to tolerate the feared stimulus to the substance.

FORM 7.5. Patient's Self-Monitoring of Fears

Patient's Name: _____ Today's Date: _____

Instructions: To collect information about your fears for treatment, please record the information below for times when you were in a feared situation. In the first column, write the date and time. In the next, describe the feared situation. Use a scale of 1–10, where 10 represents the greatest fear you can imagine. In the fourth column, describe the actual outcome: Did you avoid the situation, engage in the behavior, seek safety, etc.? What sensations and thoughts did you have? What happened? For example: "I was able to take the elevator. I thought I was going to panic, but I got up and down safely." In the last column, indicate the actual level of fear you felt in the situation, again using a scale of 0–10 where 10 represents the greatest fear you can imagine.

Date/ Time	Situation Feared and My Prediction	Expected Fear Level (0–10)	Actual Outcome	Actual Fear Level (0–10)

For full exposure to occur, the patient should be encouraged to abandon any safety behaviors, since these responses may result either in misattribution of positive results to the safety behaviors or in distraction from the stimulus (which hinders habituation). We find it helpful to ask patients directly about their safety behaviors—for example, "When you are on the plane, do you check around? Ask questions? Clench the side of your seat? Drink alcohol? Repeat any prayers, actions, images, thoughts, or sayings?" We then explain to patients that many people believe that these safety behaviors protect them, and that as long as they engage in these behaviors they are not experiencing full exposure to the stimulus. The patients are then urged to examine any signs of safety behaviors, to examine the costs and benefits of these behaviors, to review the evidence for and against the idea that these behaviors actually provide safety, and to ask themselves why they believe these behaviors are necessary to provide protection (since most people do not engage in these behaviors). We may also ask our patients to engage in an experiment in which they temporarily relinquish these behaviors, to learn what will happen.

Relaxation Training

Relaxation can be helpful for patients who experience extreme anxiety during exposure, or simply as a general coping skill for patients with specific phobia. Patients for whom relaxation training appears appropriate can be taught progressive muscle relaxation, breathing relaxation, or both (see Appendix A and the CD-ROM for detailed instructions). This can then be paired with imaginal or *in vivo* exposure to reduce the patients' anxiety. (Alternatively, patients can be instructed not to pair relaxation with exposure, in order to give them the opportunity to learn that anxiety will decrease with increased length of exposure to the feared stimulus. See the discussion of desensitization in connection with generalized anxiety disorder in Chapter 4.)

Cognitive Interventions

Most patients with specific phobia have many distorted automatic thoughts about their fears. Typical automatic thoughts include: "I'll go crazy from the anxiety," "I'll have a heart attack," "I'll never get over this," "I must be a coward," "I can't do anything right," "People will see I'm anxious," and "No one else has this problem." These automatic thoughts should be elicited and categorized (as catastrophizing, labeling, fortune-telling, overgeneralizing, dichotomous thinking, etc.—see Form B.2 in Appendix B). The therapist should then evaluate and challenge the thoughts, using any of the cognitive techniques outlined in Table B.3 of Appendix B.

A patient's thoughts that anxiety will lead to a heart attack or insanity may be examined via cognitive disputation that involves a combination of techniques. For instance, the therapist can ask "Have you ever had a heart attack [or gone crazy] before from your anxiety? Why didn't you have a heart attack [go crazy]? Is there something different about this anxiety that will be so harmful? Have you ever heard of anyone who had a heart attack [gone crazy] from fear of elevators [flying, snakes, etc.]?"

The therapist can also help the patient examine the evidence for and against his or her automatic thoughts (e.g., the evidence that flying is or is not dangerous). The therapist may need to examine the quality of this evidence as well—for example, if the patient says something like "I heard of an airplane crashing," or "I don't know how elevators stay up." Some patients reason from their anxiety ("I'm anxious; therefore, there's something dangerous"). Or the double-standard technique can be used: Patients may be asked if they know anyone else who has a phobia (preferably one that they do not have). What advice would they give this friend? Or previous instances of acting in opposition to automatic thoughts can be elicited: Have patients ever overcome a fear of anything? What did they tell themselves about the feared situation before they engaged in self-exposure, and what did they learn after they engaged in exposure? In addition, direct education about feared stimuli can be provided. For example, the therapist can say, "The reason why you feel faint when you see a needle is that your blood pressure drops. In order to increase your blood pressure, you should tense and relax your muscles 50 times. This will serve as a pump for your blood flow, increasing your blood pressure. When your blood pressure goes up, you will feel less faint."

Establishing Generalization

Throughout treatment, we attempt to encourage generalization of the effects by having patients engage in self-directed homework assignments. For example, we encourage patients to "overpractice" exposure (e.g., taking elevators twice as much as would be reasonable); this is actually a form of massed exposure, as described earlier. Moreover, although therapist modeling and direction may be helpful during the initial phase of exposure, the therapist should soon begin fading himself or herself out of the exposure experience, lest the patient attribute the effects of exposure entirely to the therapist's encouragement. In cases where patients have multiple phobias, once they have made progress on one phobia, they may be encouraged to identify others for which they would like to self-assign exposure homework.

Another way to build generalization is eventually to decrease the patient's reliance on companions who help reduce the anxiety during exposure. In fact, this may even be part of the fear hierarchy, such that facing the feared stimulus with a companion is less frightening than facing the stimulus without someone. Phasing out companions is an essential part of building the self-efficacy necessary for continued exposure.

The therapist may also troubleshoot with the patient the temptation to avoid or escape from uncomfortable situations, and may use cognitive techniques to challenge this temptation. For example, the therapist (playing the role of the negative thought) might say, "Why don't you just avoid anything that makes you uncomfortable? You don't need to prove yourself now." The patient should be encouraged to view avoidance and escape as bad habits that are self-reinforcing. We like to tell patients with specific phobia that they are not making progress unless they often do things that make them uncomfortable.

Troubleshooting Problems in Therapy

Although the treatment of specific phobia may seem straightforward, there are problems that may arise, especially during exposure. The clinician needs to maintain both structure in pursuing exposure, and flexibility and warmth in helping the patient confront his or her fears. In this section, we review some common problems in treatment.

Fear That Treatment Will Make Things Worse

Many patients believe that exposure treatment will become an ordeal that will increase their anxiety to such an intolerable level that they will either go insane or have a heart attack. We indicate to patients that the outcome for exposure treatment is very favorable, and that they have already experienced the highest levels of anxiety in the past on their own. With the reassurance of the therapist, with the use of graduated exposure and modeling (see below), and with clear explanations beforehand, a patient is usually more willing to experiment with exposure.

Some patients believe that the therapist will startle them with a "surprise stimulus" that will be a horrifying experience for them. Such patients should be told that the therapist will explain everything that will happen in the sessions before anything is done and will obtain the patients' permission beforehand.

Self-Criticism

Some patients believe that their fears are a sign of weakness or cowardice and that they should not be afraid. In the socialization phase of treatment, as noted earlier, we explain to them that most fears people have conferred greater fitness in the natural environment of our early ancestors. Consequently, rather than viewing their fears as "weaknesses," patients can reframe them as advantages in a different environment. We explain to patients that avoidance is "nature's way" of assuring safety and that they have been "quick learners" in knowing what to do. Rather than labeling fear as a "deficiency," we reconstrue it as "more rapid learning of what was initially adaptive."

Difficulties in Establishing a Fear Hierarchy

Some patients have difficulty in defining a range of feared situations, often focusing on the extreme points at the end and beginning of the scale. A therapist can assist such a patient by using imagery induction; by suggesting to the patient intermediate points on the scale; by using comparatives ("somewhat frightening," "very frightening"); by identifying points on the scale through behavior ("How much longer could you stay in the situation?" or "How often have you been willing to do that?"); by modifying the stimuli to determine "conditions" of approach ("Would you be more or less willing to approach the situation if someone were with you?" or "Would you be more or less willing if you were closer to an exit?"); and by allowing the patient to modify the hierarchy later in treatment.

Unwillingness to Engage in Exposure

As indicated above, some patients fear that exposure will produce too much discomfort. In such a case, the therapist might inquire about the patient's definition of "too much anxiety": "Exactly what do you predict will happen?" The therapist needs to explain that exposure proves to the patient that the stimulus is not dangerous, whereas avoidance maintains the fear. The patient might be asked what the costs and benefits would be of experimenting with exposure or getting rid of the fear. The therapist can indicate that there is a difference between "what you want to do and what you are willing to do," and that "being willing to do what you do not want to do is the key to making progress in therapy." The therapist can also ask the patient, "Have you ever done anything that you were reluctant or frightened of doing? If so, what was the outcome of those experiences?"

Increased willingness to engage in exposure may be enhanced by the therapist's modeling the exposure, and thus providing the patient with evidence that the stimulus is not dangerous. For example, one patient believed that all cleaning fluids contained ammonia, were dangerous, and therefore had to be avoided; this resulted in his inability to clean his kitchen without elaborate precautions against contact with such fluids. The therapist indicated that there are small traces of ammonia in the air and that cleaning fluids are highly diluted. To demonstrate this, the therapist took a bottle of a popular window-cleaning product, sprayed some of it on his hands, and left it on his hands for the entire session. The patient was encouraged to imitate this behavior. The patient complied, leaving the solution on his hands for the entire session and for hours thereafter. Although his anxiety increased dramatically during the session, it eventually abated. This assisted him in being able to overcome a phobia that had persisted for several years.

Imaginal exposure is often less anxiety-provoking than *in vivo* exposure. Using imaginal exposure, or dropping down in the patient's hierarchy to the least frightening stimuli and gradually increasing exposure from there, may be helpful in demonstrating that the patient may be able to tolerate some anxiety and to habituate during exposure. During exposure, the therapist should try to elicit the negative thoughts the patient is having, such as "I can't stand it," "It's going to drive me crazy," or "This will kill me." These thoughts augment the anxiety and can be submitted to cognitive disputation.

Demands for Certainty

Some people with specific phobia are hesitant to pursue exposure because they demand that there will be no risk. Even though it is unheard of for a patient to have a heart attack or become psychotic during exposure, it is impossible for a therapist to provide an absolute guarantee. The therapist can ask the patient to examine the costs and benefits of demanding certainty, or to examine which of the patient's other behaviors in the last week involved the outcomes that could not be completely guaranteed. Then the therapist can examine how the patient was able to pursue such "risky" behaviors, and why he or she was able to make that choice. For example, since driving confers some risk of accident, how was the patient able to tolerate this degree of risk? The patient should be encouraged to frame his or her predictions in terms of probabilities rather than possibilities—for example, "I think there's a 10% chance that the elevator will crash," rather than the unchallengeable "I think it's possible the elevator will crash."

Unavailability of Exposure Items

Therapists in private practice may not have access to the stimuli that some patients fear (such as spiders, rats, or other animals), and many therapists do not find it convenient to accompany patients for *in vivo* exposure on airplanes or in other places. Obviously, this is less than ideal, since many of the outcome studies demonstrating efficacy for treatment are based on *in vivo* exposure. However, the therapist may often overcome these obstacles by using imaginal exposure, stress inoculation in sessions, modeling exposure for the patient, using imagery and coping statements, writing down coping statements that the patient may rehearse prior to and during exposure, and taping sessions in which the therapist and patient practice imaginal exposure and relaxation. Pairing imaginal exposure with relaxation and moving gradually up the hierarchy can be very effective in preparing the patient for *in vivo* exposure. The patient may listen to a tape of the therapy session while in the presence of the feared stimulus; this can serve as a form of therapist participation.

Noncompliance with Homework

There are many reasons why patients may not engage in exposure outside of sessions. The first thing to examine is whether the therapist has made it completely clear what the patient is expected to do. Rather than tell a patient with a fear of elevators, "Take elevators this week," the therapist should specify exactly what the assignment is: "Ride up three floors and down three floors on an elevator every day. Write out your predictions before you get on the elevator, noting your anxiety level from 0 to 10, and then write out the actual outcome after you get off the elevator, noting what happened and what your anxiety level is." The therapist might also ask the patient what the costs and benefits are of doing homework, what fears or beliefs the patient has about exposure, and when he or she will schedule the homework. It can be helpful to anticipate resistance to homework and to role-play this resistance, with the therapist taking the role of the resistance and the patient challenging the therapist's negative thoughts.

If the patient still does not comply with homework, the length of exposure to *in vivo* stimuli during sessions may be increased. This may help reduce the patient's subsequent anxiety outside of sessions. Fading of the therapist assistance may be accomplished by using flash cards with coping statements about fear, taping a session and playing the tape daily, and moving down the hierarchy to less frightening situations involving the stimuli.

Therapist Fears

Some therapists have fears of inducing anxiety in patients. These countertransference cognitions need to be examined before such therapists begin using exposure. Some typical cognitions of this type are "I shouldn't make my patients anxious," "The patient will drop out of therapy," "The patient won't like me," "The patient's anxiety will get out of control," "Maybe the stimulus really is dangerous," and "I can't stand to see people who are suffering." The cognitive-behavioral model of fear reduction needs to be stressed. Exposure can only work if the patient's fear schemas are activated (Foa & Kozak, 1991), so that habituation may occur and the patient may learn that the stimulus he or she feared is tolerable. Patients do not acquire a sense of self-efficacy by dealing with trivial and unemotional situations. Our experience is that therapists who are directive and encourage patients to face their fears are far more successful and retain their patients, whereas therapists who appear apprehensive about exposure only reinforce their patients' belief that there really is something to fear. Therapists do not induce anxiety through exposure in order to satisfy sadistic needs, but rather to help the patients become liberated from their fears. Imagine what would happen if Salk did not want to give needles to children who disliked the pain of the injections, or if surgeons did not wish to inflict pain in their work. Our experience is that patients may recall the discomfort of exposure, but do not complain about it after the fact of overcoming the fear.

Phasing Out Treatment

Therapy for specific phobia can be terminated when the patient has experienced a significant decrease in anxiety, when all the items on the patient's fear hierarchy have been completed, and when the patient no longer manifests avoidance behavior.

The frequency of treatment sessions can be tapered off as the patient takes increased responsibility for doing exposure as homework. In the case example that follows, the treatment was successfully terminated after six sessions.

CASE EXAMPLE

Sessions 1–2

Presenting problem   The patient, Gail, was a 34-year-old unmarried woman who had had fears of flying for 12 years and fears of elevators for at least 15 years. Her fear of elevators was so intense that even though she lived in one of the largest cities in the United States, she would not visit people living above the 12th floor, since she refused to use an elevator and had to walk up and down the stairs. The therapist's office was on the 10th floor, so she walked up the stairs the entire distance. Because she was offered a job in an office on the 38th floor, she believed that she needed either to get over her fear of elevators or to turn down the job. This fear was so intense and chronic that she was almost certain she would not be able to overcome it.

Assessment   During the initial assessment, Gail filled out the Initial Fear Evaluation for Patients (Form 7.1), and was also asked by the therapist about a number of situations that might provoke fear. This indicated that she had fears of not only elevators, but of flying, public speaking, authority, heights, snakes, rats, and fire.

However, she stated that at this time she was interested only in treatment for the fear of elevators. Gail was also administered the standard intake battery (see Form 7.2), but this indicated no diagnoses other than specific phobia. She was taking no psychiatric medications at present and denied use of other substances. The therapist gave her the information handouts on specific phobia (Form 7.3) and cognitive-behavioral therapy in general (Form B.1, Appendix B), and assured her that effective short-term treatment for her fears was available.

Socialization to treatment

Session 2

Further socialization to treatment

Psychoeducation

The therapist discussed the behavioral, cognitive, and ethological models of fears and phobias with Gail. Like many patients with specific phobia, Gail expressed particular interest in the ethological model, so the therapist described it in some detail. He also provided some direct psychoeducation about elevators: "Did you know that Otis, the man who invented the elevator brake, actually had them suspend an elevator in a building and cut the cables, and the Otis brake held the elevator in place? And did you know that elevators are the safest means of transportation?" (At a later date, to treat her fear of flying, the therapist asked, "Did you know that 65 million passengers flew out of O'Hare airport in Chicago without a single death in one year?" and "Did you know that commercial airplanes can fly upside down and that their wings bend?")

Assessing motivation to change

In order to examine Gail's motivation to change, the therapist then told Gail about exposure treatment and indicated that about 85% of people with fears of elevators get over these fears with such treatment. However, the exposure would necessarily make her anxious, so that she would learn that the things making her anxious are in fact safe. She was asked to indicate the costs and benefits of doing the exposure treatment; she indicated that the costs (increased anxiety) were outweighed by the benefits (getting over her fear, being able to take elevators to see her friends and pursue work, and feeling more like a normal person).

Constructing a fear hierarchy

The therapist next indicated to Gail that she would need to construct a hierarchy of her feared situations related to elevators. The therapist explained to her that she could also rate how anxious she felt if she just had to imagine getting on an elevator, rather than actually doing it. This yielded the following hierarchy of least to most feared situations:

SUDs	Feared situation
2	Sitting in therapist's office thinking of elevator at home
2.5	Imagining standing outside an elevator
3	Imagining being on an elevator
4	Standing outside elevator thinking of getting in
6	Getting into elevator with therapist with door open, knowing I can get out
7.5	Being in the elevator, with therapist, as door closes
8.5	Going down on the elevator
9	Going up on the elevator
9.5	Going up to a very high floor on the elevator
10	Being stuck in an elevator between high floors

Eliciting automatic thoughts

Psychoeducation

Challenging automatic thoughts

The therapist then asked, "Specifically, what do you think is going to happen when you get in an elevator?" Gail indicated that she feared that the elevator would get stuck and that she would suffocate from lack of air. Again, psychoeducation was useful: "Elevators are not hermetically sealed like tombs in the shaft. There are vents; the ceiling can be removed; there is a call box and an alarm." The therapist also challenged her thoughts by asking, "Have you ever heard of someone suffocating in an elevator? Why not?" and "If you did not suffocate in the elevator, what is the worst thing that you imagine happening?" Gail indicated that she feared (1) that no one would know that she was stuck, and (2) that the elevator would crash. The therapist and Gail examined the possibility that no one would know that an elevator was stuck in an office or apartment building in Manhattan—she indicated that this was extremely improbable. Next, we examined why the elevator would crash. She could not identify any reason. "Have you ever noticed that when they shut the power off in an elevator to work on the elevator it does not go crashing to the basement?"

Sessions 3–4

Eliciting more automatic thoughts

Developing coping responses

First, more of Gail's automatic thoughts were elicted. This time she said, "My anxiety will make me go crazy. I can't stand my anxiety." The therapist offered rational responses—coping responses: "You've been anxious before. Fear doesn't kill you. You don't go crazy from anxiety. Remember that elevators are safe. Remember that they are not sealed tombs. They don't crash. If you get stuck between floors, the elevator will start up again. There is an escape hatch in the ceiling of the elevator. There's a doorman downstairs, and there's an alarm button." The therapist

Role-playing negative thoughts

then indicated that Gail would need to learn how to challenge her negative thoughts on her own. Consequently, the therapist and Gail engaged in a reverse role play, with the therapist playing the negative thoughts and Gail playing the rational response. This helped Gail learn that she could adequately challenge her negative thoughts.

Training in progressive muscle relaxation

After this, the therapist trained Gail in progressive muscle relaxation. Then the therapist indicated to Gail that during the initial exposure experience, he would ask Gail to imagine some of the things that she was afraid of and then practice the progressive muscle relaxation (see Appendix A). Beginning with the image of standing outside the elevator, Gail imagined this situation and practiced relaxation until her SUDs rating decreased to 1.5. Gail then moved on to imagining being on the elevator, with her fear level rising to 4.5; with repeated exposure to this image, however, her fear level dropped to 1.5 again.

Imaginal exposure and relaxation

Sessions 3–4

Behavioral rehearsal and in vivo exposure

The therapist decided at the beginning of Session 5 to have Gail engage in direct exposure to the stimulus—that is, *in vivo* exposure. When she accompanied the therapist outside to the elevator on the 10th floor, her fear level was 9.5. Her automatic thoughts were "I can't stand it. I'm too anxious. I'll go crazy. It's dangerous." The therapist challenged these thoughts, reminding her of the role plays. Next the door opened and the therapist got inside, holding the "Open" button. Gail then got in, while the therapist got out, with the door still open. She got out and then back in. Her SUDs rating at this point was about 9. The therapist asked her whether she was ready to take a ride down to the first floor. She indicated that she was extremely anxious, but she knew she had to do it. The door closed, and she closed her eyes and held onto the side of the elevator. The therapist again asked Gail what her thoughts were. "It's going to crash. I can't stand it." The therapist reminded her again that elevators do not crash, that they have brake systems and extra cables, and that the anxiety she felt now would become less. As the elevator descended to the first floor, she became visibly less anxious.

Eliciting and challenging automatic thoughts

More in vivo exposure

The therapist and Gail walked outside of the building and stood on the sidewalk. Gail admitted that the experience was not as bad as she had thought it would be. The therapist asked her what she thought would happen going up the elevator again. She thought she'd be anxious, but less so because she had faced it once. They then got back onto the elevator. Her SUDs rating was

6.5. As the elevator went up she asked, "What's that sound?", referring to the "whooshing" sound in elevators. The therapist asked her whether she thought it was dangerous. She said, "It might be." When they arrived on the 10th floor, her SUDs rating was 4.5.

Gail and the therapist got off and stood in the hall outside the elevator. She indicated that she was feeling better for having faced it. The therapist asked her whether she'd be willing to try it a third time, to see whether the experience would become less frightening still. She indicated she would. Her SUDs rating was 5 as she got back into the elevator. Again she closed her eyes and held onto the side of the elevator. The therapist indicated that she would get more out of the experience if she gave up these safety behaviors. She did so, but her SUDs level rose to 7.5. The therapist and Gail got out again, got back on, and headed up to the 10th floor. This time her SUDs level dropped to 4.5. By the time they got off and went back to the therapist's office, her SUDs level was 3.

Eliminating safety behaviors

It was important that Gail learn that elevators were safe even if the therapist was not with her. Her homework assignment after Session 5 was to take the elevator by herself to the first floor after the session and to take the elevator to the seventh floor where she lived. The therapist urged Gail to note exactly what she was predicting and what the actual outcome was—for example, before the Session 5 exposure she was predicting that the elevator would get stuck or would crash, but the outcome was that the elevator arrived at its destination. She was urged to give herself rewards (both praise and tangible rewards) for any exposure that she did. With daily exposure homework, she decided to take the elevator to the 38th floor of her new office building. Much to her surprise and pleasure, she was able to do this without escape or avoidance. Her final "test" was to take the elevator to the top of the tallest building in the city—which she was able to accomplish 3 weeks after she began exposure.

Identifying and challenging negative thoughts

Self-reward

DETAILED TREATMENT PLAN FOR SPECIFIC PHOBIA

Treatment Reports

Tables 7.2 and 7.3 are designed to help you in writing managed care treatment reports for patients with specific phobia. Table 7.2 shows sample specific symptoms; select the symptoms that are appropriate for your patient. (As always, Zuckerman's [1995] *Clinician's Thesaurus* is another source of appropriate words and phrases.) Be sure also to specify the nature of the patient's impairments, including any dysfunction in academic,

TABLE 7.2. Sample Symptoms for Specific Phobia

Specify feared object or situation

Anxiety

Specify physical symptoms of anxiety:
    Palpitations
    Difficulty breathing
    Chest pain
    Nausea
    Dizziness
    Feeling faint
    Sweating
    Shaking
    Mind going blank
    Derealization
    Depersonalization

Numbness
Tingling
Chills
Hot flashes

Specify cognitive symptoms:
    Mind going blank
    Difficulty speaking
    Loss of concentration
    Derealization
    Depersonalization

Specify behavioral symptoms:
    Avoidance (specify)
    Panic attacks

work, family, or social functioning. Table 7.3 lists sample goals and matching interventions. Again, select those that are appropriate for the patient.

Session-by-Session Treatment Options

Table 7.4 shows the sequence of interventions for a six-session course of treatment for specific phobia. Patients with more severe symptoms may require longer treatment.

TABLE 7.3. Sample Treatment Goals and Interventions for Specific Phobia

Treatment goals	Interventions
Reducing physical symptoms of anxiety	Relaxation training
Stating reduced fear of phobic object/ situation	Cognitive restructuring
Reporting anxiety level of 0–1 on a scale of 0–10 when encountering phobic object	Exposure
Modifying schemas of danger and vulnerability (or other schemas—specify)	Cognitive restructuring, cost–benefit analysis
Eliminating all avoidance behavior	Exposure
Eliminating impairment (specify—depending on impairments, this may be several goals)	Cognitive restructuring, problem-solving training, or other skills training (specify)
Eliminating all anxiety symptoms (SCL-90-R scores in normal range)	All of the above
Acquiring relapse prevention skills	Reviewing and practicing techniques as necessary

TABLE 7.4. Session-By-Session Treatment Options for Specific Phobia

Session 1

Assessment

Elicit objects or situations feared, as well as degree of avoidance
Note onset of fear, level of fear, duration, episodic nature
Elicit beliefs about feared stimulus/response
Identify safety behaviors
Assess impairment in social, occupational, and educational functioning
Have patient complete Initial Fear Evaluation for Patients (Form 7.1)
Administer standard battery of intake measures (see Form 7.2), plus additional anxiety
    questionnaires as appropriate
Evaluate for comorbid conditions (e.g., major depression, other anxiety disorders)
Evaluate substance use; evaluate need for counseling or detoxification if patient has
    substance abuse or dependence
Assess need for medication

Socialization to Treatment

Indicate that fears and phobias are common and that brief treatment is available
Provide patient with information handouts on specific phobia (Form 7.3) and on cognitive-
    behavioral therapy in general (Form B.1, Appendix B)

Session 2

Assessment

Provide feedback on evaluation
Explain costs–benefits of eliminating fears

Socialization to Treatment

Explain to patient the evolutionary, behavioral, and cognitive models of fear acquisition and
    of fear maintenance through avoidance
Explain need for exposure treatment

Behavioral Interventions

Construct fear hierarchy (see Form 7.4) and train patient in use of SUDs
Train patient in relaxation during session

Cognitive Interventions

Begin identifying patient's distorted automatic thoughts

Homework

Have patient engage in and self-monitor relaxation

Sessions 3–4

Note: All sessions involving exposure may be double-length.

Assessment

Review homework

Behavioral Interventions

Elicit imagery of feared stimuli

Review fear hierarchy

Begin imaginal exposure in session

Begin *in vivo* exposure in session, if possible (or therapist may model exposure)

Identify safety behaviors during exposure

Encourage patient to eliminate safety behaviors

[Exposure may be concentrated in one session (massed exposure) or spaced over several sessions, with homework exposure in between sessions.]

Cognitive Interventions

Elicit patient's negative automatic thoughts during exposure

Begin to challenge patient's automatic thoughts

Homework

Have patient engage in and self-monitor *in vivo* exposure and relaxation experiences (provide Form 7.5 for self-monitoring exposure)

Have patient identify and challenge automatic thoughts

Sessions 5–6

Assessment

Review homework

Behavioral Interventions

Continue exposure (imaginal or *in vivo*) during session

Encourage "overpractice" of exposure

Encourage decreased reliance on companions

Discuss possible future problems and ways of coping with them

Cognitive Interventions

Practice stress inoculation during session (develop coping cards, model arguing against negative thoughts, model making coping/self-reinforcing statements, have patient imitate therapist's coping statements, plan stress inoculation as homework)

Examine patient's explanations for improvement (e.g., presence of therapist, exposure, disconfirmation of negative beliefs, safety behaviors, luck)

Encourage self-efficacy statements

Discuss possible future problems and ways of coping with them

Homework

Encourage patient to continue eliminating safety behaviors

Have patient plan further *in vivo* exposure and relaxation experiences, and encourage self-monitoring of these

Encourage continuing work on automatic thoughts

CHAPTER 8

Obsessive–Compulsive Disorder

DESCRIPTION AND DIAGNOSIS

Symptoms

Obsessive–compulsive disorder (abbreviated OCD in the text of this chapter) is a condition in which the patient has either "obsessions" (recurring thoughts, impulses, or images that cause anxiety or distress), "compulsions" (repetitive behaviors or mental acts that the patient feels driven to do in order to reduce distress or to avoid some feared event or situation), or both. Typical obsessions include fears of being contaminated by germs or poison, fears of causing harm to oneself or others, and fears of committing some unacceptable action. Often the obsessive thoughts are in direct contradiction to the patient's value system (e.g., a highly religious woman fears she will commit blasphemy; a loving father fears he will kill his child). Compulsions, which are also known as "rituals," can be either overt acts (such as repeatedly checking that a stove has been turned off) or mental acts (such as silently repeating a prayer). Typical compulsions include excessive washing and cleaning, checking, seeking reassurance, hoarding objects, and insisting that things be put in a specific order or pattern.

The majority of patients with OCD have both obsessions and compulsions. Some patients appear to suffer only from obsessions; however, careful inquiry will generally reveal that although these patients do not display overt rituals, they do perform covert mental acts intended to neutralize their obsessive thoughts. People with OCD have some recognition that their obsessions and compulsions are exaggerated and unrealistic. Nevertheless, they find themselves unable to stop thinking the obsessive thoughts and feel driven to perform the compulsive behaviors in order to control their anxiety and distress.

OCD can be a debilitating disorder. Some patients feel compelled to perform rituals for hours at a time; this often interferes with their ability to fulfill social roles, such as work or parenting. Many patients avoid situations that provoke obsessive thoughts, and some become homebound. Often patients involve other family members in their compulsive behaviors; for example, a mother may have her children engage in elaborate washing rituals before they are allowed to enter the house.

Prevalence and Life Course

OCD was once thought to be a rare disorder. However, community samples have found prevalence rates between 1.9% and 3.2% (Salkovskis & Kirk, 1997). The Epidemiologic Catchment Area study (Karno, Golding, Sorenson, & Burnam, 1988) found a lifetime prevalence for OCD of approximately 2.5% and a 6-month prevalence rate of 1.6%, making OCD the fourth most common psychiatric problem in the United States.

The typical ages of onset are the late teens or early 20s, although onset in childhood is sometimes seen. The course of the disorder is generally chronic, with waxing and waning of symptoms. Stress appears to exacerbate the condition. About 15% of cases show progressive deterioration (American Psychiatric Association, 1994).

Checking and cleaning are the most common rituals, being reported by 53% and 50% of OCD sufferers, respectively. Reported rates of other rituals are 36% for counting, 31% for needing to ask or confess, 28% for symmetry rituals, and 18% for hoarding; 19% of patients report obsessions only. Multiple rituals are reported by 48% of people with OCD, while 60% report multiple obsessions (Ball, Baer, & Otto, 1996).

Genetic/Biological Factors

Several different lines of research point to a role for biological factors in the development of OCD. Monozygotic twins have a higher concordance rate for OCD than dizygotic twins do (65% vs. 15%). First-degree relatives of patients with OCD are more likely to suffer from OCD than are the relatives of psychiatric controls; however, the occurrence of the disorder in first-degree relatives is under 25%. Often obsessive or compulsive features are present rather than the full-blown disorder. Overall, the evidence suggests that genetic factors play a small but significant role in the disorder (Steketee, 1993).

Patients with OCD have higher than average rates of birth abnormalities, history of head trauma, epilepsy, encephalitis, meningitis, and Sydenham's chorea, suggesting a possible role for early trauma. A higher frequency of neurological "soft signs" has also been reported (Steketee, 1993).

Abnormalities in brain functioning have been observed via positron emission tomography in patients with OCD. These patients have been found to have higher than normal glucose metabolic rates in the head of the caudate nucleus, and to have increased correlation in metabolic activity between elements of the orbital prefrontal cortex, caudate nucleus, and thalamus. The caudate nucleus is believed to be involved in procedural learning and implicit memory. Interestingly, patients who have been successfully treated for OCD, either with fluoxetine (Prozac) or with behavior therapy, show a decrease in activity in the caudate nucleus (Schwartz, Stoessel, Baxter, Martin, & Phelps, 1996).

Coexisting Conditions

Between 28% and 38% of patients diagnosed with OCD have been found to meet criteria for major depression. Anxiety disorders are also common, especially specific phobia and panic disorder (Steketee, 1993). Eating disorders are sometimes present. Between

5% and 7% of OCD patients meet criteria for Tourette's disorder. Alcohol abuse and other forms of substance abuse are often found (American Psychiatric Association, 1994).

The most common comorbid personality disorders are avoidant, dependent, and histrionic. Obsessive–compulsive personality disorder occurs in fewer than 25% of OCD patients (Steketee, 1993). Patients with comorbid personality disorders generally have poorer outcome and may require longer treatment (Jenike, 1995).

Major depression in the mild to moderate range does not appear to have a negative impact on the outcome of standard cognitive-behavioral treatment for OCD. In fact, depression often improves as OCD symptoms decrease. However, patients with severe depression may require medication and/or cognitive therapy before being able to participate in treatment. Comorbid substance abuse must be addressed before treatment for OCD can be initiated (Steketee, 1993).

Differential Diagnosis

The obsessive thinking that characterizes OCD must be distinguished from the ruminations that are typical in depression and from the worrying that marks generalized anxiety disorder. In depression the ruminations are mood-congruent and ego-syntonic, and in generalized anxiety disorder they are experienced as realistic concerns about actual life events. In contrast, the obsessions in OCD are ego-dystonic and therefore resisted. They are also generally recognized as being unrealistic.

If the obsessive thoughts focus only on a subject that is related to another mental disorder, that diagnosis should be given instead of OCD (e.g., body dysmorphic disorder, specific phobia, or hypochondriasis). If additional obsessions or compulsions are present, OCD may also be diagnosed.

If the obsessive thoughts are not recognized as exaggerated or unrealistic, and if they take on a bizarre quality, a diagnosis of delusional disorder should be considered. Stereotyped behaviors that are ego-syntonic and are not recognized as unrealistic may be manifestations of schizophrenia rather than OCD (American Psychiatric Association, 1994).

A diagnostic flow chart for OCD (Figure 8.1) illustrates the differential diagnosis of this disorder.

UNDERSTANDING OBSESSIVE–COMPULSIVE DISORDER IN COGNITIVE-BEHAVIORAL TERMS

Behavioral Factors

The Behavioral Model

The behavioral conceptualization of OCD emphasizes the role of conditioning in the development and maintenance of the disorder (Salkovskis & Kirk, 1989). Suppose a person has intrusive thoughts that for some reason cause feelings of distress, such as anxiety, guilt, shame, or disgust. Over time, the feelings of distress can become linked with the

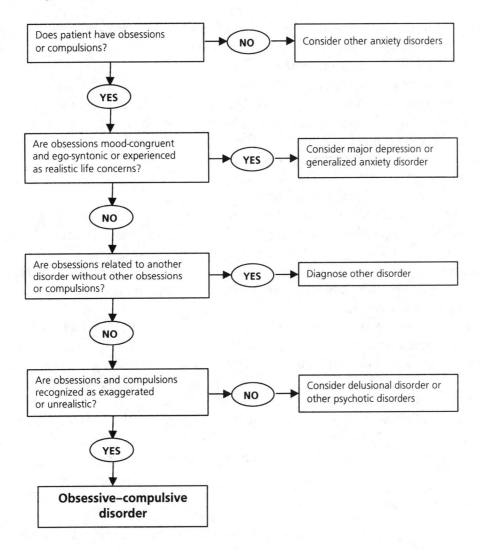

FIGURE 8.1. Diagnostic flow chart for obsessive–compulsive disorder.

thoughts (through classical conditioning), so that having the thoughts automatically triggers distress. In essence, the person becomes afraid of his or her own thoughts.

The problem with being afraid of a thought (as opposed to an object or animal) is that thoughts are rather difficult to avoid. One approach commonly attempted by OCD sufferers is to try not to think the troubling thoughts. However, the more one tries *not* to think about something, the more one winds up thinking about it (Wegner, 1989). This can easily be demonstrated to patients by asking them to try *not* thinking about a pink elephant. Of course, a pink elephant is the first thing that comes to mind. The result, therefore, of trying to avoid thinking obsessive thoughts is that patients wind up thinking them more, thereby exacerbating their distress.

Unable to control their anxiety by avoiding their thoughts, OCD sufferers typically turn to other strategies. For example, if they are afraid of contamination, they may wash their hands. If they are afraid of a blasphemous thought, they may say a prayer. Such actions generally make the patients feel better for the moment. This temporary reduction in distress is rewarding to the patients, which makes it more likely that the actions will be repeated. (In operant conditioning terms, the actions are negatively reinforced.) The problem is that the reduction of distress is short-lived: When the obsessive thoughts occur again, the actions must be done again. Before long, the actions have become rituals. Although OCD sufferers are generally distressed by their rituals, which can become time-consuming and often seem senseless, they feel compelled to continue to perform them because of the temporary relief they provide.

Another way OCD sufferers attempt to reduce their distress is by avoiding situations that are likely to trigger obsessive thoughts. For example, a woman who fears being contaminated by pesticides may avoid all stores where she thinks pesticides might be sold. As with rituals, this avoidance is reinforced because it provides temporary relief. Many OCD suffers go to great lengths to avoid anxiety-provoking situations, and this often results in significant restriction of their lives.

In essence, OCD may be seen as a phobia of certain thoughts, which, like all phobias, is maintained by avoidance. The association between the obsessive thoughts and emotional distress can be extinguished if patients allow themselves to experience the thoughts without attempting to avoid them or neutralize them with rituals. However, patients are generally afraid to do this because they fear that (1) their feelings of distress will continue unabated; (2) the distress will be unbearable; and/or (3) thinking the thoughts will cause them to perform some unacceptable action. The result is that they continue the endless cycle of obsessive thoughts and compulsive rituals.

Behavioral Treatments

For many years OCD was considered to be resistant to treatment. In 1966, Meyer reported successfully treating OCD patients with a procedure he called "exposure and response prevention." The treatment consisted of repeatedly exposing patients to their obsessive thoughts while preventing them from carrying out their rituals. In the years since Meyer's paper was published, the combination of exposure and response prevention has been extensively studied; it is currently regarded as the "gold standard" in treatment for OCD.

The goal of exposure and response prevention is to break the cycle of conditioning that maintains the disorder. Just as a person with a specific phobia of dogs needs to be exposed repeatedly to dogs without experiencing any negative consequences in order to reduce the association between dogs and fear, so a person with OCD must be exposed to his or her obsessive thoughts. If exposure is done long enough and frequently enough, the patient's anxiety will decrease, and the patient will come to realize that he or she can tolerate the obsessive thoughts without avoidance. For exposure to be effective, however, patients must be prevented from performing rituals. Otherwise, they will use the rituals to manage their anxiety during exposure. Neither exposure alone nor response prevention alone has been found to be as effective as the two together (Foa & Kozak, 1997).

Cognitive Factors

Until recently, more attention has been paid to behavioral factors than to cognitive factors in the formulation and treatment of OCD. This is due to the fact that the efficacy of behavioral interventions for OCD has been well established. However, in the past decade there has been increasing interest in the role of cognition in the disorder. On a theoretical level, cognitive factors may help explain why some people are more prone than others to react to intrusive thoughts with distress. On a practical level, it has been proposed that integrating cognitive techniques into the treatment of OCD may help decrease dropout, improve compliance, increase the efficacy of standard behavioral treatment, and help those patients who do not respond to behavioral interventions (Salkovskis, 1989).

Cognitive Models

Salkovskis (Salkovskis, 1989; Salkovskis & Kirk, 1997) and van Oppen and Arntz (1994) have proposed similar cognitive models of OCD. Both models regard intrusive thoughts as normal phenomena. In fact, 90% of nonclinical subjects report intrusive thoughts similar to those experienced in OCD (Salkovskis & Kirk, 1997). What distinguishes patients with OCD, according to these models, is their evaluation of the thoughts. OCD patients overestimate (1) the likelihood of the occurrence of negative events; (2) the damage that would result if the events occurred; (3) the degree of responsibility that they would bear for the events; and (4) the consequences of being held responsible. In other words, OCD sufferers have overactive schemas of danger and responsibility. These schemas, and the assumptions that accompany them, lead to automatic thoughts that trigger anxiety and obsessive behaviors. Salkovskis and Kirk (1997) place particular emphasis on responsibility, pointing out that schemas of danger, in the absence of perceived responsibility, will lead to other forms of anxiety but not to OCD. Patients with OCD have been found to have higher scores on two measures of perceived responsibility than either normal controls or patients with anxiety disorders other than OCD (Salkovskis & Kirk, 1997). Table 8.1 lists automatic thoughts, assumptions, and schemas that are typical for patients with OCD.

Foa and Kozak (1991) cite several processing errors OCD sufferers make in their inferences about harm: (1) They tend to assume that in the absence of evidence for safety, events are dangerous; (2) they often have insufficient knowledge of the laws of probability; (3) they tend to make an "availability" error, judging events as dangerous on the basis of immediately available but limited information (e.g., sensational news stories) rather than complete information; (4) they exaggerate the risk of minute amounts of potentially dangerous substances; (5) they ignore the source of information about risk in evaluating its accuracy; and (6) they focus exclusively on reducing the risk of harm and ignore the more likely losses associated with their avoidance and ritualistic behavior. Similarly, Guidano and Liotti (1983) emphasize OCD sufferers' cognitive need for perfect certainty. Since it is almost impossible to rule out all risk or doubt, they are unable to decide that an event or situation is safe. The processing errors described by these authors may be seen as maintaining the schemas of danger and responsibility.

TABLE 8.1. Examples of Three Types of Cognitive Distortions in Obsessive–Compulsive Disorder

<u>Distorted automatic thoughts</u>

Danger

"There are germs everywhere."

"This object is dirty."

"I've been contaminated."

"I just know I have cancer."

"You can't trust doctors. What if he's wrong? Something terrible could happen."

"I can't stand my anxiety."

"I have to clean this right now or I'll go crazy."

"What if I need this sometime in the future and I don't have it?"

"Something terrible could happen to someone I love."

"I could do or say something unacceptable without realizing it."

Responsibility

"If I don't wash my hands I could spread germs to my whole family."

"What if I forgot to lock the door?"

"I have to be sure."

"I'd better check."

"I'll feel better if I do this."

"Better safe than sorry."

"I can't let myself think that or I'll lose control."

"I'm a terrible person for having such thoughts."

"If anything bad happens it's my fault."

"That horrible thought will come true unless I do something to stop it right now."

"This has to be perfect."

<u>Maladaptive assumptions</u>

Danger

"All risk must be avoided."

"You must be absolutely sure things are safe, otherwise you are in danger."

"Anxiety is bad and must be avoided."

"Thoughts are powerful and can cause bad things to happen."

"Safety is the more important than anything else."

Responsibility

"I should be able to control my thoughts."

"If I can't control my thoughts, I won't be able to control my actions."

"If anything bad happens, it's my fault."

"I am to blame if I don't take all possible precautions."

"Things must be perfect to be good enough."

"I must work very hard to keep myself under control or I could do something terrible."

<u>Dysfunctional schemas</u>

Danger

"The world is full of dangers (germs, contaminants, accidents, etc.)."

"The probability of something bad happening is high."

"I'm a bad person with thoughts and impulses that are dangerous."

Responsibility

"Other people cannot be relied on for safety."

"I am the only one I can truly count on."

"I am responsible for keeping myself and others safe."

"I'm inherently irresponsible unless I try very hard."

Cognitive Treatments

Two forms of cognitive therapy have been tested in the treatment of OCD: rational–emotive therapy (Ellis, 1962) and Beck-style cognitive therapy based on the work of Salkovskis (1989). Cognitive therapy targets patients' beliefs about their intrusive thoughts rather than the thoughts themselves. Various techniques are aimed at modifying patients' schemas related to responsibility and danger. Patients are encouraged to take an alternative view of their thoughts, so that rather than seeing them as inherently dangerous, they conclude that—however distressing they may be—the thoughts are irrelevant to further action. As a result, they come to see that efforts to control them are unnecessary and counterproductive (Salkovskis & Kirk, 1997).

Outcome Studies for Behavioral and Cognitive Treatments

Foa and Kozak (1997) reviewed 13 controlled studies of exposure and response prevention, and found that an average of 83% of patients showed moderate to marked improvement (generally defined as a 30% or greater reduction in symptoms). Even patients who were much improved usually had some residual symptoms. When followed up at periods averaging over 2 years after termination, an average of 76% of patients continued to be improved (Foa & Kozak, 1997). However, Salkovskis and Kirk (1997) point out that treatment refusal and dropout are common in behavior therapy for OCD. When these factors are taken into account, the average rate of positive outcome drops to about 50%.

Three studies have compared cognitive therapy to exposure and response prevention. All three found slight superiority for cognitive therapy (Abramowitz, 1997).

The average length of treatment in the review by Foa and Kozak (1997) was 15 sessions, with a typical session lasting 2 hours. Abramowitz (1997) found a large and significant correlation ($r = .87$) between the amount of therapist-assisted exposure and outcome.

Patients who are much improved at termination have been found to have lower relapse rates than patients who have significant residual symptoms. Long rather than brief exposure sessions improve outcome. The addition of imaginal exposure to *in vivo* exposure improves long-term but not short-term outcome (Foa & Kozak, 1997).

Hiss, Foa, and Kozak (1994) examined the effectiveness of a relapse prevention program following 15 sessions of exposure and response prevention. The program consisted of four additional 90-minute sessions and nine 15-minute follow-up phone contacts. The training included instruction in cognitive restructuring, self-exposure, and changes in lifestyle. The treatment was compared to an attention control procedure. At follow-up, 50% of the attention control patients had relapsed, compared to 14% of the relapse prevention group.

ASSESSMENT AND TREATMENT

Rationale and Plan for Treatment

The treatment package described in this chapter emphasizes exposure and response prevention. Cognitive restructuring is included to help build motivation, improve compliance, and reinforce the lessons learned during exposure. Relaxation training is also included

Exposure targets patients' obsessive thoughts and the distress they trigger. Exposure weakens the link between the thoughts and the distress, so that patients are able to tolerate their thoughts without feeling so upset. When patients allow themselves to think their feared thoughts rather than attempting to push them away, the occurrence of the thoughts decreases. Response prevention directly targets patients' compulsions. As patients discover that the anxiety associated with their obsessive thoughts can be decreased without the use of compulsive behaviors, they are often able to give up those behaviors.

Cognitive restructuring targets the distress associated with the obsessions and compulsions. By modifying patients' assumptions and schemas of danger and responsibility, cognitive restructuring helps patients see that their obsessive thoughts do not pose a threat and need not lead to action. Cognitive techniques also help patients develop and maintain motivation for treatment and cope with life stresses that might otherwise exacerbate their OCD symptoms. Relaxation training gives patients an alternative means to deal with anxiety and can be a useful coping strategy for dealing with life stress.

The package provides 20 sessions of treatment, including assessment. Most of the sessions are 45 minutes, except for the first exposure sessions, which are 90 minutes.

This provides somewhat fewer hours of therapist contact than the average of the studies reviewed by Foa and Kozak (1997). However, for patients with mild to moderate symptoms, 20 sessions will often be sufficient. Patients with more severe symptoms are likely to require longer treatment.

The treatment package for OCD is outlined in Table 8.2.

Assessment

The goals of assessment include making the differential diagnosis; evaluating comorbid conditions that require prior or additional treatment; exploring motivation for treatment; establishing a baseline level of distress and impairment that can be used in assessing progress; and identifying the specific obsessions, rituals, and avoided situations that will become the targets of treatment.

Initial Clinical Evaluation of Obsessions and Compulsions

The primary means of assessment is the clinical interview. The details of patients' obsessive thoughts, the rituals they perform, and the situations they avoid should be obtained. The ways in which patients' symptoms interfere with daily functioning should be explored, as well as the history and development of the symptoms.

Patients are often reluctant to reveal their obsessions. Because the thoughts are so distressing to them, they may assume that others will react with disgust or condemnation. They may even fear that if they reveal their thoughts, they will be hospitalized against their will or have their children taken away from them. Normalizing the obsessive thoughts will often help patients talk more freely. Among the techniques that can be useful are (1) informing patients that, according to research, most people have thoughts

---

TABLE 8.2. General Plan of Treatment for Obsessive–Compulsive Disorder

Assessment
    Initial clinical evaluation of obsessions and compulsions
    Tests and other evaluations
    Consideration of medication

Socialization to treatment

Building motivation

Relaxation training

Exposure

Response prevention

Cognitive restructuring

Relapse prevention

Phasing out treatment

at times that they find very upsetting; (2) reassuring patients that nothing bad can happen as a result of discussing their thoughts; (3) giving examples of thoughts that others have reported, and asking patients whether they have any similar thoughts; and (4) pointing out to patients that most people are distressed by thoughts that run contrary to their values, and that the fact that they find their thoughts so upsetting means they are *less* likely, not *more* likely, to act on them.

It is also important to assess whether patients recognize that their obsessive thoughts are to some extent unrealistic. It is often helpful to ask patients how strongly they believe their fears will come true when they are not actually in the situations that provoke their fears—for example, "When you are not in a public restroom, how likely do you think it is that you will get AIDS from touching the faucet handle?" Alternatively, patients may be asked how likely they think it is that their feared consequences would happen to someone else.

If patients cannot, on inquiry, express some recognition that their fears are exaggerated, this indicates the presence of "overvalued ideas." Patients with overvalued ideas generally do not respond well to exposure and response prevention. In such cases, it is advisable to attempt to reduce beliefs in the obsessive fears via cognitive techniques before proceeding (Steketee, 1993).

Another important source of information is self-monitoring by the patient. As homework after the initial assessment, patients are asked to monitor their obsessive thoughts, rituals, and avoided situations on a daily basis. Self-monitoring provides detailed information that may not emerge during the initial assessment and can serve as a baseline measure to assess progress. Self-monitoring is also a preliminary intervention that often leads to some reduction in symptoms. Form 8.1 is a form for self-monitoring obsessions and rituals.

Tests and Other Evaluations

In addition to the clinical interview, self-report measures may be helpful in the assessment of patients with OCD. The Obsessive–Compulsive Questionnaire (OCQ) is a symptom checklist we have developed for assessing our patients. Patients' responses to individual items can help in making a diagnosis, and when the scale is readministered later, they can be used to evaluate therapeutic progress. The OCQ is shown in Form 8.2.

The SCL-90-R (which is part of the standard intake battery described in previous chapters) has an Obsessive–Compulsive subscale, although it has been found not to discriminate between OCD and general distress. Other measures from the standard battery (the BAI, BDI, GAF, SCID-II, and Locke–Wallace), as well as other anxiety questionnaires (the ADIS-R, etc.), may be used as appropriate. Form 8.3 provides space for recording scores on the standard intake battery and additional anxiety questionnaires. It also enables a therapist to record a patient's medication, alcohol, and other drug use; to record (at intake only) the nature of any previous episodes of anxiety (the nature of these should be specified); to note (on later evaluations) which obsessions and compulsions the patient is still engaging in and which have been overcome; and to indicate treatment recommendations.

FORM 8.1. Patient's Obsession/Ritual Log

Patient's Name: _____   Week: _____

Instructions: During the next week, please write down any obsessions you have and any rituals you do. If you have an obsession without doing a ritual, leave the "Ritual" column blank. For rituals without obsessions, leave the "Obsession" column blank. Be sure to note how much time you spent in the ritual (or how long the obsession lasted) and how much distress you felt, from 0 (no distress) to 10 (maximum distress).

Date	Time	Obsession	Ritual	Time Spent	Distress (0–10)

FORM 8.2. Obsessive–Compulsive Questionnaire (OCQ) for Patients

Patient's Name: _____ Today's Date: _____

Obsessions

Listed below are some common fears people have. Please check how much you have been bothered by each one in the past week. If you have additional fears that are not listed, please write them in and rate how much they bother you.

Fear	None (0)	A little (1)	Moder-ately (2)	A lot (3)
Fear of germs	____	____	____	____
Fear of getting or having a disease	____	____	____	____
Fear of contact with poisonous or dangerous substances	____	____	____	____
Fear of dirt	____	____	____	____
Fear of making a mistake or doing something wrong	____	____	____	____
Fear of forgetting to do something (e.g., lock a door, turn off a stove)	____	____	____	____
Fear of hurting or killing someone (in the past or future)	____	____	____	____
Fear of someone being injured or dying	____	____	____	____
Fear of being killed or injured	____	____	____	____
Fear of doing or saying something bad, immoral, or embarrassing	____	____	____	____
Fear of not having something available or on hand when you need it	____	____	____	____
Fear of having things out of order	____	____	____	____
Fear of things not being perfect	____	____	____	____
Other obsessions: _____	____	____	____	____
_____	____	____	____	____
_____	____	____	____	____

(cont.)

Compulsions

Listed below are typical compulsions or rituals. An action is considered a compulsion if you do it more often than it is commonly done by others or if it is done to make you feel less anxious. Please check how much time or effort you have spent on each compulsion in the past week. If you have additional compulsions, please add them.

Compulsions	None (0)	A little (1)	Moder-ately (2)	A lot (3)
Washing hands, showering, or other personal cleansing	____	____	____	____
Cleaning (objects, surfaces, rooms, etc.)	____	____	____	____
Checking to make sure you did (or didn't do) something	____	____	____	____
Checking to make sure things are right or perfect	____	____	____	____
Repeating actions	____	____	____	____
Hoarding or collecting things	____	____	____	____
Putting or keeping things in a certain order	____	____	____	____
Saying things to yourself repeatedly (such as prayers, lists, or other phrases)	____	____	____	____
Asking for reassurance from others	____	____	____	____
Other compulsions: _____	____	____	____	____
_____	____	____	____	____
_____	____	____	____	____

FORM 8.3. Further Evaluation of Obsessive–Compulsive Disorder: Test Scores, Substance Use, History, Treatment Progress, and Recommendations

Patient's Name: _____ Today's Date: _____

Therapist's Name: _____ Sessions Completed: _____

Test data/scores

Beck Depression Inventory (BDI) _____   Beck Anxiety Inventory (BAI) _____

Global Assessment of Functioning (GAF) _____   Locke–Wallace Marital Adjustment Test _____

Symptom Checklist 90-Revised (SCL-90-R) _____

Structured Clinical Interview for DSM-III-R, Axis II (SCID-II) _____

Anxiety Disorders Interview Schedule—Revised (ADIS-R) _____

Other anxiety questionnaires (specify) _____

Substance use

Current use of psychiatric medications (include dosage) _____

_____

Who prescribes? _____

Use of alcohol/other drugs (kind, frequency, amount, consequences) _____

_____

History (intake only)

Previous episodes of anxiety (specify nature):

    Onset   Duration   Precipitating events   Treatment

Treatment progress (later evaluations only)

Obsessions and compulsions still engaged in:_____

_____

Obsessions and compulsions no longer engaged in:_____

_____

Recommendations

Medication evaluation or reevaluation:

Increased intensity of services:

Behavioral interventions:

Cognitive interventions:

Interpersonal interventions:

Marital/couple therapy:

Other:

Consideration of Medication

The most extensively researched medication for OCD is clomipramine, a tricyclic antidepressant that selectively targets serotonin. Clomipramine has repeatedly been found to be more effective than placebo, with 51–60% of patients showing moderate to marked improvement. Other tricyclic antidepressants have been found to be minimally effective (Foa & Kozak, 1997).

Recent studies have provided evidence for the effectiveness of SSRIs, including fluoxetine, fluvoxamine, and sertraline. However, the effect sizes for SSRIs have not been as large or as consistent as those for clomipramine (Abramowitz, 1997).

Studies comparing behavior therapy and clomipramine have generally found behavior therapy to be superior. In addition, relapse rates as high as 95% have been reported when medication is discontinued. The addition of medication to behavior therapy has been found to improve short-term outcome. However, this improvement disappears once medication is stopped (Foa & Kozak, 1997).

Socialization to Treatment

Once the diagnosis is established, patients should be educated regarding the cognitive and behavioral models of OCD and the rationale for exposure and response prevention. Having an explanation of the disorder will reduce demoralization and increase motivation to undergo treatment. Form 8.4 is an information handout about OCD that can be given to patients. In addition, the handout about cognitive-behavioral therapy in general (Form B.1, Appendix B) can be provided. Finally, patients can be assigned to read one of the self-help books that are available for OCD, such as Foa and Wilson's (1991) *Stop Obsessing!*, Baer's (1991) *Getting Control*, or Steketee and White's (1990) *When Once Is Not Enough*.

Several key points should be made in the process of educating patients: (1) It is normal to have unpleasant, intrusive thoughts; (2) the strategies patients are currently using (i.e., attempting to avoid thinking these thoughts or neutralizing them with rituals) actually make their anxiety worse; and (3) allowing themselves to have the thoughts without ritualizing will lead to a decrease in their anxiety, in the frequency of the thoughts, and in urges to ritualize. Patients should be told that cognitive-behavioral treatment for OCD provides substantial relief and improved quality of life for most patients, but that it is typical for patients to continue to have some residual symptoms. This creates hope while also setting realistic expectations.

Building Motivation

Cognitive-behavioral treatment for OCD is demanding; it requires considerable time and the toleration of significant anxiety. Premature dropout and noncompliance are common problems and are the biggest reasons for treatment failure. It is crucial, therefore, to establish strong motivation before initiating exposure and response prevention. If motivation is initially low, extra time will be required for this step. Patients can be asked to list

FORM 8.4. Information for Patients about Obsessive–Compulsive Disorder

What Is Obsessive–Compulsive Disorder?

People with obsessive–compulsive disorder (OCD) have obsessions, compulsions, or both. "Obsessions" are thoughts, mental pictures, or impulses that are upsetting but that keep coming back. "Compulsions" are actions that people feel they have to perform to keep from feeling anxious or to prevent something bad from happening. Most people with OCD suffer from both obsessions and compulsions.

Common obsessions include:

- **Fears of getting a disease,** such as AIDS or cancer.
- **Fears of touching poisons,** such as pesticides.
- **Fears of hurting or killing someone,** often a loved one.
- **Fears of forgetting to do something,** such as turn off a stove or lock a door.
- **Fears of doing something embarrassing or immoral,** such as shouting obscenities.

Compulsions are also called "rituals." Common compulsions include the following:

- **Excessive washing or cleaning,** such as washing one's hands many times a day.
- **Checking,** such as looking at a stove repeatedly to make sure it is off.
- **Repeating actions,** such as always turning a light switch on and off 16 times.
- **Hoarding or saving things,** such as keeping old newspapers or scraps of paper.
- **Putting objects in a set pattern,** such as making sure everything in a room is symmetrical.

Most people with OCD know that their fears are not completely realistic. They also feel that their compulsions do not make sense. However, they find themselves unable to stop.

OCD is a common problem. During any 6-month period, over 4 million people in the United States suffer from OCD. One person in every 40 will have OCD at some point during his or her life.

OCD can cause serious problems. People with OCD often spend hours a day doing rituals. This makes it hard to work or take care of a family. Many people with OCD also avoid places or situations that make them anxious. Some become homebound. Often they have family members help them perform their rituals.

What Are the Causes of Obsessive–Compulsive Disorder?

The exact causes of OCD are not known. Genes play a role. Family members of people with OCD often have OCD and other anxiety problems. However, genes alone do not explain OCD; learning and life stress also appear to contribute to the disorder.

How Does Obsessive–Compulsive Disorder Develop?

Studies show that 90% of people have thoughts similar to those that trouble people with OCD. However, people with OCD appear to be more upset by these thoughts than other people are. Often the thoughts that worry people with OCD go against their beliefs and values—for example, a very religious man fears that he will commit blasphemy, or a loving mother fears harming her child.

(cont.)

Because people who develop OCD are upset by these thoughts, they try to avoid them. Often they try to force themselves to stop thinking the thoughts. The problem is that the more you try not to think about something, the more you end up thinking about it. You can try this yourself: Try *not* thinking about a pink elephant for the next 60 seconds. The chances are good that the first thing that comes to your mind will be just what you are trying to avoid thinking about—a pink elephant.

When people find that they cannot avoid upsetting thoughts, they often turn to other ways to feel less anxious. They may begin to perform some action, such as washing a lot or saying a silent prayer. This usually relieves their anxiety. The problem is that the relief is only *temporary*. Soon they must perform the action more often in order to feel better. Before long, the action has become a compulsion.

How Does Cognitive-Behavioral Treatment for Obsessive–Compulsive Disorder Work?

People with OCD are afraid that if they let themselves think their feared thoughts without doing any compulsions, they will get more and more anxious, and they won't be able to stand it. They often worry that they might go crazy.

Cognitive-behavioral treatment is aimed at helping you learn that you can control your anxiety without compulsions. You will learn coping strategies such as relaxation exercises, and ways of thinking that can help you feel less anxious. You will also learn that if you face your fears rather than avoid them, they will go away. This may be hard to believe, but it's true. Your therapist will help you gradually face the things that you fear most, until you are confident that you can handle your fears without compulsions.

Cognitive-behavioral treatment for OCD usually takes about 20 sessions. Treatment may take longer for people with severe symptoms.

Studies show that over 80% of people who complete cognitive-behavioral treatment for OCD are moderately to greatly improved. It is common to have occasional obsessions and urges to ritualize, even after treatment. However, patients usually feel much more in control and able to enjoy their lives. The studies also show that most people continue to feel better after therapy has stopped.

Can Medications Help?

The medications that work best for OCD increase the level of the chemical serotonin in the brain. Your physician or a psychiatrist can suggest the medication that would be best for you. Studies show that 50–60% of patients improve with these medications. However, most patients find that their symptoms return if the medication is stopped. For this reason, cognitive-behavioral therapy should always be used in addition to medication. For some patients, the combination of medication and therapy will give the best results.

What Is Expected of You as a Patient?

It is common to feel anxious at the beginning of therapy and to have doubts about whether you can be helped. All that is required is that you be willing to give therapy a try. Your therapist will teach you new ways of dealing with your anxiety and will help you begin to face the things you fear. You will be asked to practice these new skills between sessions. If you work on the exercises your therapist gives you and complete the treatment, and your chances for feeling better are excellent.

the advantages and disadvantages of undergoing treatment. Advantages should include activities they would be able to engage in with the time they now spend ritualizing; reduced anxiety; and improved relationships and occupational functioning. Disadvantages may include such problems as disruptions to family systems, as well as the need to face situations and decisions that the patients do not currently have to deal with because they are preoccupied with their OCD. Careful questioning may be necessary to help a patient make a complete list of advantages and disadvantages, and cognitive distortions on either side of the equation should be attended to. If motivation seems low after this procedure, it may be advisable to suggest that the patient wait before undergoing treatment, or consider an alternative such as medication.

Relaxation Training

Early in treatment, patients are taught simple breathing relaxation exercises and progressive muscle relaxation. (Detailed descriptions of these techniques can be found in Appendix A and the CD-ROM that accompanies this book.) The purpose of these techniques is to increase patients' sense of self-efficacy in dealing with their anxiety.

Although it is helpful for patients to use relaxation to deal with general anxiety, relaxation techniques are *not* used during exposure. In treating OCD, the aim is to expose the patients to their own anxiety, in order to help them recognize that they can tolerate the anxiety and that it will eventually decline without any special effort on their part. Having a patient practice relaxation during an exposure exercise is contrary to this goal. In addition, there is a danger that relaxation could become a new ritual.

Exposure

The purpose of exposure is to weaken the association between obsessive thoughts and emotional distress. Patients must come to understand that if they allow themselves to think their obsessive thoughts, without attempting to avoid or neutralize them through ritualizing, their anxiety will eventually decrease.

The first step in exposure is to create a hierarchy of a patient's obsessive thoughts. This is done by taking all of the obsessive thoughts reported by the patient on the self-monitoring form (Form 8.1) and having the patient rate (on the usual SUDs scale of 0–10) how anxious each thought makes him or her. The thoughts are then listed in order from the least anxiety-provoking to the most. A second hierarchy should be created of situations that are avoided. Forms 8.5 and 8.6 are hierarchy forms for patients with OCD.

For some patients, the hierarchy of obsessive fears will be largely distinct from that of avoided situations. In such cases, exposure should start with the obsessive thoughts; avoided situations should then be added, either in sessions or as homework. For other patients, however, it may be difficult to distinguish between the obsessive fears and the situations that provoke them. For example, a patient may fear contamination from pesticides and avoid going to grocery stores. Exposure may consist of having the patient go to a store and purchase pesticides. Being near pesticides will trigger the patient's fear of con-

FORM 8.5. Patient's Hierarchy of Obsessions

Patient's Name: _____ Today's Date: _____

Please list your feared thoughts, images, and impulses in order from least to most distressing. In the last column, note how upset each one makes you from 0 (no distress) to 10 (maximum distress).

Rank	Thought/Image/Impluse	Distress (0–10)

FORM 8.6. Patient's Hierarchy of Anxiety-Provoking/ Avoided Situations

Patient's Name: _____ Today's Date: _____

Please rank your anxiety-provoking and avoided situations in order from least to most distressing. In the last column, note how upset each one makes you, from 0 (no distress) to 10 (maximum distress).

Rank	Situation	Avoided (Yes/No)	Distress (0–10)

tamination; consequently, exposure to the situation and exposure to the obsessive thought occur simultaneously.

Once the hierarchies are constructed, exposure can begin. The patient is initially exposed to the lowest-ranking item on the hierarchy in the presence of the therapist, either in the consulting room or in an actual situation. Throughout the exposure, the patient is asked to rate his or her anxiety or distress every 5 minutes on the 0–10 SUDs scale. Exposure is continued until the patient's anxiety is reduced, ideally by at least half. Since it may take as long as an hour for a patient to habituate during an initial exposure, early exposure sessions should be scheduled for 90 minutes. The patient is then assigned to repeat the exposure daily as homework until it evokes minimal anxiety. After the first item on the hierarchy has been mastered, exposure to the next item is begun. Detailed instructions for conducting exposure are included in Appendix A and the CD-ROM. Forms A.1 and A.2 in Appendix A are forms for recording exposure homework.

Some obsessions are most easily addressed via imaginal exposure. This will be true, for example, when the patient fears some catastrophe (e.g., a family member's being killed) or fears committing some unacceptable action (e.g., murdering a child). In these cases, a scenario can be created in which the patient's worst fears come true. This should be tape-recorded during an therapy session, so that the patient can listen to it repeatedly—first in the session and then as homework—until he or she has habituated.

Other obsessions are most easily accessed with *in vivo* exposure. This is common when patients have fears of contamination or of failing to perform some action, such as locking a door. In such cases, putting the patient in contact with a feared situation (e.g., using a public restroom or walking away from the house without checking) will effectively activate the obsessional fears.

In all cases, however, it is important to include both *in vivo* and imaginal exposure in the treatment, as this will lead to the best outcome. Patients whose obsessive fears can only be accessed in imagination should nonetheless be encouraged to do *in vivo* exposure to situations that they avoid and that evoke obsessive fears. Patients whose fears are activated by *in vivo* exposure should be encouraged to imagine their worst fears' coming true as a result of the action. For example, a woman whose exposure consists of leaving the house without checking the door can be asked to imagine a burglar's breaking into the house, stealing her most prized possessions, and burning the house down, and then her husband's blaming her for the disaster and divorcing her.

Patients whose obsessions consist of specific thoughts or images and whose rituals are covert mental acts present a special problem. Such patients have traditionally not responded as well as other OCD patients to behavioral treatment. However, effective exposure can be accomplished by having these patients record their obsessive thoughts on a 30-second loop tape (the kind used in answering machines). The tape should include only the feared thoughts without any neutralizing thoughts. Patients are then assigned to listen to the tape for extended periods until they habituate.

Modeling may be useful early in treatment in order to facilitate exposure. The therapist models the exposure behavior—for example, "contaminating" himself or herself with a feared substance—before asking the patient to do so. This can encourage the patient to begin exposure. However, modeling should be discontinued as soon as possible, as it may also reduce the patient's anxiety and therefore prevent full exposure.

Two additional notes regarding exposure for OCD are in order. First, exposure is generally carried further than a person might act in everyday life. For example, a person who has a fear of being contaminated by newspapers might be asked not only to read a newspaper, but to rub it over his or her clothes and kitchen countertops. Second, therapists should avoid giving reassurance to patients during exposure. For many patients, seeking reassurance is one way of managing their anxiety and constitutes a form of ritualizing. It is also important as therapy progresses to have patients design and carry out their own exposure assignments. This will counteract their tendency to reduce anxiety by assigning responsibility to their therapists.

Response Prevention

Once exposure has begun, it is important to block the performance of rituals. Patients should be prevented from ritualizing not only during exposure sessions, but throughout the day. Otherwise, they may manage their anxiety during exposure by planning to ritualize later.

Prior to beginning formal exposure work, therapists may prepare patients for response prevention by instructing them to engage in behaviors that disrupt their rituals. Useful techniques include (1) performing a ritual very slowly (which interferes with the intensity of the ritual); (2) repeating the activity an unusual number of times (e.g., if a patient always does sets of four repetitions, have him or her try sets of three); and (3) postponing the ritual. With postponing, the patient starts by putting off ritualizing for a minute, and then gradually increases the time to up to several hours. After the specified time has elapsed, the patient is asked to decide either to perform the ritual or to postpone it again. Many patients are surprised to find that if they resist the initial impulse to ritualize, the urge will go away. Patients should be encouraged to experiment and find the technique that works best for them.

The preferred method of response prevention is to have a patient go "cold turkey" (i.e., give up all ritualizing at the beginning of the exposure phase of treatment). If properly prepared, patients will often agree to this. For many patients, however, it may be necessary to eliminate rituals gradually. This is done by having the patients stop all rituals associated with obsessions they have already been exposed to, while still allowing ritualizing to items higher on the hierarchy.

It is common for patients to have some lapses in response prevention during treatment. A patient should continue to log all rituals, and the therapist should inquire about any lapses in each session. Reasons for a lapse should be explored, including the patient's thoughts that led to the lapse (e.g., "I can't stand the anxiety," or "Just a little won't hurt"). Advantages and disadvantages of having engaged in the ritual should then be explored. Over time, patients generally come to realize that ritualizing increases the occurrence of obsessive thoughts, while response prevention actually decreases them. In some cases, it may be helpful to engage family members to remind patients to forgo rituals. Certainly, family members should be instructed to refuse to help patients perform rituals and to avoid providing reassurance.

Cognitive Restructuring

Cognitive interventions may be useful in several ways as adjuncts to exposure and response prevention: (1) to weaken belief in the possibility of danger before initiating exposure work, thereby improving compliance; (2) to challenge the automatic thoughts, assumptions, and schemas of danger and responsibility that contribute to the patient's anxiety; and (3) to challenge the processing errors that maintain the assumptions and schemas.

Assumptions about the dangerousness of obsessive thoughts can be challenged in a number of ways. The occurrence of intrusive thoughts can be normalized by informing patients that the vast majority of people experience thoughts similar to those of people with OCD. Possible advantages of some intrusive thoughts (e.g., creative ideas or pleasant fantasies) can be discussed, along with the difficulty of inhibiting some thoughts while allowing others.

Fears of catastrophe can be challenged by having patients compare their estimates of risk for themselves to how often the feared events actually occur. For example, a patient who initially states that the chance of hitting a pedestrian while driving to work is 70% can be asked whether 7 out of 10 people have such accidents every morning. When patients are not aware of the base rates of feared events, such as a plane crash, they can be asked to research them. van Oppen and Arntz (1994) suggest having a patient (1) list the probability of each step leading to a feared outcome, and then (2) calculate the cumulative probability. For example, if there are six steps between failing to unplug a toaster at night and the house's burning down (i.e., the toaster catches fire, the fire spreads, the fire alarm doesn't work, no one smells smoke, etc.) and each step has a one in ten probability, the cumulative probability becomes one in a million.

Behavioral experiments can also be useful. Patients who fear that their obsessive thoughts will cause a catastrophe or lead them to commit some unacceptable action may be asked to make something happen just by thinking it—for example, "Try willing yourself to die right now." Patients can also be asked to experiment with trying to avoid and neutralize their obsessive thoughts on some days, allowing themselves to think these thoughts on others, and tracking how often they have thoughts and how distressed they feel on the different days. This will generally lead patients to realize that avoiding and neutralizing actually make their obsessions worse (Salkovskis & Kirk, 1997).

A number of techniques can also be used to challenge assumptions of responsibility. For example, patients can be asked to create a "pie chart" showing the portion of responsibility held by all relevant parties. If patients put in everyone else's responsibility first, they usually realize that very little of the "pie" is left for them. The double standard technique may also be useful. For example, if a patient assumes that he or she will be held responsible if the patient's mother dies in a plane crash after the two of them have had an argument, the patient can be asked what he or she would say to a friend in similar circumstances.

In the later stages of treatment, cognitive restructuring can be used to help patients cope with possible sources of stress or anxiety that might lead to a relapse of OCD. It can also help patients overcome the anxiety associated with facing life challenges that have been avoided or put off because of their OCD symptoms.

Troubleshooting Problems in Therapy

As noted earlier, the most common problems encountered in treating OCD are premature dropout and noncompliance. If the treatment is considered from a patient's point of view, this makes sense. The principles of exposure and response prevention are counterintuitive. Therapists are, in fact, asking patients to do the very things that they most fear doing and have believed would lead to disaster.

The first step in preventing premature dropout is properly preparing a patient. The cognitive-behavioral conceptualization of OCD must be explained in a way the patient can understand. Any fears the patient has should be elicited and discussed. It may also be helpful to have the patient read stories by people who have successfully undergone treatment. *Stop Obsessing!* (Foa & Wilson, 1991) provides a number of such stories.

Ultimately, however, it is helpful to acknowledge that some doubt and anxiety are to be expected before treatment begins. If the patient continues to hesitate, behavioral experiments may be used before full exposure and response prevention are initiated. For example, the patient may be asked to try purposely thinking an obsessive thought and observing the results. Similarly, the patient may be asked to attempt to postpone rather than forgo rituals. If the patient continues to resist full exposure, adding medication to the treatment may be helpful.

Premature dropout sometimes happens after a patient has done enough exposure and response prevention to get some relief, but before he or she has completed the exposure hierarchy. This too makes sense from the patient's point of view: The extreme distress that motivated the patient to seek treatment has subsided, but the fear associated with the highest items on the hierarchy still remains to be faced. It is helpful to warn patients about the risks of premature dropout and to inform them that according to the research, patients who continue to have substantial symptoms are at greater risk of relapse. If a patient suddenly stops coming to sessions, it is important to establish contact and discuss his or her fears. If the patient does not return, the message should be conveyed that the therapist is available if the patient should desire further treatment at any point in the future. It has been our experience that a number of patients will return after premature dropout because they have experienced a relapse; such patients may then have the motivation to complete treatment.

Noncompliance presents a more subtle problem. It is common for patients to engage in covert forms of avoidance during exposure. For example, they may distract themselves from the exposure cues; they may perform covert mental rituals; or they may promise themselves that they will ritualize later. The best way to detect covert avoidance is to monitor a patient's SUDs levels throughout the exposure. If the patient fails to experience significant anxiety, inquiry should be made about any actions he or she may be taking to feel less anxious. The patient should then be reminded of the need for full exposure. In some cases, it may be necessary to contract with the patient to proceed more slowly with exposure, in exchange for a promise to forgo covert avoidance.

Failure to do homework is another problem. Simply asking patients to record their practice on the forms provided in Appendix A (Forms A.1 and A.2) should increase compliance. If a patient fails to habituate over time to exposure items, noncompliance with homework should be suspected. Again, the patient's fears should be explored, and the patient encouraged to experiment on his or her own to determine the results of doing or avoiding self-directed exposure.

Noncompliance with response prevention is also common. The patient should be encouraged to discuss any ritualizing he or she has engaged in during the week. Lapses should be approached nonjudgmentally as learning opportunities. The advantages and disadvantages of having ritualized can be explored, along with the automatic thoughts that led to the lapse. If the patient continues to have difficulty refraining from ritualizing, family members may be recruited to help remind the patient of the need to forgo rituals and to monitor any rituals that are performed. Patients with severe OCD who are incapable of response prevention may need to undergo treatment in an inpatient setting.

Relapse Prevention

Before ending treatment, it is important to help patients predict possible sources of stress that might lead to a relapse. This serves two functions: (1) it gives patients tools to deal with such stressors; and (2) it helps them see a temporary return of symptoms as a natural occurrence, which, rather than indicating that treatment has failed, provides an opportunity to practice the skills they have learned. It is also important to deal with any stressors that might be related to the reduction in OCD symptoms, such as the need to fill extra time that is now available or family conflict that has heretofore taken a back seat to the OCD symptoms.

Once possible stressors are identified, ways of coping with these stressors are reviewed, including relaxation and cognitive restructuring. Finally, each patient is asked to write out a list of procedures to follow if a relapse does occur, including self-directed exposure and response prevention, as well as calling the therapist for booster sessions if the patient is not able to bring the symptoms under control.

Phasing Out Treatment

The last few sessions should be scheduled at intervals of 2 weeks to a month. In addition, patients should be asked to design their own exposure homework. This will give patients increased confidence in their ability to cope with their symptoms on their own.

CASE EXAMPLE

The following example of the treatment of a patient with OCD is based on a case previously described in less detail in Holland (1997).

Sessions 1–2

Presenting problem   Robert was a 25-year-old single white male. He presented in the first session specifically requesting treatment for OCD. He had been previously diagnosed by a psychiatrist, who had prescribed Prozac. Robert never took the medication, however; he had read that one of the side effects was nausea, and as it turned out, vomiting was one of his obsessive fears.

Robert lived with his mother. His parents had divorced 5 years earlier. He was employed as the office manager of a small company. He aspired to be a photographer, but had yet to seek work in his chosen profession.

Rituals

When asked about his symptoms, Robert complained of a history of ritualizing since the age of 10. His rituals involved repeating actions, often hundreds of times. He reported that his condition had worsened in the last 3 years. He had rituals for dressing, showering, and shaving that often took several hours a day. Many of his rituals involved going from one part of a room to another, tapping objects. He often did this so rapidly and intensely that he would sweat. At his job, Robert would open and close computer files hundreds of times. When working in his darkroom, he often reprinted the same photograph repeatedly until he felt he had done the procedure without thinking any "bad" thoughts.

Obsessions

Robert's obsessions included a fear of vomiting, especially in anxiety-provoking situations such as job interviews; fears of being injured or killed in a car or plane accident; and fears of family members' dying. He was afraid that if he allowed himself to have one of these thoughts, the feared event might actually occur. Robert avoided subways, buses, and airplanes, as well as walking down streets where he had once had an obsessive thought. He avoided buying books or CDs that he associated with vomiting or plane crashes. In addition, he sometimes avoided eating for fear of being nauseated; consequently, he was slightly underweight.

Impairment

When asked how his OCD had interfered with his life, Robert reported a number of problems. His college girlfriend had broken up with him because of his ritualizing, and he had not dated or been sexually active in almost 2 years. Although he did hold a job that was unstructured enough for him to hide most of his ritualizing, he was not functioning at his optimal level at work. He said he was afraid to pursue work as a photographer for fear he would become anxious and his OCD would get worse. He continued living at home in spite of a stated desire to be on his own.

Family history

Robert reported that his mother had been treated for anxiety. He described her as overprotective and said that she actively discouraged him from moving out of the house. In spite of wishing for more independence, Robert was very close to his mother. Robert's father, an attorney, was largely an absent figure.

Socialization to treatment

Robert was administered the OCQ (Form 8.2), and the standard intake battery (see Form 8.3). The therapist educated Robert

Homework

concerning the effectiveness of cognitive-behavioral therapy for OCD, and provided him with the information handouts on OCD (Form 8.4) and on cognitive-behavioral therapy in general (Form B.1). The option of combining therapy and medication was also discussed, but Robert stated a strong preference to try therapy without medication. For homework, he was assigned to write out his goals for therapy and to begin reading *Stop Obsessing!* Robert expressed fear that reading the book would make his symptoms worse, but he was assured that this was not likely.

Sessions 3–4

Further socialization to treatment

Building motivation

Homework

In the third session, the therapist and Robert further discussed the cognitive–behavioral model of OCD and the steps involved in treatment. Robert was advised that although his chances for improvement were excellent, some minor symptoms would probably remain. In the session, Robert was asked to list the ways his life would become better if his OCD symptoms improved. For homework, he was assigned to make a list of advantages and disadvantages of proceeding with treatment, as well as to begin logging his obsessions and rituals (Form 8.1).

Obsession/ ritual log

Building motivation

Breathing relaxation training

The log Robert presented in the fourth session revealed almost constant obsessing and ritualizing. He reported that recording his rituals had made him more aware of what he was doing and had led to a decrease in the time he spent ritualizing. Robert was pleased, because he felt this indicated he was already making progress. The advantages and disadvantages of treatment were reviewed further. Although Robert expressed the desire to proceed, he said he was afraid that exposure would make his anxiety worse. The therapist told Robert that exposure would actually lessen his anxiety, and suggested that Robert experiment in the coming week with allowing himself to think one of his obsessive thoughts instead of trying to avoid it. Robert was then taught breathing relaxation, and was assigned to practice this during the week. He was also asked to continue logging his obsessions and rituals.

Sessions 5–6

Progressive muscle relaxation training

In the next session, Robert reported that his ritualizing had continued to decrease. He had tried allowing himself to think one of his obsessive thoughts and was pleased to discover that, as the therapist had predicted, his anxiety had decreased. He was then taught progressive muscle relaxation. For homework, he was assigned to experiment with altering and postponing his rituals, and to practice progressive muscle relaxation as well as breathing relaxation.

Response prevention

In the sixth session, Robert reported that he had found postponing his rituals very helpful. Indeed, he found (much to his surprise) that when he did postpone, his urge to ritualize went away. Robert continued to express fears that exposure would make his anxiety worse, however. The therapist used Socratic dialogue to challenge these thoughts. Robert was assigned to continue practicing relaxation and to continue to experiment with altering rituals.

Cognitive restructuring; homework

Sessions 7–10

Exposure hierarchies

The next three sessions were devoted to preparing Robert to begin exposure. This involved developing hierarchies of obsessive thoughts and avoided situations and continuing to respond to Robert's fears about exposure. This process took somewhat longer than expected because of the extensive nature of Robert's symptoms; for example, his logs reflected over 50 distinct rituals.

Plan for exposure

In the ninth session Robert was presented with a schedule for the next 3 weeks, consisting of one 90-minute session each week for exposure. An additional 45-minute session was scheduled the first week for troubleshooting any problems that arose. Imaginal exposure would be used in sessions to target Robert's obsessive fears. In between sessions, Robert would repeat the imaginal exposure and would do self-directed *in vivo* exposure to his avoided situations. Robert was told to set aside an hour a day for homework. The options of either stopping rituals "cold turkey" or phasing them out as he moved up his hierarchies were discussed. Robert was asked to think about which method he preferred prior to the next session. Robert's exposure hierarchies are shown in Tables 8.3 and 8.4.

Response prevention

Response prevention

At the start of the 10th session, Robert reported that he had gone "cold turkey" and had not ritualized for the past week. He was very pleased by this and said, "I don't want to ritualize, and no one can make me." He was praised for this, but was also warned that relapse was likely.

Imaginal exposure

Imaginal exposure was then initiated to the first thought from Robert's hierarchy (i.e., that his face would be disfigured in a car accident). His SUDs rating never increased above 4 and he habituated quickly. Therefore, exposure was begun for the second item (his fear of vomiting).

Exposure scenario

The imaginal exposure scenario used for Robert's fear of

TABLE 8.3. Patient's Hierarchy of Obsessions (Form 8.5), as Completed by Robert

Patient's Name: _Robert_   Today's Date: _10/15_

Please list your feared thoughts, images, and impulses in order from least to most distressing. In the last column, note how upset each one makes you from 0 (no distress) to 10 (maximum distress).

Rank	Thought/Image/Impluse	Distress (0–10)
1	Car accident—face damaged	4
2	Getting sick—throwing up	5
3	The number 13	5
4	Throwing up at a job interview	8
5	Car accident—family member hurt	9
6	Helicopter accident—I'm killed	9.5
7	Plane accident—I'm killed	9.5
8	Family member dying	10

vomiting is described below. It contains a number of specific elements that were taken from Robert's hierarchy of avoided situations. For example, Robert's fear of vomiting had increased following his becoming ill after eating scallops at age 12. He had avoided scallops ever since.

THERAPIST: You get a call from your friend Larry saying that there is a party a week from now at his house, and that he really wants you to come because one of the guests is an agent who might be interested in your photographs. He also mentions that Sally [a woman the patient worked with and liked] is going to be there. She just broke up with her boyfriend and said she's looking forward to seeing you. What are you thinking and feeling?

ROBERT: I'm feeling anxious. Why did he have to call so far in advance? Now I'm going to be nervous all week. I want to call and cancel.

TABLE 8.4. Patient's Hierarchy of Anxiety-Provoking/Avoided Situations (Form 8.6), as Completed by Robert

Patient's Name: _Robert_   Today's Date: _10/15_

Please rank your anxiety-provoking and avoided situations in order from least to most distressing. In the last column, note how upset each one makes you, from 0 (no distress) to 10 (maximum distress).

Rank	Situation	Avoided (Yes/No)	Distress (0–10)
1	Bus	No	3
2	Car	No	3
3	Touch something touched by someone sick	Yes	4
4	Walk down block after obsession	Yes	8
5	Print picture associated with obsession	Yes	8
6	The number 13	Yes	8
7	Complete layouts so things line up	Yes	8
8	Purchase and use items associated with obsession	Yes	8
9	Boats	Yes	9
10	Eat when I might vomit	Yes	9
11	Certain CDs	Yes	9.5

THERAPIST: What do you feel physically?

ROBERT: I feel a knot in my stomach and maybe, yes, I think a little nauseated.

THERAPIST: Good. And you have an urge to ritualize to control the anxiety, but you promised to go "cold turkey," so you don't. What are you feeling?

ROBERT: I'm really anxious, 'cause I think that if I don't ritualize, I might vomit when I get to the party.

THERAPIST: OK. Now it's a week later. It's the morning of the party, and you started feeling a little sick last night. There's been a flu going around, and you think you might have it. How are you feeling?

ROBERT: Well, I'm a little light-headed. I feel just a bit queasy, and I'm really worried I'm going to get sick before this party.

THERAPIST: Now you go to get dressed, and you realize that the only jacket you have that isn't at the cleaner's is the green one, the one you never wear because it reminds you of vomit. So you put it on. What's going through your mind?

ROBERT: Why don't I have anything else to wear? Maybe I can just wear a nice sweater.

THERAPIST: OK, but you decide that you have to look professional to meet this agent, so you put on the green jacket and go to work. [Note the attempted avoidance by the patient even in the fantasy, and the move by the therapist to block it.]

As the exposure continued, Robert was told that he went to work, but felt sicker as the day went on. He didn't have time to get lunch, and all that was available was someone's leftover chicken and cashews from the local Chinese restaurant. While he was eating it, he noticed that the chicken looked slightly undercooked. It was raining when he left, so he couldn't get a cab. He had to take a bus. It was very crowded, and the exhaust system didn't work, so it smelled. By the time he got to the party, he was feeling very nauseated. However, Sally greeted him warmly and said she was very glad he was there because she had cooked her special dish, scallops marinara, and wanted him to try it.

THERAPIST: What are you feeling now?

ROBERT: I'm really sick and I don't want to eat anything.

THERAPIST: But you really like this girl, and she's looking right at you as you sit there with the food in front of you. So you start to take a bite. What does it taste like?

ROBERT: The scallop is kind of rubbery, and it smells like seaweed. I don't like it. I try to swallow a little, but it feels like my throat is closing. I'm feeling really nauseated.

Robert's SUDs rating, which had climbed slowly during this exposure, suddenly jumped to 9 when he was asked to imagine eating the scallop. He was only able to habituate slightly, reducing his anxiety to 7. Because insufficient time was left to allow Robert to habituate further, a distraction exercise—asking him to count the items in the office that were blue—was used to help reduce his anxiety before the session ended. Robert was assigned to listen to

Homework

the tape of the vomit exposure as homework.

Sessions 11–16

Troubleshooting

As planned, the next session was held 2 days after the first exposure session. Robert reported that he had felt very anxious after the prior session and had begun ritualizing again. He had not lis-

Cognitive restructuring

tened to the tape. He also reported being afraid that he would become so anxious he would vomit. The therapist asked whether he had ever vomited when he felt anxious. Robert answered, "No," and seemed surprised by his own answer. It had never occurred to him that although he constantly feared vomiting from anxiety, this had never happened.

Resumption of exposure

The therapist apologized for having started a new exposure scenario in the preceding session when there was not sufficient time to allow Robert to habituate, and suggested that the best way to deal with the anxiety Robert was feeling was to resume the exposure. The therapist offered to extend the present session, which had been planned for 45 minutes, as long as necessary to allow Robert to habituate. He also suggested that Robert inform him immediately if his SUDs rating got above 7, and they would then wait for his anxiety to decrease before proceeding with new elements of the scenario.

Robert agreed, and exposure was resumed. All of the elements from the scenario were repeated, and new ones were added until Robert had imagined eating an entire bowl of scallops and vomiting in front of the agent. At no time did Robert's SUDs rating climb above a 3. Robert was amazed. The therapist explained that Robert had habituated, probably because of his thinking about the exposure between sessions. Robert was assigned to listen to the tape of the exposure scenario every day, and to begin self-directed exposure to items on his hierarchy of avoided situations.

Completion of hierarchy

Sessions 12 and 13 were again 90 minutes long. Robert was exposed to the rest of his obsessive thoughts. In addition to imaginal exposure, he was asked to do things such as writing the thoughts "I will die in a plane crash," and "My mother will die," 13 times each (since he was also obsessed with the number 13). Robert habituated easily to these exposures. All future sessions were planned for 45 minutes.

Effects of exposure

In Session 14 Robert indicated that he was very pleased with his progress. He reported that he was now able to say the word "vomit" and to watch a TV show that involved vomiting without feeling anxious. He had also exposed himself to a number of avoided situations that had not been on his original hierarchy (it was becoming apparent that both his rituals and his avoidance were even more extensive than he had reported). He stated, "If I challenge myself, nothing can bother me."

Response prevention

Robert did report some minor ritualizing, accompanied by the automatic thought "Just let me do that." He usually followed these rituals with some new exposure. However, he also reported that he was avoiding listening to the exposure tapes made during

Homework

In vivo exposure

sessions, because he didn't feel "clean" afterward. It was pointed out that this was a form of avoidance, and the advantages and disadvantages of exposure were reviewed. Robert was again assigned to listen to the tapes daily.

The next two sessions were primarily spent planning and discussing self-directed *in vivo* exposure. Robert exposed himself to a variety of previously avoided situations. He also reported progress in areas that had not been direct targets of therapy: He said that he was expressing disagreement with his mother more often without feeling guilty, and that he was apologizing less often at his job. In addition, he had begun putting together a portfolio so that he could solicit jobs as a free-lance photographer.

Sessions 17–20

Cognitive restructuring

Work during the 17th through 20th sessions focused on areas of functioning that had been problematic for Robert; various cognitive techniques were employed. Robert was having trouble completing his portfolio, and his automatic thought was "It has to be perfect." This thought was challenged, with the therapist emphasizing the impossibility of achieving perfection and the advantages of starting to show his work even if it was not yet perfect. The following week Robert reported that he had completed the portfolio and made some appointments to show it. Robert then stated that his goal was to feel no anxiety during these appointments. This led to a discussion of the advantages and disadvantages of trying to feel no anxiety versus accepting anxiety. Robert's underlying assumption was that any anxiety was dangerous. The therapist pointed out that mild anxiety actually enhances performance.

Further response prevention

Robert again reported some minor bouts of ritualizing, accompanied by the thought "Just one for safety." The advantages and disadvantages of performing "just one" ritual were discussed, and Robert concluded that rather than making him less anxious, continued ritualizing only served to reinforce his obsessive fears.

Continuation of therapy

By the 20th session, Robert was ritualizing minimally and was far less troubled by his obsessive thoughts. The possibility of terminating therapy was discussed. If Robert had opted to stop treatment at this point, three or four more sessions would have been held, spaced every other week, to focus on relapse prevention. However, Robert felt that there were several areas of life functioning that he wished to work on, including pursuing his career as a photographer, dating, and resolving his conflict about moving out of his mother's house. Therapy was therefore continued once a week on an open-ended basis. The extended treatment of this case has been described in Holland (1997).

DETAILED TREATMENT PLAN
FOR OBSESSIVE–COMPULSIVE DISORDER

Treatment Reports

Tables 8.5 and 8.6 are designed to help you in writing managed care treatment reports for patients with OCD. Table 8.5 shows sample specific symptoms; select the symptoms that are appropriate for your patient. (Once again, Zuckerman's [1995] *Clinician's Thesaurus* can be consulted for additional words and phrases.) Be sure also to specify the nature of the patient's impairments, including any dysfunction in academic, work, family, or social functioning. Table 8.6 lists sample goals and matching interventions. Again, select those that are appropriate for the patient.

Session-by-Session Treatment Options

Table 8.7 shows the sequence of interventions for a 20-session course of treatment for OCD. As noted above, patients with severe symptoms may require longer treatment.

TABLE 8.5. Sample Symptoms for Obsessive–Compulsive Disorder

Obsessions (specify)—for example:
    Fear of contracting disease (specify)
    Fear of contamination (specify)
    Fear of hurting someone (specify)
    Fear of failure to do something (specify)
    Fear of losing control (specify)
Compulsions (specify)—for example:
    Excessive washing or cleaning (specify)
    Checking (specify)
    Repeating (specify)
    Hoarding (specify)
    Ordering (specify)
Anxious mood
Specify physical symptoms of anxiety:
    Palpitations
    Difficulty breathing
    Chest pain

Nausea
Dizziness
Feeling faint
Sweating
Shaking
Numbness
Tingling
Chills
Hot flashes
Specify cognitive symptoms:
    Mind going blank
    Difficulty speaking
    Loss of concentration
    Derealization
    Depersonalization
Avoidance (specify)

TABLE 8.6. Sample Treatment Goals and Interventions for Obsessive–Compulsive Disorder

Treatment goals	Interventions
Reducing physical anxiety symptoms	Relaxation
Reducing intrusive thoughts (images, impulses)	Imaginal exposure
Reporting obsession-related distress less than 2 on a scale of 0–10	Exposure
Eliminating compulsions (specify)	Response prevention
Stating belief that anxiety is not dangerous and can be tolerated	Cognitive restructuring, exposure
Stating understanding that seeking perfect certainty exacerbates symptoms	Cognitive restructuring
Modifying schemas of danger and responsibility (or other schemas—specify)	Cognitiving restructuring, developmental analysis
Engaging in previously avoided behaviors (specify)	*In vivo* exposure
Eliminating impairment (specify—depending on impairments, this may be several goals)	Cognitive restructuring, problem-solving training, or other skills training (specify)
Eliminating all anxiety symptoms (SCL-90-R and/or OCQ scores in normal range)	All of the above
Acquiring relapse prevention skills	Reviewing and practicing techniques as necessary

TABLE 8.7. Session-by-Session Treatment Options for Obsessive–Compulsive Disorder

Sessions 1–2

Assessment

    Ascertain presenting problems

    Inquire regarding all symptoms

    Assess presence of obsessions and compulsions

    Assess avoidance behaviors

    Assess impairment in social, educational, and occupational functioning

    Assess social supports and involvement of family members in rituals

    Have patient complete OCQ (Form 8.2)

    Administer standard battery of intake measures (see Form 8.3), plus additional anxiety
        questionnaires as appropriate

    Evaluate for comorbid conditions (e.g., major depression, other anxiety disorders)

    Evaluate substance use; evaluate need for counseling or detoxification if patient has
        substance abuse or dependence

Socialization to Treatment

    Inform patient of diagnosis

    Educate patient regarding treatment options, including medication

    Provide patient with handouts on OCD (Form 8.4) and on cognitive-behavioral therapy in
        general (Form B.1, Appendix B)

    Begin developing short-term and long-term goals for therapy

Homework

    Have patient begin reading *Stop Obsessing!* or other self-help book

    Have patient write out goals for therapy

Sessions 3–4

Assessment

    Evaluate homework

    Evaluate anxiety (BAI) and depression (BDI)

    Assess motivation for treatment

Socialization to Treatment

    Discuss cognitive-behavioral conceptualization of OCD and describe cognitive-behavioral
        treatment

    Educate patient regarding outcome research

    Build motivation for treatment, as needed

Behavioral Interventions

    Teach breathing relaxation

Homework

    Have patient list advantages and disadvantages of proceeding with treatment

    Have patient begin to log all obsessions and rituals (Form 8.1)

    Assign breathing relaxation practice

Sessions 5–6

Assessment

As in Sessions 3–4

Socialization to Treatment

Obtain patient's commitment to proceed with treatment
Educate family members regarding diagnosis and their role in treatment, if appropriate

Behavioral Interventions

Teach progressive muscle relaxation
Help patient construct hierarchies of obsessions, avoided situations
Plan initial exposure sessions
Teach response prevention techniques: postponing, slowing, and changing repetitions

Cognitive Interventions

Educate patient regarding intrusive thoughts as normal phenomena
Help patient devise behavioral experiments (e.g., avoiding or not avoiding thoughts and tracking results; attempting to influence events by thoughts)

Homework

Have patient continue to log obsessions/rituals
Assign relaxation practice (breathing and progressive muscle relaxation)
Have patient conduct behavioral experiments
Assign practice in disrupting rituals

Sessions 7–10

Note: Initial exposure sessions should be 90 minutes to allow for habituation; it may be advisable, after the first exposure session, to schedule a 45-minute session later in the week to monitor any problems with exposure homework

Assessment

As in Sessions 3–4

Behavioral Interventions

Exposure (both imaginal and *in vivo*) to initial items on hierarchy of obsessions
Help patient block all rituals, or rituals associated with current exposure items

Homework

Assign daily repetition of exposure
Have patient continue logging obsessions/rituals
Assign continued relaxation practice

Sessions 11–16

Assessment

As in Sessions 3–4

(cont.)

TABLE 8.7 *(cont.)*

Behavioral Interventions
 Complete exposure to hierarchy of obsessions
 Begin exposure to hierarchy of avoided situations
 Monitor any avoidance of exposure homework
 Continue to help patient block rituals
 Examine any lapses in response prevention

Cognitive Interventions
 Examine and challenge any thoughts related to avoidance of exposure
 Examine and challenge any thoughts related to lapses in rituals
 Help patient evaluate advantages/disadvantages of rituals
 Examine and challenge automatic thoughts, assumptions, and schemas related to danger
  and responsibility

Homework
 Have patient continue logging obsessions/rituals
 Have patient record automatic thoughts related to any lapses
 Assign continued daily repetition of exposure
 Assign continued relaxation practice

Sessions 17–20 (Scheduled Biweekly or Monthly)
Assessment
 As in Sessions 3–4
 Assess and address any residual symptoms
 Assess any life problems related to OCD or patient improvement

Behavioral Interventions
 Have patient apply relaxation to life stressors
 Complete all exposure hierarchies
 Continue helping patient block all rituals
 Monitor any lapses in response prevention

Cognitive Interventions
 Continue challenging automatic thoughts, assumptions, and schemas of danger and
  responsibility
 Help patient apply cognitive skills to life stressors

Relapse Prevention
 Educate patient regarding likelihood of residual symptoms and use of lapses as opportunity
  to practice skills
 Evaluate possible future stressors
 Review coping skills and develop strategies for future stressors
 Address current life problems
 Have patient prepare list of skills learned in therapy
 Encourage patient to call if booster sessions are needed

Homework
 Have patient self-assign exposure homework
 Encourage patient to continue practicing all skills learned

Review of
Selected Behavioral Techniques

BEHAVIORAL ACTIVATION (REWARD PLANNING
AND ACTIVITY SCHEDULING)

Behavioral activation is used primarily in the treatment of depression, although it may also be applied to the treatment of some anxiety disorders, such as generalized anxiety disorder (see Chapter 4) and posttraumatic stress disorder (see Chapter 6, Table 6.3). The overall goal is to increase behaviors that are likely to result in a patient's being rewarded in some way. Rewards may be internal (such as pleasure or a sense of accomplishment) or external (such as social attention). Increasing rewards helps to lift patients' moods. A secondary goal is to decrease depressive rumination by having patients focus on other activities (Beck, Rush, Shaw, & Emery, 1979).

There are four steps to implementing behavioral activation: (1) monitoring current activities, (2) developing a list of rewarding activities, (3) planning such activities, and (4) completing these activities.

1. *Monitoring.* The patient is asked to list all activities he or she engages in during the day on an hour-by-hour basis. The Patient's Weekly Activity Record (Chapter 2, Form 2.5) can be used for this. The patient rates each hour's activity on two dimensions: (1) pleasure and (2) mastery. Each dimension is rated from 0 (no pleasure/mastery) to 10 (maximum pleasure/mastery). "Mastery" is defined as a feeling of effectiveness or accomplishment. This monitoring typically reveals that the patient is engaging in very few rewarding activities. Often the patient spends hours in activities with low reward, such as watching television or sitting and ruminating. Alternatively, the patient may be engaging in some activities that seem likely to bring pleasure or mastery, but do not because he or she is having negative thoughts that interfere with enjoyment. These negative thoughts can be elicited and challenged by means of cognitive techniques (see Appendix B, Table B.3).

2. *Developing a list of rewarding activities.* The next step is to list activities the patient can engage in that are likely to be rewarding. Included on the list should be activities the patient

currently enjoys, activities the patient has enjoyed in the past when not depressed, and activities the patient has thought about trying but never has.

3. *Planning rewarding activities.* Next, the patient is assigned to schedule some activities from the activity list each day. The patient may be asked to predict in advance how much he or she will enjoy or experience mastery from the activity, again using a 0–10 scale. The Patient's Weekly Planning Schedule (Chapter 2, Form 2.6) can be used for this purpose.

4. *Completing planned activities.* Finally, the patient engages in the planned activities according to schedule, and records the actual ratings for mastery and pleasure. The Patient's Weekly Activity Record (Form 2.5) can again be used for this.

DISTRACTION

The purpose of distraction is temporarily to interrupt the flow of negative thoughts that leads to patients' feelings of anxiety or depression. It can be used before patients have learned rational responding, when thoughts and emotions are so overwhelming that a patient is unable to cope by other means, or when a patient is flooded with intrusive memories or images (as in posttraumatic stress disorder) and is not in a situation where exposure is appropriate. We emphasize that distraction should be used only as a temporary solution. Eventually the negative thoughts or intrusive memories or images must be dealt with via other techniques.

Any activity that absorbs a patient's attention can be useful for distraction. Patients should be encouraged to experiment and find what works for them. Doing crossword puzzles, reading a book, seeing a movie, talking to a friend, daydreaming about pleasurable times in the past, or playing a sport all may be helpful. Activities that are routine and do not require mental concentration, such as doing household chores or watching television, may not be effective.

Distraction can be demonstrated in a session by first having a patient think about an upsetting thought or image until the patient becomes depressed or anxious, and then asking him or her to engage in some mentally absorbing activity, such as counting backward by 7 from 1,000 out loud, or counting the number of objects of a certain color in the therapist's office. Patients are often surprised to find that their distress level decreases rapidly.

Patients should be told that when they first attempt distraction, they may find that the negative thoughts or emotions continue to intrude. However, if they persist in returning their attention to the distracting activity, they will eventually become absorbed in it. Like all skills, distraction takes practice, and the more often the patient uses it the better it will work.

One contraindication for distraction should be noted: It should not be used for the obsessive thoughts of patients with obsessive–compulsive disorder, as it could become another ritual.

EXPOSURE

Exposure is the most important behavioral technique for the treatment of anxiety disorders. It is based on the assumption that anxiety is maintained by avoidance of the thing feared. The essence of exposure is for patients to come deliberately into contact with the cues that evoke their anxiety, and to remain in contact with those cues until they begin to realize that the negative consequences they expect do not occur and their anxiety diminishes. The process of diminishing anxiety is referred to as "habituation."

The types of cues that evoke anxiety vary from disorder to disorder. For specific phobia, the cue is the feared object. For social phobia, the cues are various social situations. For posttraumatic stress disorder, the cues are memories of the traumatic event and stimuli that remind the patient of the event. For panic disorder, the cues are bodily sensations that trigger panic attacks. For agoraphobia, the cues are situations that the patient avoids. For obsessive–compulsive disorder, the cues may be the patient's thoughts or mental images, or they may be situations that trigger obsessive fears.

Types of Exposure

There are two main types of exposure: *in vivo* and imaginal. *In vivo* exposure consists of patients' coming into contact with cues in real-life situations. In imaginal exposure, patients come into contact with cues in their imaginations.

In Vivo *Exposure*

Whenever possible, *in vivo* exposure should be used. Unless the cue is portable (e.g., a specific object, a bodily sensation), this means that exposure will generally have to take place outside the therapist's office. The therapist may accompany the patient during the exposure, or the patient may be assigned to do exposure on his or her own as homework. Research suggests that therapist-directed exposure is generally no more effective than self-directed exposure (Al-Kubaisy et al., 1992). In practice, we find that most patients are able to do self-directed *in vivo* exposure. When patients are too anxious to initiate such exposure on their own, initial exposure may be done with the therapist. But therapist involvement should be quickly faded out, and the patients should be encouraged to repeat *in vivo* exposure on their own as homework.

With an extremely anxious patient, it may be helpful for the therapist to model exposure before asking the patient to do it. Thus, the therapist will first contact the feared cue (e.g., getting on an elevator) while the patient watches. Then the patient is asked to do the same. Again, modeling should be quickly discontinued, with the patient then doing the exposure entirely on his or her own.

Imaginal Exposure

Sometimes *in vivo* exposure is not practical. This may be because the cues are internal (e.g., memories, thoughts), are not immediately available (e.g., public performance), or cannot practically be evoked (e.g., catastrophic fears such as the death of a family member). In addition, some patients may be too anxious to start with *in vivo* exposure. In such cases, imaginal exposure may be used.

Imaginal exposure involves having patients imagine themselves coming in contact with external cues, or, into cases where the cues are memories or thoughts, having patients deliberately evoke internal cues. This is typically done with a patient sitting in a relaxed position with eyes closed, speaking into a tape recorder while attempting to visualize the cues.

When doing exposure to a memory, the patient is asked to narrate the sequence of events. In order to help the patient contact the relevant anxiety-provoking cues, the therapist may prompt the patient by asking about specific sensations and emotions experienced at the time. In the case of an imagined scenario (e.g., the house has burned down because the patient forget to check that the stove was off), the therapist narrates the scenario while periodically asking the patient what he or she would be thinking, feeling, sensing, or doing, as a way to help the patient visualize. Such a scenario should include all of the patient's catastrophic fears. Patients who fear specific thoughts may be asked to speak the thoughts onto a 30-second loop tape (the kind used in answering machines) and to listen to the tape repeatedly.

Forms of imaginal exposure other than tape-recorded scenarios include having the patient write about a feared cue or memory, or draw or paint something related to the cue. Another form of imaginal exposure, particularly useful for patients with social phobia, is role playing. The therapist and the patient can act out imaginary social interactions that are similar to the social situations that the patient fears.

Steps in Conducting Exposure

There are four steps in doing either imaginal or *in vivo* exposure with patients: (1) preparation, (2) creation of an exposure hierarchy, (3) initial exposure, and (4) repeated exposure.

1. *Preparation.* Exposure is a demanding treatment that requires patients to tolerate fairly high initial levels of anxiety. Patients need to be prepared before exposure is initiated. The rationale for exposure and its procedures should be clearly explained. Any concerns patients have should be discussed. Advantages and disadvantages of doing exposure may be reviewed. Finally, a commitment to proceed with exposure should be obtained. For some patients, this process may be very brief; for more fearful patients, it may extend over several sessions.

2. *Creation of an exposure hierarchy.* The beginning of the next step is for the patient to describe all of the cues that evoke anxiety in him or her. The patient is then taught to rate his or her anxiety on a scale from 0 (no anxiety) to 10 (the most anxiety the patient has ever felt). These are called "subjective units of distress" or "SUDs" ratings. The patient assigns a SUDs rating to each cue based on the anxiety he or she feels when encountering the cue, or, if it is a cue that is always avoided, the anxiety the patient imagines he or she would feel upon coming in contact with it. The cues are then listed and ranked from least to most anxiety-provoking. Such a list is referred to as an "exposure hierarchy." Several chapters of this book provide forms that enable patients with different anxiety disorders to develop exposure hierarchies (see Forms 3.5, 7.4, 8.5, and 8.6).

The cues on an exposure hierarchy may all be different but related to a central theme. For example, a man with social phobia may have diverse items on his hierarchy all related to his fears of being judged or rejected, such as calling a friend to make plans, attending a party with strangers, and asking someone for a date. Alternatively, a hierarchy may consist of progressively closer approaches to a single highly feared situation. For example, a woman with a specific phobia of elevators may have a hierarchy consisting of imagining being on an elevator, standing in front of an elevator, getting on an elevator with the doors open, riding the elevator one floor, and riding an elevator to the top of a tall building.

3. *Initial exposure.* If all of the items on a patient's hierarchy evoke substantial fear, the least anxiety-provoking item is chosen for the initial exposure. If some items provoke only minimal fear (SUDs ratings of 3 or less), it is best to start with an item that evokes moderate anxiety (SUDs rating of 4 or greater).

The initial exposure should take place during a therapy session. Because patients can take an hour or more to habituate to a new cue, the first exposure session should be scheduled for at least 90 minutes. If patients habituate more quickly, as they often do once they are used to the procedure, subsequent exposure sessions may be shortened to 45 minutes.

During the initial exposure, a patient is introduced to an anxiety-provoking cue and asked to remain in contact with it. If the cue is an object, the patient stays in contact with the object until he or she habituates. If the cue is a situation, memory, or scenario that lasts a discrete period of time, the cue is repeated until the patient habituates.

The patient is asked for SUDs ratings every 5 minutes during the exposure. Typically, patients' SUDs ratings will rise initially, plateau, and then begin to decline. Exposure should continue until the SUDs rating has dropped by at least half. It is important that exposure not be terminated before a patient's anxiety has dropped; otherwise, the connection between the cue and the anxiety response will be strengthened rather than weakened.

4. *Repeated exposure.* After the initial exposure, the patient is assigned to repeat the exposure on his or her own as homework, usually daily. The patient tracks his or her own SUDs ratings and continues each exposure session until the SUDs rating decreases by half. Forms A.1 and A.2 can be given to patients for tracking exposure practice, both in sessions and as homework. With repetition, the peak SUDs rating obtained during each exposure exercise will decline. Exposure should be repeated until the cue evokes minimal anxiety. An exposure that the patient has been practicing at home may be repeated in the next therapy session to assess the degree to which the patient has habituated. Once the cue no longer evokes anxiety, the patient moves up to the next item on the exposure hierarchy.

Problems with Exposure

Exposure is most effective when it consists of clearly specified tasks that (1) evoke anxiety, (2) are prolonged until habituation takes place, and (3) are repeated until the fear response decreases across repetitions (Foa & Kozak, 1986). When exposure is not effective, it is usually because one or more of these criteria have not been met.

An initial exposure may fail to evoke anxiety for one of two reasons: (1) The exposure task does not include the relevant anxiety-provoking cues; or (2) the patient is engaging in some subtle form of avoidance, such as attempts at self-distraction (e.g., daydreaming) or not fully engaging with the cues (e.g., attending a party but avoiding talking to anyone). If the task does not include anxiety provoking cues, new tasks should be tried. If the patient is avoiding contact with the cues during exposure, he or she should be encouraged to attend actively to and interact with the cues.

If patients' SUDs rating do not drop during exposure, it is generally because exposure has not continued long enough. Even when the therapist extends exposure sessions to allow time for habituation, patients will often fail to allow enough time during exposure homework. Patients should be told to continue exposures until their SUDs ratings decline by half, regardless of the time taken. It is better to do fewer exposures of sufficient length than to do many short exposures during which habituation does not occur.

Finally, when patients fail to show a reduction of anxiety in response to a cue over time, it is likely that exposure has not been repeated sufficiently. Exposure should continue until the peak anxiety evoked by the cue on any given day is minimal. (See Chapters 3, 5, 6, 7, and 8 for case examples using exposure.)

FORM A.1. Patient's Imaginal Exposure Practice Record

Patient's Name: _____ Week: _____

Instructions: Each day that you do exposure, please note the imagined situation practiced. Then note the highest level of distress you feel for each trial (repetition) of the exposure. Repeat the exposure until the highest distress on the last trial is less than half the highest distress on the first trial for that day.

Date: _____		Date: _____		Date: _____	
Exposure: _____		Exposure: _____		Exposure: _____	
_____		_____		_____	
Trial	Maximum Distress (0–10)	Trial	Maximum Distress (0–10)	Trial	Maximum Distress (0–10)
1		1		1	
2		2		2	
3		3		3	
4		4		4	
5		5		5	
6		6		6	
7		7		7	
8		8		8	
9		9		9	
10		10		10	
Date: _____		Date: _____		Date: _____	
Exposure: _____		Exposure: _____		Exposure: _____	
_____		_____		_____	
Trial	Maximum Distress (0–10)	Trial	Maximum Distress (0–10)	Trial	Maximum Distress (0–10)
1		1		1	
2		2		2	
3		3		3	
4		4		4	
5		5		5	
6		6		6	
7		7		7	
8		8		8	
9		9		9	
10		10		10	

FORM A.2. Patient's *In Vivo* Exposure Practice Record

Patient's Name: _____ Week: _____

Instructions: Each day that you practice exposure, please note the trigger or situation you are working on. Then note the level of distress when you feel when you first begin the exposure and every 5 minutes after that. Continue the exposure until the distress level has dropped by at least half.

Date: _____ Exposure: _____ _____	Date: _____ Exposure: _____ _____	Date: _____ Exposure: _____ _____
Time Distress (0–10)	Time Distress (0–10)	Time Distress (0–10)
Initial	Initial	Initial
:05	:05	:05
:10	:10	:10
:15	:15	:15
:20	:20	:20
:25	:25	:25
:30	:30	:30
:35	:35	:35
:40	:40	:40
:45	:45	:45
:50	:50	:50
:55	:55	:55
:60	:60	:60

Date: _____ Exposure: _____ _____	Date: _____ Exposure: _____ _____	Date: _____ Exposure: _____ _____
Time Distress (0–10)	Time Distress (0–10)	Time Distress (0–10)
Initial	Initial	Initial
:05	:05	:05
:10	:10	:10
:15	:15	:15
:20	:20	:20
:25	:25	:25
:30	:30	:30
:35	:35	:35
:40	:40	:40
:45	:45	:45
:50	:50	:50
:55	:55	:55
:60	:60	:60

Contraindications

Because of the high levels of initial anxiety that may be experienced during exposure, it should not be undertaken with patients who are currently in crises, abusing drugs or alcohol, or psychotic.

For some disorders, such as social phobia, it is common to have patients practice relaxation during exposure (see "Application Practice" under "Relaxation" in this appendix). However, relaxation should not be used during exposure when the patient's own anxiety symptoms are cues that trigger anxiety and are, therefore, subjects of exposure. For example, a patient with social phobia who fears being seen with his hand shaking in a social situation needs to deliberately make his hand shake during exposure in order to discover that there are no negative consequences to this behavior. Using relaxation to suppress the hand shaking would prevent complete exposure. Similarly, relaxation should never be used during exposure for OCD patients, as they are likely to turn relaxation into another ritual rather than realize that their anxiety will decrease on its own.

GRADED TASK ASSIGNMENT

Graded task assignment may be used when a patient feels too depressed and hopeless or too anxious to begin a complex or demanding task (Beck et al., 1979). The therapist helps the patient break the task into smaller components. The patient is then asked to attempt only one small step at a time. For example, a patient who feels paralyzed at the thought of writing a résumé can be asked to write down the name of one company he or she used to work for. When that is done, the patient can be asked next to write down as many others as he or she can remember. Then he or she can write down approximate dates of employment. After succeeding at these very simple tasks, the patient can be given greater challenges, such as writing a rough draft of the resumé. These activities start in a session (especially for very depressed patients), but are then extended as homework. Typically patients feel less hopeless and overwhelmed and more motivated as they discover they can succeed with small steps. Often they will proceed to complete the task on their own.

REBREATHING

Rebreathing is used for patients with panic disorder who hyperventilate when they are anxious. Since many of their symptoms are the result of increased oxygen intake, the purpose of rebreathing is to decrease oxygen and increase CO_2. Patients are taught to "rebreathe" air they have already exhaled. This is accomplished by having the patients cup their hands over their mouths and breathe into their hands. Alternatively, patients may be asked to breathe into a paper lunch bag. Rebreathing is continued until the symptoms of hyperventilation, such as light-headedness, decrease. The technique should be practiced first in a session, by having a patient deliberately hyperventilate and then use rebreathing. The technique is then practiced as homework.

Rhythmic breathing, described below under "Breathing Relaxation," may also be used to restore oxygen balance. When used for this purpose, the exhalation should be made slightly longer than the inhalation (e.g., a patient may inhale to a count of 4 and exhale to a count of 5 or 6).

RELAXATION

Almost any form of relaxation can benefit patients, from commercially prepared tapes to meditation. Most research-based relaxation treatments have been based on variations of progressive muscle relaxation, which was first developed by Jacobson (1938). Typically, patients are taught a series of progressively shorter exercises designed to condition a relaxation response that can ultimately be evoked in a matter of seconds. The full sequence of progressive muscle relaxation exercises is described below, followed by a description of breathing relaxation exercises, which can be taught in less time and may be used when teaching the entire progressive muscle sequence does not appear necessary or practical.

Progressive Muscle Relaxation

Relaxation training should start with providing the patient with a rationale for the treatment. Relaxation is presented as a method for counteracting the patient's physiological responses to anxiety. This should be tied to the symptoms that most concern the patient (e.g., palpitations, sweating, insomnia, etc.). Relaxation should be described as a skill that the patient can learn to gain greater control of his or her own bodily responses. Like all skills, relaxation requires practice to master. The patient should be told that the goal is to provide him or her with a rapid, reliable, and portable means for coping with anxiety. The sequence of exercises described below is based on those of Barlow and Cerny (1988), Ost (1987), and Clark (1989).

Twelve-Muscle-Group Relaxation

Before starting the exercise, you, the therapist, should explain to the patient that you will be asking him or her first to tense and then to relax different groups of muscles. The purpose is to help the patient notice the difference between tension and relaxation. Describe the full exercise, and demonstrate the 12 muscle groups as follows:

1. Lower arms: Tightening the fists and pulling them up.
2. Upper arms: Tensing the arms by the side of the body.
3. Lower legs: Extending the legs and pointing the feet up.
4. Thighs: Pushing the legs together.
5. Stomach: Pushing it back toward the spine.
6. Upper chest and back: Inhaling into the upper lungs and holding for a count of 10.
7. Shoulders: Picking them up toward the ears.
8. Back of the neck: Pushing the head back.
9. Lips: Pursing the lips without clenching the teeth.
10. Eyes: Squinting with eyes closed.
11. Eyebrows: Pushing them together.
12. Upper forehead and scalp: Raising the eyebrows.

Next have the patient assume a comfortable seated position, with both legs on the floor, while you narrate the relaxation exercise. This should be audiotaped so that the patient can practice the exercise at home. The patient may keep his or her eyes open during the training in order to follow you, but should close the eyes when practicing.

Tell the patient to focus on his or her breathing. After two or three breaths, begin the instructions for tensing each muscle group. Name the muscle group and instruct the patient to tense it while you count to 5 and then say, "Release." You can demonstrate by doing the exercise along with the patient. There should be a pause of 15 to 20 seconds between each muscle group, during which time you should give suggestions for relaxation, such as the following:

"Notice the difference between the tension and the relaxation."
"Feel the muscles grow more relaxed."
"Let the muscles grow soft and warm."
"Continue breathing easily."

After completing all 12 muscle groups, instruct the patient to focus again on his or her breathing. Then say, "I am now going to count you down from 5 to 1. With each count, you will grow more relaxed." Begin counting, timing each count with an exhalation if possible, and allowing one or two breaths between each count. Between each count, give further suggestions for relaxation, such as these:

"Feel the relaxation spreading down from the top of your head, through your face and neck."
"Feel it spreading down through your shoulders and your arms, down through your torso."
"Feel it going down through your legs and feet."
"Feel the relaxation spreading through your whole body. You are growing more and more deeply relaxed."

After reaching the count of 1, instruct the patient to focus again on breathing and to say "Relax" to himself or herself with each exhalation. After a minute or two, tell the patient, "I am now going to count you up from 1 to 5. With each count you will become a little more alert, while staying very relaxed, until on 5 you open your eyes." Then count the patient up from 1 to 5, again timing the count with the patient's breathing. On 5, instruct the patient to open his or her eyes.

The patient should be assigned to practice relaxation twice a day. Practice at first should *not* take place during stressful situations. Emphasize that relaxation is a skill, and that as with any skill, it takes time to get good at it. The patient may not feel much relaxation at first, but will find that over time he or she is able to become deeply relaxed.

Some patients have difficulty with this exercise, because they become so focused on trying to relax that they make themselves more tense. These patients should be told that their goal is not to relax; rather, it is simply to follow the instructions on the tape. Other patients report muscle soreness after trying the exercise. They are usually applying too much tension. They should be instructed to use only three-quarters tension when tightening their muscles. Patients with abuse histories sometimes have difficulty letting go of enough control to relax. They can be assigned to practice a few muscle groups for a week in order to get used to the exercise, and then to build up to all 12 muscle groups.

After practicing for a week with the tape, the patient should be instructed to begin doing the exercise without the tape and to practice it in various positions and times of day (e.g., sitting with feet up, lying in bed, sitting in an office chair).

Eight-Muscle-Group Relaxation

Once the patient has mastered the full-length muscle relaxation procedure described above (generally 1–3 weeks), eight-muscle-group relaxation can be taught. The patient is told that the goal is to help him or her achieve the same level of relaxation in a briefer time. The instructions are the same as for 12-muscle-group relaxation, except that only the groups listed below are used.

1. Whole arms: Slightly extended, elbows bent, fists tightened and pulled back.
2. Whole legs: Extended, toes pointed up.
3. Stomach: Pushing it back toward the spine.
4. Upper chest and back: Inhaling into the upper lungs and holding for a count of 10.
5. Shoulders: Picking them up toward the ears.
6. Back of the neck: Pushing the head back.
7. Face: Squinting eyes, scrunching features toward tip of the nose.
8. Forehead and scalp: Raising eyebrows.

The time between tensing each muscle group should be lengthened to a minimum of 30 seconds. The rest of the exercise (i.e., counting down, breathing while saying "Relax," counting up) remains the same. This exercise may be audiotaped, but patients should be encouraged to practice without the tape as soon as they have learned the sequence.

Four-Muscle-Group Relaxation

Relaxation with just four muscle groups further shortens the time needed to relax. Proceed as with the eight-muscle-group relaxation, but use only the following muscle groups:

1. Whole arms: Slightly extended, elbows bent, fists tightened and pulled back.
2. Upper chest and back: Inhaling into the upper lungs and holding for a count of 10.
3. Shoulders and neck: Slightly hunching the shoulders and pushing the head back.
4. Face: Squinting eyes, scrunching features toward tip of the nose.

For homework, have the patient practice this exercise in a variety of positions and settings (e.g., waiting for a bus, walking, sitting at a desk).

Release-Only Relaxation

The purpose of the release-only exercise is to have patients begin to relax without first using tension. The same four muscle groups are used as in the prior exercise. The patient is asked to focus on the first muscle group, noticing any tension that is present. He or she is then asked to recall the sensation of relaxation and to relax the muscles. Allow 30 to 45 seconds and give relaxation suggestions, as before. Then ask the patient to signal if the muscles are not fully relaxed by raising one finger. If they are fully relaxed, proceed to the next muscle group. If not, repeat the instructions. If a muscle group is still not fully relaxed, have the patient tense and then release that muscle group. After all four muscle groups are relaxed, follow the usual procedure for counting down, repeating "Relax," and counting up.

If the patient is able to relax all four muscle groups without first tensing, have him or her practice this exercise during the next week. If not, have the patient continue to practice the four-muscle-group relaxation, occasionally trying release-only relaxation until he or she is able to master it.

Cue-Controlled Relaxation

Cue-controlled relaxation is the final exercise in progressive muscle relaxation. To teach it, have the patient do release-only relaxation and signal when he or she is fully relaxed. Then instruct the patient to take one to three deep breaths and think "Relax" with each exhalation, while scanning the body for any tension and releasing it. "Relax" becomes the cue to signal the patient's body to relax. Once the patient has learned this exercise, it should be repeated in session without being preceded by the release-only procedure. Patients are then instructed to practice cue-controlled relaxation 10 to 15 times each day, in a variety of settings. Certain cues may be established as reminders to relax (e.g., looking at a watch, stopping at a red light, hearing the phone ring, etc.). Patients may also stick small colored dots in various places (on a mirror, on a desk, on the phone, etc.) as prompts for relaxation.

Application Practice

At each stage of training, patients are instructed to practice relaxation in non-anxiety-provoking situations. However, in order to be most effective, the relaxation exercises must be applied in situations where the patients feel anxious. Patients should be taught to recognize early warning signs of anxiety, and to apply the techniques before they become highly anxious. Application practice should be done daily.

Breathing Relaxation

Breathing relaxation exercises are brief and may be used when the more extensive muscle relaxation training described above is not practical. These exercises may also be particularly helpful for patients whose anxiety manifests itself as difficulty breathing. For some patients, a combination of progressive muscle relaxation (with 12 or 8 muscle groups) plus one or two breathing relaxation exercises can be very effective.

Before patients are taught any of the breathing exercises, they should be taught diaphragmatic breathing. Often patients are used to breathing only into their upper chests, sucking their abdomens in as they breathe. This can lead to hyperventilation and other breathing difficulties. In diaphragmatic breathing, the diaphragm at the base of the lungs is distended, which pushes the abdomen out and draws air into the lower lungs. You should first model diaphragmatic breathing for a patient by placing your hand on your own abdomen, and then pushing it in as you exhale and out as you inhale. The patient is then asked to do the same, continuing breathing in and out for approximately 2 minutes. Patients should be instructed to take normal-size breaths while doing this, rather than unusually large breaths, in order to avoid hyperventilation. Some patients will need to practice diaphragmatic breathing for a week before they can be taught the relaxation exercises. Once taught, the exercises should be practiced several times a day.

Holding the Breath

Inhale through the nose for a count of 3, drawing air into the lower lungs. Hold the breath for a count of 3. Then release the breath through pursed lips, while saying "Relax" to yourself.

Rhythmic Breathing

Inhale through the nose for a count of between 3 and 6. Choose a count that feels comfortable to you. Exhale through the nose for the same count. Do not hold the breath in between. Continue breathing in this rhythm for up to several minutes.

Counting Breaths

The breath-counting exercise is adapted from Zen meditation, and can be particularly helpful for patients who find that their minds race when they are anxious. This exercise may be used for a minute or two as a brief form of relaxation, or it may be extended for 15 minutes or longer as a form of meditation.

Sit in a comfortable position, with the back relatively straight. Keep the eyes open and allow them to focus on the floor a yard or two in front of you. Breathe through the nose. Count each exhalation silently to yourself. When you reach 10, start again at 1. If your mind wanders and you lose track of the count (which is likely to happen), simply return to counting at 1.

SELF-REWARD

Many depressed or anxious patients fail to reward themselves for positive behaviors, with predictable consequences: low motivation and depressed or anxious mood. They often believe that they should punish themselves (e.g., with self-critical thoughts) for failures rather than rewarding themselves for successes. Providing them with information about basic principles of reinforcement can be very helpful. In addition, patients should be told that it is important that rewards be administered as soon after positive behaviors as possible.

The steps in teaching self-reward are (1) listing possible rewards, (2) setting criteria for rewards, and (3) administering rewards.

1. *Listing rewards.* Patients are asked to make a list of possible rewards. One of the most effective rewards, of course, is self-praise. Tangible rewards may also be used, such as having a pleasurable snack, watching a favorite TV program, or talking on the phone to a friend. Larger rewards for greater accomplishments may also be used, such as getting a massage or going out to a fancy dinner. (If a patient is also engaging in behavioral activation, the list of rewarding activities developed for that purpose can be used, and other rewards that are not activities per se can be added to it. See "Behavioral Activation," above.)

2. *Setting criteria for rewards.* Next, patients should list positive behaviors with specific, identifiable criteria to be met in order to earn a reward. Patients should be encouraged to reward themselves for steps toward larger goals, rather than waiting until an entire task is complete. Thus, a patient might decide to reward himself or herself with a 10-minute break for every hour worked on a paper, and then with a favorite dessert once the paper is done.

3. *Administering rewards.* Finally, patients are asked to write down the rewards they give themselves. Patients should also be encouraged to reward themselves, especially with self-praise, for unplanned tasks or accomplishments.

Although self-reward is most often used with depressed patients, anxious patients can use self-reward to provide motivation for accomplishing treatment goals, such as facing a particularly difficult exposure task or going for a week without ritualizing.

THOUGHT STOPPING

Thought stopping may be used when a patient is overwhelmed by ruminative thinking or intrusive images. It is useful as a temporary coping measure until the patient can be taught to respond effectively to the negative thoughts or to do exposure to the intrusive images. It will often be helpful to follow thought stopping with a distracting activity. The steps for teaching thought stopping are (1) description of the technique, (2) demonstration, and (3) practice.

1. *Description of the technique.* The therapist should first describe the procedure to the patient and explain the rationale for its use.

2. *Demonstration.* Next, the patient is asked to bring to mind some upsetting thought or image. After a few moments, the therapist says "Stop!" in a loud voice and claps his or her hands. The patient is then asked what happened to the thought; generally, patients will report that they stopped thinking about it. This procedure is repeated several times. The patient is then asked to attempt the procedure independently, first by saying "Stop!" out loud and clapping his or her hands. After a few repetitions, the patient is asked to try saying "Stop!" silently and picturing a large stop sign.

3. *Practice.* The patient should then be assigned to practice this technique several times daily, or whenever he or she has intrusive or ruminative thoughts.

One contraindication for thought stopping should be noted: It is not recommended for patients with obsessive–compulsive disorder, as it is contrary to the goal of helping these patients tolerate rather than avoid their thoughts.

VISUALIZATION

Visualization combines elements of relaxation and distraction. During visualization, patients imagine themselves in a place or situation they find pleasant and relaxing. It may be a place they have really been (such as a favorite vacation spot or a place they loved in childhood), or it may be an imaginary scene. As in teaching thought stopping, the steps in teaching visualization are (1) description of the technique, (2) demonstration, and (3) practice.

1. *Description of the technique.* The therapist first explains the procedure. The patient is then asked to choose a place or image to use.

2. *Demonstration.* The therapist next has the patient engage in either progressive muscle relaxation or breathing relaxation. Relaxation is deepened by counting the patient down from 5 to 1 while the patient focuses on his or her breathing. During this count, suggestions may be given for relaxation, or the patient may be asked to imagine himself or herself descending a flight of stairs. When 1 is reached, the patient is asked to imagine that he or she is in the scene. The therapist may give prompts to aid visualization, such as "Imagine what you smell, what feelings you have on your skin, what you see," and so on. After several minutes, the therapist counts the patient up from 1 to 5 and has the patient open his or her eyes. This procedure may be audiotaped for use by the patient in practice.

3. *Practice.* Patients are assigned to practice visualization as homework. At first, they may listen to the audiotape made by the therapist. Eventually, they should practice the technique without the tape, doing relaxation and counting themselves down before entering the image. They may then continue the image as long as they like.

APPENDIX B

Review of Selected
Cognitive Concepts and Techniques

INTRODUCTION TO COGNITIVE AND COGNITIVE-BEHAVIORAL THERAPY

The basic premise of cognitive approaches to therapy is that dysfunctional or distorted ways of thinking can cause or exacerbate dysfunctional emotions and behaviors. Cognitive interventions identify and target specific distorted automatic thoughts, maladaptive assumptions, and negative or otherwise dysfunctional schemas. The cognitive-behavioral therapist also utilizes behavioral interventions (e.g., behavioral activation and exposure) to assist the patient in testing and challenging cognitive distortions. An information handout for patients about cognitive-behavioral therapy is provided in Form B.1.

THE THREE LEVELS OF COGNITIVE DISTORTIONS

Beck identifies cognitive distortions at three levels of thinking: "automatic thoughts," "assumptions," and "schemas." Automatic thoughts are thoughts that come spontaneously and seem plausible to a person, but they may become distorted in depressed or anxious patients. Distorted automatic thoughts can be associated with negative affect or dysfunctional behavior. They can be arranged into specific categories (see Form B.2, which is also a handout for patients).

Assumptions are at a deeper cognitive level than automatic thoughts; they are more abstract and generalized. In depressed or anxious patients, assumptions can become maladaptive: They take the form of a set of rules, "shoulds," imperatives, or "if–then" statements that can have disabling effects. Examples of some maladaptive assumptions are provided in Form B.3 (another patient handout).

Schemas exist at a still more fundamental level than assumptions; they reflect deep-seated models of the self and others. Depressed or anxious patients may have a selective focus on certain schemas that mark their vulnerability. Beck, Freeman, and Associates (1990) have identified a variety of negative or otherwise dysfunctional schemas that characterize the various personality disorders (see Table B.1), as well as various types of attempts to avoid or compensate for these

FORM B.1. General Information for Patients about Cognitive-Behavioral Therapy

Issues	Answers
General description	Cognitive-behavioral therapy is a relatively short-term, focused psychotherapy for a wide range of psychological problems, including depression, anxiety, anger, marital conflict, fears, and substance abuse/ dependence. The focus of therapy is on how you are thinking (your "cognitions"), behaving, and communicating *today,* rather than on your early childhood experiences. Numerous studies have demonstrated that cognitive-behavioral therapy is as effective as medication for depression, anxiety, obsessions, and other fears. Furthermore, because patients learn self-help in therapy, they are often able to maintain their improvement after therapy has been completed.
Evaluation of patients	When you begin cognitive-behavioral therapy, your therapist will ask you to fill out several self-report forms that assess a range of symptoms and problems. These forms evaluate depression, anxiety, anger, fears, physical complaints, personality, and relationships. The purpose of this evaluation is to gather as much information on you as possible, so that you and your therapist can learn quickly what kinds of problems you do (or do not) have and the extent of your problems.
Treatment plans	You and your therapist will work together to develop a plan of therapy. This might include how often you need to come; the relevance of medication; your diagnosis; your goals; skill acquisition; needed changes in the way you think, behave, and communicate; and other factors.
What are therapy sessions like?	Some other forms of therapy are unstructured, but in cognitive-behavioral therapy you and your therapist will set an agenda for each meeting. The agenda might include a review of your experience in the previous session, your homework, one or two current problems, a review of what you've accomplished in this session, and homework for the next week. The goal is to solve problems, not just complain about them.
Self-help homework	If you went to a personal trainer at a health club, you would expect to get guidance on how to exercise when the trainer is not there. The same thing is true in cognitive-behavioral therapy. What you learn in therapy is what you practice *outside* of therapy on your own. Research demonstrates that patients who carry out homework assignments get better faster and stay better longer. Your self-help homework might include keeping track of your moods, thoughts, and behaviors; scheduling activities; developing goals; challenging your negative thoughts; collecting information; changing the way you communicate with others; and other assignments.

(cont.)

FORM B.1. General Information about Cognitive-Behavioral Therapy (p. 2 of 2)

Issues	Answers
Aren't my problems due to my childhood experiences?	*Part* of your problems may be due to how your parents, siblings, and peers treated you, but your solutions to your problems lie in what you are thinking and doing *today.* However, with many people we do find it useful at times to review the sources of your problems and help you learn how to change the way you think about them now.
Aren't my problems due to biochemistry?	*Part* of your problems may be due to biochemistry, but many other factors—such as the way you think, behave, and relate, as well as current and past life events—are important. Using cognitive-behavioral therapy does not rule out the use of medication. For most psychiatric disorders, there is considerable evidence that cognitive-behavioral therapy is as effective as medication. For very serious levels of depression and anxiety, we believe that it may be best to combine medication with therapy. An advantage of cognitive-behavioral therapy is that you also learn ways to solve your problems on your own.
How will I know if I'm getting better?	You and your therapist can identify specific goals at the beginning of therapy—and you can modify these goals as you continue. Then you can evaluate whether you are becoming less depressed, anxious, angry, or the like. You should feel free to give your therapist feedback on your progress. This feedback from you is useful in order to figure out what works and what doesn't work.
How can I learn more about cognitive-behavioral therapy?	Depending on the problems that you want to solve, your therapist can recommend a number of books or other readings for you. We believe that the more you know about yourself, the better off you will be. We hope that you can learn to become your own therapist.

FORM B.2. Categories of Distorted Automatic Thoughts: A Guide for Patients

1. **Mind reading:** You assume that you know what people think without having sufficient evidence of their thoughts. "He thinks I'm a loser."
2. **Fortunetelling:** You predict the future negatively: Things will get worse, or there is danger ahead. "I'll fail that exam," or "I won't get the job."
3. **Catastrophizing:** You believe that what has happened or will happen will be so awful and unbearable that you won't be able to stand it. "It would be terrible if I failed."
4. **Labeling:** You assign global negative traits to yourself and others. "I'm undesirable," or "He's a rotten person."
5. **Discounting positives:** You claim that the positive things you or others do are trivial. "That's what wives are supposed to do—so it doesn't count when she's nice to me," or "Those successes were easy, so they don't matter."
6. **Negative filtering:** You focus almost exclusively on the negatives and seldom notice the positives. "Look at all of the people who don't like me."
7. **Overgeneralizing:** You perceive a global pattern of negatives on the basis of a single incident. "This generally happens to me. I seem to fail at a lot of things."
8. **Dichotomous thinking:** You view events or people in all-or-nothing terms. "I get rejected by everyone," or "It was a complete waste of time."
9. **Shoulds:** You interpret events in terms of how things should be, rather than simply focusing on what is. "I should do well. If I don't, then I'm a failure."
10. **Personalizing:** You attribute a disproportionate amount of the blame to yourself for negative events, and you fail to see that certain events are also caused by others. "The marriage ended because I failed."
11. **Blaming:** You focus on the other person as the *source of* your negative feelings, and you refuse to take responsibility for changing yourself. "She's to blame for the way I feel now," or "My parents caused all my problems."
12. **Unfair comparisons:** You interpret events in terms of standards that are unrealistic—for example, you focus primarily on others who do better than you and find yourself inferior in the comparison. "She's more successful than I am," or "Others did better than I did on the test."
13. **Regret orientation:** You focus on the idea that you could have done better in the past, rather on what you can do better now. "I could have had a better job if I had tried," or "I shouldn't have said that."
14. **What if?:** You keep asking a series of questions about "what if" something happens, and you fail to be satisfied with any of the answers. "Yeah, but what if I get anxious?" or "What if I can't catch my breath?"
15. **Emotional reasoning:** You let your feelings guide your interpretation of reality. "I feel depressed; therefore, my marriage is not working out."
16. **Inability to disconfirm:** You reject any evidence or arguments that might contradict your negative thoughts. For example, when you have the thought "I'm unlovable," you reject as *irrelevant* any evidence that people like you. Consequently, your thought cannot be refuted. "That's not the real issue. There are deeper problems. There are other factors."
17. **Judgment focus:** You view yourself, others, and events in terms of evaluations as good–bad or superior–inferior, rather than simply describing, accepting, or understanding. You are continually measuring yourself and others according to arbitrary standards, and finding that you and others fall short. You are focused on the judgments of others as well as your own judgments of yourself. "I didn't perform well in college," or "If I take up tennis, I won't do well," or "Look how successful she is. I'm not successful."

FORM B.3. Examples of Maladaptive Assumptions: A Guide for Patients

"I should be successful at everything I try."

"If I am not successful, then I am a failure."

"If I fail, then I'm worthless [I'm unlovable, life is not worth living, etc.]."

"Failure is intolerable and unacceptable."

"I should get the approval of everyone."

"If I am not approved of, then I am unlovable [ugly, worthless, hopeless, alone, etc.]."

"I should be certain before I try something."

"If I am not certain, then the outcome will be negative."

"I should never be anxious [depressed, selfish, confused, uncertain, unhappy with my partner, etc.]."

"I should always keep my eye out for any anxiety."

"If I let my guard down, something bad will happen."

"If people see that I am anxious, they will think less of me [reject me, humiliate me, etc.]."

"My sex life [feelings, behaviors, relationships, etc.] should be wonderful and easy at all times."

schemas. For example, patients with obsessive–compulsive personality disorder (which, incidentally, is *not* the same thing as the anxiety disorder called obsessive–compulsive disorder) attempt to compensate for their problems by trying to achieve perfection, or, in some cases, they may avoid any tasks in which mistakes appear probable. These compensatory and avoidant strategies are also targets for cognitive therapy.

These three levels of cognitive distortions are related in a hierarchical fashion, such that distorted automatic thoughts are the most directly and easily accessible, followed by maladaptive assumptions and then dysfunctional schemas. For example, consider a female patient who goes to a party and thinks of approaching a man. Her automatic thought might be "He'll reject me." The underlying assumption could be "I need to be approved of by men in order to like myself." The patient's schema about herself might be "I'm unlovable," and her schema about men might be "Men are rejecting." These different levels are depicted in Table B.2.

In therapy with a depressed or anxious patient, the therapist may elicit cognitive distortions at any level and intervene at any level. For example, the therapist may challenge automatic thoughts or focus on underlying assumptions or schemas. Or, if the therapist takes a more behavioral approach, he or she may wish to modify the environment to avoid specific "activating events."

IDENTIFYING AND CHALLENGING COGNITIVE DISTORTIONS

As just indicated, the essence of cognitive therapy is intervening with a patient's cognitive distortions at any level required. The therapist takes an active role in inquiring about and challenging the patient's thinking. The usual procedure in practice is to begin by working with the patient's distorted automatic thoughts, and then to do the same with maladaptive assumptions and dysfunctional schemas as needed.

Once the therapist has educated the patient about the nature of automatic thoughts and the various categories into which distorted thoughts can be classified (Form B.2 is helpful in this regard), the patient is told that moods (such as sadness or anxiety) are related to the thoughts he or she is having at the time. The patient is therefore asked to keep regular records of events in his or her life and the moods and thoughts related to them, as well as to rate the intensity of these moods. The Patient's Event–Mood–Thought Record (Form B.4) can be used for this purpose; the Patient's Daily Record of Dysfunctional Automatic Thoughts (see Form 2.7 in Chapter 2) can also be used, once the patient has received some coaching in methods of developing rational responses to automatic thoughts (see below). The identification of maladaptive assumptions and dysfunctional schemas is usually not as easy for a patient as the identification of distorted automatic thoughts; therefore, these two types of cognitive distortions are usually identified by the patient and therapist working together in sessions.

Once a patient's automatic thoughts, assumptions, or schemas have been identified, they are subjected to any of a wide variety of cognitive (and sometimes behavioral) challenges. In each case, the ultimate goal of this process of challenging is the production of a "rational response"— that is, a new, more logical, more realistic, and more adaptive version of the original thought, assumption, or schema. For example, the maladaptive assumption "Something is wrong with me if I am anxious" can be replaced by the rational response "Anxiety is normal; everyone has anxiety."

TABLE B.1. Dysfunctional Schemas in Personality Disorders

Personality disorder	View of self	View of others	Main beliefs	Main compensatory/ avoidant strategies
Avoidant	Vulnerable to depreciation, rejection Socially inept Incompetent	Critical Demeaning Superior	"It's terrible to be rejected [put down]." "If people know the real me, they will reject me." "I can't tolerate unpleasant feelings."	Avoid evaluative situations Avoid unpleasant feelings or thoughts
Dependent	Needy Weak Helpless Incompetent	Idealized Nurturant Supportive Competent	"I need people to survive [be happy]." "I need a steady flow of support and encouragement."	Cultivate dependent relationships
Passive–aggressive	Self-sufficient Vulnerable to control, interference	Intrusive Demanding Interfering Controlling Dominating	"Others interfere with my freedom of action." "Control by others is intolerable." "I have to do things my own way."	Passive resistance Surface submissiveness Evade, circumvent rules
Obsessive–compulsive	Responsible Accountable Fastidious Competent	Irresponsible Casual Incompetent Self-indulgent	"I know what's best." "Details are crucial." "People should be better [try harder]."	Apply rules Perfectionism Evaluate, control Use "shoulds," criticize, punish

Disorder	View of self	View of others	Main beliefs	Main strategy
Paranoid	Righteous Innocent, noble Vulnerable	Interfering Malicious Discriminatory Abusive motives	"Motives are suspect." "Be on guard." "Don't trust."	Be wary Look for hidden motives Accuse Counterattack
Antisocial	Loner Autonomous Strong	Vulnerable Exploitative	"I'm entitled to break rules." "Others are patsies [wimps]." "Others are exploitative."	Attack, rob Deceive Manipulate
Narcissistic	Special, unique Deserving special rules, superior Above the rules	Inferior Admirers	"Since I'm special, I deserve special rules." "I'm above the rules." "I'm better than others."	Use others Transcend rules Be manipulative Be competitive
Histrionic	Glamorous Impressive	Seducible Receptive Admirers	"People are there to serve or admire me." "They have no right to deny me my just deserts."	Use dramatics, charm Throw temper tantrums, cry Make suicide gestures
Schizoid	Self-sufficient Loner	Intrusive	"Others are unrewarding." "Relationships are messy [undesirable]."	Stay away

Note. Adapted from Beck, Freeman, and Associates (1990). Copyright 1990 by The Guilford Press. Adapted by permission.

FORM B.4. Patient's Event–Mood–Thought Record

Patient's Name: _____

Date/time	**Event:** Describe what happened. What were you doing at the time?	**Mood:** Describe your feelings (sad, anxious, angry, hopeless, etc.), and rate their intensity on a 0–100% scale.	**Thought:** Write down your automatic thoughts at the time.

TABLE B.2. Relationship between Cognitive Levels

Event	Automatic thought	Maladaptive assumption	Schema (self and other)
Approaching man at a party.	He'll reject me.	I need the approval of men to like myself.	I'm unlovable. Men are rejecting.

Tables, forms, and in-text examples in several chapters of this book (see Tables 2.5 and 2.6; the examples given in the "Cognitive Interventions" section of Chapter 3; Form 3.6 and Table 3.3; Form 4.5 and Table 4.3; Tables 5.3 and 5.4; and Table 6.3) provide practical demonstrations of how cognitive distortions can be challenged and rational responses can be produced.

Table B.3 summarizes the cognitive techniques that can be used to identify and challenge cognitive distortions. More details about these are provided in the CD-ROM that accompanies this book.

TABLE B.3. Summary of Cognitive Techniques

Technique	Description or example
Socializing patient	
Establishing therapeutic contract	Directly ask the patient about commitment to therapy, such as willingness to come regularly and do homework.
Bibliotherapy	Assign readings, such as patient information handouts or books (e.g., Burns's *The Feeling Good Handbook*).
Indicating how thoughts create feelings	Example: "I feel anxious [mood] because I think I'll fail [thought]."
Distinguishing thoughts from facts	Example: "I can believe that it is raining outside, but that doesn't mean it's a fact. I need to collect evidence—go outside—to see whether it's raining."
Identifying and categorizing distorted automatic thoughts	
Identifying negative thoughts that come spontaneously and seem plausible	Examples: "I think I'll fail," "I always fail," "It's awful to fail."
Identifying the emotions these thoughts create	Examples: Sadness, anxiety.
Rating confidence in accuracy of thoughts, as well as intensity of feelings	Example: "I feel anxious [80%] because I think I'll fail [95%]."
Categorizing thoughts (see Form B.2 for complete list of categories)	Examples: "I think I'll fail" (fortunetelling), "I always fail" (dichotomous/all-or-nothing thinking), "It's awful to fail" (catastrophizing).
Challenging distorted automatic thoughts	
Providing direct psychoeducation	Example: Give information about elevator safety to a patient with a specific phobia of elevators.
Defining the terms (semantic analysis)	Example: Ask patient, "How would you define 'failure' and 'success'?"
Examining testability of thoughts	Can patient make any real-world observations that will confirm or refute thoughts?
Examining logic of thoughts	Is patient jumping to conclusions that don't follow logically from premises (e.g., "I'm a failure because I did poorly on that test")?
Examining limits on patient's information	Is patient jumping to conclusions without sufficient information? Is patient only looking for evidence that supports his or her thoughts, not evidence that might refute them?

Technique	Description or example
Vertical descent	Ask, "What would it mean [what would happen, why would it be a problem] if X occurred? What would happen next? And what would that mean [what would happen, why would it be a problem]?"
Double standard	Ask, "Would you apply the same thought [interpretation, standard] to others as you do to yourself? Why/why not?"
Challenging recursive self-criticism	Is patient locked in a loop of self-criticism for being self-critical (e.g., "I think I'm a loser because I'm depressed and I'm depressed because I think I'm a loser")?
Examining internal contradictions	Does patient have contradictory thoughts (e.g., "I'd like to meet as many people as possible, but I never want to be rejected")?
Reductio ad absurdum	Are implications of patient's thought absurd (e.g., "If I'm single, I'm unlovable; all people who are married were once single; therefore, all married people are unlovable")?
Distinguishing behaviors from persons	Example: Indicate how failing on an exam is different from being a failure as a person.
Challenging reification	In self-criticisms, is patient making "real" something that is abstract/unobservable (e.g., worthlessness)? Can patient change reifications into "preferences" (e.g., "I prefer doing better at exams")?
Examining variability/degrees of behavior	Help patient examine evidence that his or her behavior varies across time, situations, and persons, and that it occurs to varying degrees (not in all-or-nothing ways).
Weighing the evidence for and against a thought	Example of thought: "I'll get rejected." Evidence in favor: "I'm anxious [emotional reasoning]," "Sometimes people don't like me." Evidence against: "I'm a decent person," "Some people like me," "There's nothing rude or awful about saying hello to someone," "People are here at the party to meet other people." For: 25%. Against: 75%. Conclusion: "I don't have much convincing evidence that I'll get rejected. Nothing ventured, nothing gained."
Examining quality of evidence	Would patient's evidence stand up to scrutiny by others? Is patient using emotional reasoning and selective information to support arguments?
Keeping a daily log	Have patient keep a daily log of behaviors/events that confirm or disprove a thought.
Surveying others' opinions	Have patient survey others for their opinions and see whether these confirm or disprove a thought. *(cont.)*

TABLE B.3 *(cont.)*

Technique	Description or example
Cost–benefit analysis	Example of thought: "I need people's approval." Costs: "This thought makes me shy and anxious around people, and lowers my self-esteem." Benefits: "Maybe I'll try hard to get people's approval." Costs: 85%. Benefits: 15%.
Alternative interpretations	Example: Ask patient, "If someone doesn't like you, might it simply be that the two of you are different? Or perhaps the other person is in a bad mood, or shy, or involved with someone else? Or perhaps there are many other people who can and do like you?"
Negation of problems	Have patient list all the reasons why the current situation is not a problem, rather than all the reasons why it is a problem.
Defense attorney	Tell patient, "Imagine that you have hired yourself as an attorney to defend yourself. Write out the strongest case you can in favor of yourself, even if you don't believe it."
Carrying out an experiment	Have patient test a thought by engaging in behavior that challenges the thought (e.g., for the thought "I'll be rejected," approaching 10 people at a party).
Continuum technique	Have patient place current situation or event on a 0–100 continuum of negative outcomes and examine what would be better and worse than this situation/event.
Putting situation/event into perspective	What would patient still be able to do even if a negative thought were true? Or how does patient's situation compare to that of someone with, say, a life-threatening illness?
"Pie" technique	Have patient draw a "pie chart" and divide up responsibility for situation/event.
Examining mitigating factors; reattribution	Are there other causes for a situation/event that should be considered (e.g., provocation, duress, lack of knowledge or preparation, lack of intention, failure on others' part, task difficulty, lack of clear guidelines)? If so, can patient reattribute some of the responsibility for the situation/ event to these causes?
Externalizing both sides of a thought through role play	Take the "con" aspects of a thought while patient takes the "pro" aspects, and engage in a role-play argument (e.g., say, "You'll fail the exam"; patient replies, "There's no evidence that I'll fail"; and continue in this manner).
Using role play to apply a negative thought to a friend	Take the role of a friend to whom patient applies a negative thought. How does it sound?

Technique	Description or example
Acting "as if"	First in role play and then in actual situations, have patient act as if he or she does not believe negative thoughts.
Challenging absolutistic thinking	Example: Ask patient, "If you believe that no one will like you, is it plausible that no one in the whole world will?"
Setting a zero point for comparisons; depolarizing comparisons	If patient always compares himself or herself to the best, how does he or she compare to the worst? And how does patient compare to people in the middle of the distribution?
Positive reframing (finding positives in negatives)	Is there a more positive way of interpreting patient's behavior or situation (e.g., instead of saying, "I really bombed on the exam," can patient say, "I learned I can't procrastinate" or "Thank God that course is over")?
Decatastrophizing	Ask patient, "Why would X not be so awful after all?"
Examining the "feared fantasy"	Ask patient, "Imagine the worst possible outcome of X. How would you handle it? What behaviors could you control even if it happened?"
Anticipating future reactions	Ask patient, "How will you [or others] feel about X 2 days, a week, a month, and a year from now?"
Examining past predictions, failure to learn from false predictions, and self-fulfilling prophecies	Has patient generally made negative predictions in the past that have not come true? If so, has patient failed to learn that these predictions have been distorted and biased? Have these predictions turned into self-fulfilling prophecies (i.e., has patient behaved as if they will come true and thus ensured that they will come true)?
Testing predictions	Have patient make a list of specific predictions for the next week and keep track of the outcomes.
Examining past worries	Has patient worried about things in the past that he or she no longer thinks about? If so, have him or her list as many of these as possible and ask, "Why are these no longer important to me?"
Examining future distractions	What are all the other events (unrelated to current event) that will transpire over the next day, week, month, and year and that will cause patient not to care as much about the current event?
Distinguishing possibility from probability	Example: Ask patient, "It may be possible that you will have a heart attack if you are anxious, but what is the probability?"

(cont.)

TABLE B.3 *(cont.)*

Technique	Description or example
Calculating sequential probabilities	Have patient multiply the probabilities of a predicted sequence of negative events.
Fighting overgeneralization	Ask patient, "Just because X happened once, does that mean it will inevitably happen?"
Challenging the need for certainty	Tell patient, "You can't have certainty in an uncertain world. If you are trying to rule out absolutely all possibility of negative outcomes, you will be unable to act."
Advocating acceptance	Suggest to patient, "Rather than trying to control and change everything, perhaps there are some things you can learn to accept and make the best of. For example, perhaps you won't be perfect in your job, but perhaps you can learn to appreciate what you can do."
Using "point–counterpoint" with difficult thoughts	For difficult thoughts that are resistant to other techniques, engage in "point–counterpoint" role play with patient.
Reexamining original negative thought and emotion, confidence in accuracy of thought, and intensity of emotion	Example: "I feel anxious [15%] because I think I'll fail [20%]."
Developing rational response to thought (new, more realistic, more adaptive thought)	Example: "There isn't much actual evidence that I'll fail; therefore, there's no real reason for me to think I'll fail, and no real reason for me to be anxious."

Identifying maladaptive assumptions

Determining contents of patient's "rule book" ("shoulds," "musts," "if–then" statements underlying distorted automatic thoughts)	Examples: "I should succeed at everything I do," "If people don't like me, it means there's something wrong with me," "I must be approved by everyone."

Challenging maladaptive assumptions

Using techniques for challenging distorted automatic thoughts	See above.
Evaluating patient's standards	Ask patient, "Are you setting unrealistic expectations for yourself? Are your standards too high? Too low? Too vague? Do your standards give you room for a learning curve?"

Technique	Description or example
Examining patient's value system	Ask patient, "What is your hierarchy of values? For example, do you place success above everything else? Are you trying to accomplish everything simultaneously?"
Examining social standards	Ask patient, "Are you trying too hard to measure up to society's standards—for example, beauty and thinness for women, or power and status for men? If you don't exactly meet these standards, do you think this makes you a bad or worthless person?"
Distinguishing progress from perfection	Help patient examine the advantages of trying to improve, rather than trying to be perfect.
Challenging idealization of others	Have patient try to list all the people he or she knows who are completely perfect. Since it's unlikely that there will be any, what does this mean about patient's achieving perfection? Or have patient ask an admired person whether he or she has ever made any mistakes or had any problems, and consider what this person's response implies about patient's idealization of others and devaluation of self.
Advocating adaptive flexibility	Help patient examine the benefits of being more flexible in standards and behaviors.
Borrowing someone else's perspective	Ask patient, "Instead of getting trapped by your way of reacting, try to think of someone you know who you think is highly adaptive. How would this person think and act under these circumstances?"
Emphasizing curiosity, challenge, and growth rather than perfection	Example: Suggest to patient, "If you do poorly on an exam, work on how you can develop curiosity about the subject matter or feel challenged to do better in the future, rather than focusing on your grade as a final measure of your worth."
Reexamining maladaptive assumptions and substituting new, more adaptive assumptions	Example: "I'm worthwhile regardless of what others think of me," instead of "If people don't like me, it means there's something wrong with me."
Examining costs and benefits of more adaptive assumptions	Example of more adaptive assumption: "I'm worthwhile regardless of what others think of me." Costs: "Maybe I'll get conceited and alienate people." Benefits: "Increased self-confidence, less shyness, less dependence on others, more assertiveness." Costs: 5%. Benefits: 95%. Conclusion: "This new assumption is better than the one that I have to get other people to like me in order to like myself."

(cont.)

TABLE B.3 *(cont.)*

Technique	Description or example
Identifying dysfunctional schemas	
Identifying negative or otherwise dysfunctional views of self and others underlying distorted automatic thoughts and maladaptive assumptions	Examples: "I'm incompetent," "I'm no good," "I must be admired," "Others are rejecting," "Others are all-powerful," "Others must pay tribute to me."
Explaining schematic processing	Indicate how dysfunctional schemas are formed and how they systematically bias the ways events are attended and responded to.
Identifying strategies of avoiding/compensating for schemas	Help patient determine how he or she avoids challenging a schema (e.g., "If you think that you are unlovable, do you avoid getting involved with people?") or compensates for a schema (e.g., "If you believe you are inferior to others, do you attempt to become perfect in order to overcome your 'inferiority'?").
Challenging dysfunctional schemas	
Using techniques for challenging distorted automatic thoughts and maladaptive assumptions	See above.
Activating early memories to identify sources of schemas	Ask patient, "Who taught you to think in this dysfunctional way? Was it your parents? Teachers? Friends? Do you think that their teaching was valid? Were they poor role models?"
Challenging the sources of schemas through role play	Have patient role-play himself or herself challenging the source of a schema and arguing vigorously against this person.
Imagery restructuring; rewriting life scripts	Have patient imagine going back in time and confronting a schema's source. Or have patient revise his or her negative life script so that it has a positive outcome (e.g, for a negative early image of humiliation, have patient write a script in which he or she rejects or criticizes the person responsible for the humiliation).
Writing letters to the source	Have patient write letters to a schema's source (which need not be sent) expressing his or her anger and frustration.
Imagery and emotion	Have patient close eyes, evoke a negative feeling (e.g., loneliness), and then associate a visual image with this feeling. Ask patient to complete this sentence: "This image bothers me because it makes me think . . ."

Technique	Description or example
Coping imagery	Help patient to develop an image of himself or herself coping competently with a feared person or situation.
Miniaturizing the frightening image	Help patient to develop an image of a feared person or thing as much smaller and weaker than patient, instead of bigger and more powerful.
Desensitizing images	Have patient engage in repeated exposure to a feared image or situation, in order to diminish its capacity to elicit fear.
Nurturant self-statements	Have patient imagine himself or herself as a child and make nurturing statements to the child of the kind he or she wishes had actually been made.
"Bill of rights"	Help patient compose a personal "bill of rights" (e.g., the right to make mistakes, to be human, etc.).
Reexamining original schemas and developing new, more adaptive schemas	Examples: "I am competent" and "Others are only human," instead of "I am incompetent" and "Others are all-powerful."

Problem solving and self-control

Technique	Description or example
Identifying a problem	Is there a problem that needs to be solved? For example, if patient does poorly on an exam, perhaps he or she needs to study more.
Accepting the problem	Help patient to accept the existence of the problem and begin working toward its solution, instead of being self-critical or catastrophizing.
Examining the goal; generating alternative goals	What is patient's goal in the situation? If one goal has not worked, can patient modify the goal or generate alternative goals (e.g., replace "to be liked by everyone" with "to meet some new people" or "to learn how well I can do")?
Anti-procrastination steps	Guide patient through a series of steps to minimize procrastination (specifying a goal; breaking it down into smaller steps; examining costs and benefits of first step vs. an alternative; scheduling a specific time, place, and duration for the activity; role-playing resistance to engaging in the activity; carrying out the activity).
Self-correction	Encourage patient to learn from any mistakes instead of engaging in self-criticism.

(cont.)

TABLE B.3 *(cont.)*

Technique	Description or example
Developing self-instructional statements; creating a "coping card"	Have patient develop self-instructions for use in times of difficulty (e.g., "Don't worry about my anxious arousal. It's arousal. It's not dangerous. Anxiety doesn't mean I'm going crazy. I can tolerate it"). Put these statements, along with reminders and so on, on a "coping card" that patient can refer to easily.
Delaying a decision	For an impulsive patient, it may be useful to delay making a decision on a thought until a certain amount of time has passed or until the patient has had two good nights' sleep.
Canvassing friends	To reduce compulsiveness, a patient can be asked to survey five friends for their advice on the intended thought or action.
Anticipating problems	Have patient list the kinds of problems that might come up and develop rational responses to these.
Inoculation	With the patient, role-play the worst negative thoughts and problems that might come up, and have patient indicate how he or she would challenge them.
Self-reward statements	Encourage patient to list positive thoughts about himself or herself after doing something positive.
Problem solution review	Have patient review past problems and the solutions he or she has used.

APPENDIX C

Overview of Contents
of Companion CD-ROM

DISORDERS

For each of the seven disorders covered in the book, the CD-ROM provides a brief outline of treatment, sample symptoms and goals with related interventions, specific techniques, therapist forms, and patient forms and handouts.

Depression
Panic Disorder and Agoraphobia
Generalized Anxiety Disorder
Social Phobia
Posttraumatic Stress Disorder
Specific Phobia
Obsessive–Compulsive Disorder

APPENDIX A (EXPANDED FOR CD-ROM): BEHAVIORAL TECHNIQUES

The CD-ROM provides a detailed reference to behavioral techniques, including forms, handouts, and step-by-step guidelines. Again, many techniques are included here that are not covered in detail in the book's text.

Assertiveness Training
Behavioral Activation (Reward Planning and Activity Scheduling)
Communication Skills Training
Distraction
Exposure

Note: The CD-ROM contains PDF files, for which a copy of Adobe Acrobat Reader 4.0 is provided as well. Acrobat® Reader 4.0 ©1987–1999 Adobe Systems, Incorporated. All rights reserved. Adobe, Acrobat, and Acrobat logo are trademarks of Adobe Systems, Incorporated which may be registered in certain jurisdictions.

Graded Task Assignment
Modeling
Problem Solving
Rebreathing
Relaxation
Self-Reward
Social Skills Training
Thought Stopping
Visualization

APPENDIX B (EXPANDED FOR CD-ROM): COGNITIVE CONCEPTS AND TECHNIQUES

The CD-ROM provides a detailed reference to cognitive techniques, including forms, handouts, and step-by-step guidelines. Topics and techniques are included here that are not covered in the book's text.

Introduction to Cognitive and Cognitive-Behavioral Therapy
The Three Levels of Cognitive Distortions
Identifying and Challenging Cognitive Distortions
Examples of Challenges to Specific Negative Automatic Thoughts
Examining Maladaptive Assumptions
Examining the Content of Dysfunctional Schemas
Self-Instruction and Self-Control
Conclusion

MEDICATIONS

The CD-ROM includes detailed information on the various medications used to treat the specific disorders. It covers information on both trade and generic drug names, usual daily dosages, disorders for which each drug is prescribed, and common side effects.

Antidepressants—monoamine oxidase inhibitors (MAO)
Antidepressants—tricyclics
Antidepressants—selective serotonin reuptake inhibitors (SSRIs)
Antidepressants—miscellaneous
Anxiolytics—benzodiazepines
Anxiolytics—miscellaneous
Stimulants
Antipsychotics—phenothiazines
Antipsychotics—miscellaneous
Antimanics
Hypnotics

References

Abramowitz, J. S. (1997). Effectiveness of psychological and pharmacological treatments for obsessive–compulsive disorder: A quantitative review. *Journal of Consulting and Clinical Psychology*, *65*(1), 44–52.

Abramson, L. Y., Metalsky, G. I., & Alloy, L. B. (1989). Hopelessness depression: A theory-based subtype of depression. *Psychological Review, 96*, 358–372.

Abramson, L. Y., Seligman, M. E. P., & Teasdale, J. D. (1978). Learned helplessness in humans: Critique and reformulation. *Journal of Abnormal Psychology, 87*, 102–109.

Acierno, R., Hersen, M., Van Hasselt, V. B., Tremont, G., & Meuser, K. T. (1994). Review of the validation and dissemination of eye-movement desensitization and reprocessing: A scientific and ethical dilemma. *Clinical Psychology Review, 14*, 287–299.

Akiskal, H. S. (1995). Mood disorders. In H. I. Kaplan & B. J. Sadock (Eds.), *Comprehensive textbook of psychiatry* (6th ed., Vol. 1, pp. 1067–1078). Baltimore: Williams & Wilkins.

Alberti, R. E., & Emmons, M. L. (1974). *Your perfect right* (2nd ed.). San Luis Obispo, CA: Impact.

Al-Kubaisy, T., Marks, I. M., Logsdail, S., Marks, M. P., Lovell, K., Sungur, M., & Araya R. (1992). Role of exposure homework in phobia reduction: A controlled study. *Behavior Therapy, 23*, 599–621.

American Psychiatric Association. (1994). *Diagnostic and statistical manual of mental disorders* (4th ed.). Washington, DC: Author.

Angst, J., & Vollrath, M. (1991). The natural history of anxiety disorders. *Acta Psychiatrica Scandinavica, 84*, 446–452.

Arntz, A., Hildebrand, M., & van den Hout, M. (1994). Overprediction of anxiety and disconfirmatory processes in anxiety disorders. *Behavior Research and Therapy, 32*, 709–722.

Arntz, A., Rauner, M., & van den Hout, M. (1995). "If I feel anxious, there must be danger": Ex-consequentia reasoning in inferring danger in anxiety disorders. *Behavior Research and Therapy, 33*, 917–925.

Baer, L. (1991). *Getting control*. Boston: Little, Brown.

Ball, S. G., Baer, L., & Otto, M. W. (1996). Symptom subtypes of obsessive–compulsive disorder in behavioural treatment studies: A quantitative review. *Behaviour Research and Therapy, 34*(1), 47–51.

Bandura, A. (1969). *Principles of behavior modification*. New York: Holt, Rinehart & Winston.

Bandura, A. (1977). *Social learning theory*. Englewood Cliffs, NJ: Prentice-Hall.

Barkham, B., Rees, A., Shapiro, D. A., Stiles, W. B., Agnew, R. M., Halstead, J., Culverwell, A., & Harrington, V. M. G. (1996). Outcomes of time-limited psychotherapy in applied settings: Replicating the second Sheffield psychotherapy project. *Journal of Consulting and Clinical Psychology, 64*(5), 1079–1085.

Barlow, D. H. (1988). *Anxiety and its disorders: The nature and treatment of anxiety and panic*. New York: Guilford Press.

Barlow, D. H. & Cerny, J. A. (1988). *Psychological treatment of panic*. New York: Guilford Press.

Barlow, D. H., & Craske, M. G. (1988). The phenomenology of panic. In S. Rachman & J. D. Maser (Eds.), *Panic: Psychological perspectives* (pp. 11–35). Hillsdale, NJ: Erlbaum.

Barlow, D. H., DiNardo, P. A., Vermilyea, B. B., Vermilyea, J. A., & Blanchard, E. E. (1986). Comorbidity and depression among the anxiety disorders: Issues in classification and diagnosis. *Journal of Nervous and Mental Diseases, 174,* 63–72.

Basco, M. R., & Rush, A. J. (1996). *Cognitive-behavioral therapy for bipolar disorder.* New York: Guilford Press.

Baucom, D. H., & Epstein, N. (1990). *Cognitive-behavioral marital therapy.* New York: Brunner/Mazel.

Baumeister, R. F., & Tice, D. M. (1990). Anxiety and social exclusion. *Journal of Social and Clinical Psychology, 9,* 165–195.

Beach, S. R. H., Arias, I., & O'Leary, K. D. (1986). The relationship of marital satisfaction and social support to depressive symptomatology. *Journal of Psychopathology and Behavioral Assessment, 8,* 305–316.

Beach, S. R. H., Jouriles, E. N., & O'Leary, K. D. (1986). Extramarital sex: Impact on depression and commitment in couples seeking marital therapy. *Journal of Sex and Marital Therapy, 11,* 99–108.

Beach, S. R. H., & O'Leary, K. D. (1986). The treatment of depression occurring in the context of marital discord. *Behavior Therapy, 17,* 43–49.

Beach, S. R. H., Sandeen, E. E., & O'Leary, K. D. (1990). *Depression in marriage: A model for etiology and treatment.* New York: Guilford Press.

Beck, A. T. (1976). *Cognitive therapy and the emotional disorders.* New York: International Universities Press.

Beck, A. T. (1988). *Love is never enough.* New York: Harper & Row.

Beck, A. T. (1996). Beyond belief: A theory of modes, personality, and psychopathology. In P. Salkovskis (Ed.), *Frontiers of cognitive therapy* (pp. 1–25). New York: Guilford Press.

Beck, A. T., Emery, G., & Greenberg, R. L. (1985). *Anxiety disorders and phobias: A cognitive perspective.* New York: Basic Books.

Beck, A. T., Epstein, N., Brown, G., & Steer, R. A. (1988). An inventory for measuring clinical anxiety: Psychometric properties. *Journal of Consulting and Clinical Psychology, 56,* 893–897.

Beck, A. T., Freeman, A., & Associates. (1990). *Cognitive therapy of personality disorders.* New York: Guilford Press.

Beck, A. T., Rush, A. J., Shaw, B. F., & Emery, G. (1979). *Cognitive therapy of depression.* New York: Guilford Press.

Beck, A. T., Ward, C. H., Mendelson, M., Mock, J. E., & Erbaugh, J. K. (1961). An inventory for measuring depression. *Archives of General Psychiatry, 33,* 561–571.

Beck, A. T., Weissman, A., Lester, D., & Trexler, L. (1974). The measurement of pessimism: The Hopelessness Scale. *Journal of Consulting and Clinical Psychology, 42,* 861–886.

Beck, J. S. (1995). *Cognitive therapy: Basics and beyond.* New York: Guilford Press.

Blazer, D., George, L. K., & Hughes, D. (1991). The epidemiology of anxiety disorders: An age comparison. In C. Salzman, B. Lebowitz, et al. (Eds.), *Anxiety in the elderly: Treatment and research* (pp. 17–30). New York: Springer.

Borkovec, T. D., & Inz, J. (1990). The nature of worry in generalized anxiety disorder: A predominance of thought activity. *Behaviour Research and Therapy, 28,* 153–158.

Borkovec, T. D., & Roemer, L. (1996). Generalized anxiety disorder. In T. D. Borkovec & L. Roemer (Eds.), *Handbook of the treatment of the anxiety disorders* (2nd ed., pp. 81–118). Northvale, NJ: Jason Aronson.

Borkovec, T. D., Shadick, R. N., & Hopkins, M. (1991). The nature of normal and pathological worry. In R. M. Rapee & D. H. Barlow (Eds.), *Chronic anxiety: Generalized anxiety disorder and mixed anxiety disorder* (pp. 29–51). New York: Guilford Press.

Borkovec, T. D., & Whisman, M. A. (1996). Psychosocial treatments for generalized anxiety disorder. In M. R. Mavissakalian & R. F. Prien (Eds.), *Long-term treatments of anxiety disorders* (pp. 171–199). Washington, DC: American Psychiatric Press.

Breslau, N., & Davis, G. C. (1985). DSM-III generalized anxiety disorder: An empirical investigation of more stringent criteria. *Psychiatry Research, 14,* 231–238.

Brown, T. A., & Barlow, D. H. (1992). Comorbidity among anxiety disorders: Implications for treatment and DSM-IV. *Journal of Consulting and Clinical Psychology, 60,* 835–844.

Brown, T. A., Moras, K., Zinberg, R. E., & Barlow, D. H. (1993). Diagnostic and symptom distinguishability of generalized anxiety disorder and obsessive–compulsive disorder. *Behavior Therapy, 24,* 227–240.

Burns, D. D. (1980). *Feeling good: The new mood therapy.* New York: New American Library.

Burns, D. D. (1989). *The feeling good handbook: Using the new mood therapy in everyday life.* New York: Morrow.

Burns, L. E., & Thorpe, G. L. (1977). The epidemiology of fears and phobias (with particular relevance to the National Survey of Agoraphobics). *International Medical Research, 5* (Suppl. 5), 1–7.

Butler, G. (1985). Exposure as a treatment for social phobia: Some instructive difficulties. *Behaviour Research and Therapy, 23*(6), 651–657.

Butler, G., Fennell, M., Robson, P., & Geldeer, M. (1991). A comparison of behavior therapy and cognitive behavior therapy in the treatment of generalized anxiety disorder. *Journal of Consulting and Clinical Psychology, 59,* 167–175.

Butler, G., & Wells, A. (1995). Cognitive-behavioral treatments: Clinical applications. In R. G. Heimberg, M. R. Liebowitz, D. A. Hope, & F. R. Schneier (Eds.), *Social phobia: Diagnosis, assessment, and treatment* (pp. 310–323). New York: Guilford Press.

Chambless, D. L., Caputo, G. C., Jasin, S. E., Gracely, E. J., & Williams, C. (1997). The mobility inventory for agoraphobia. In S. Rachman et al. (Eds.), *Best of behavior research and therapy* (pp. 83–92). New York: Pergamon/Elsevier Science.

Chambless, D. L., Renneberg, B., Goldstein, A., & Gracely, E. J. (1992). MCMI-diagnosed personality disorders among agoraphobic outpatients: Prevalence and relationship to severity and treatment outcome. *Journal of Anxiety Disorders, 6,* 193–211.

Chapman, T. F. (1997). The epidemiology of fears and phobias. In G. C. L. Davey (Ed.), *Phobias: A handbook of theory, research and treatment* (pp. 415–434). New York: Wiley.

Chapman, T. F., Mannuzza, S., & Fyer, A. J. (1995). Epidemiology and family studies of social phobia. In R. G. Heimberg, M. R. Liebowitz, D. A. Hope, & F. R. Schneier (Eds.), *Social phobia: Diagnosis, assessment, and treatment* (pp. 21–40). New York: Guilford Press.

Christensen, A., Jacobson, N. S., & Babcock, J. C. (1995). Integrative behavioral couple therapy. In N. S. Jacobson & A. S. Gurman (Eds.), *Clinical handbook of couple therapy* (pp. 31–64). New York: Guilford Press.

Clark, D. C. (1995). Epidemiology, assessment, and management of suicide in depressed patients. In E. E. Beckham & W. R. Leber (Eds.), *Handbook of depression* (2nd ed., pp. 526–538). New York: Guilford Press.

Clark, D. M. (1986). A cognitive approach to panic. *Behaviour Research and Therapy, 24,* 461–470.

Clark, D. M. (1989). Anxiety states: Panic and generalized anxiety. In K. Hawton, P. M. Salkovskis, J. Kirk, & D. M. Clark (Eds.), *Cognitive behavior therapy for psychiatric problems: A practical guide* (pp. 52–96). Oxford: Oxford University Press.

Clark, D. M. (1996). Panic disorder: From theory to therapy. In P. M. Salkovskis (Ed.), *Frontiers of cognitive therapy* (pp. 318–344). New York: Guilford Press.

Clark, D. M., Salkovskis, P., & Chalkley, A. J. (1985). Respiratory control as a treatment for panic attacks. *Journal of Behavior Therapy and Experimental Psychiatry, 16,* 23–30.

Clark, D. M., & Wells, A. (1995). A cognitive model of social phobia. In R. G. Heimberg, M. R. Liebowitz, D. A. Hope, & F. R. Schneier (Eds.), *Social phobia: Diagnosis, assessment, and treatment* (pp. 69–93). New York: Guilford Press.

Coyne, J. C. (1989). Thinking post-cognitively about depression. In A. Freeman, K. M. Simon, L. E. Butler, & H. Arkowitz (Eds.), *Comprehensive handbook of cognitive therapy* (pp. 227–244). New York: Plenum Press.

Craske, M. G., & Rowe, M. K. (1997). Nocturnal panic. *Clinical Psychology: Science and Practice, 4,* 153–174.

Dattilio, F., & Padesky, C. (1990). *Cognitive therapy with couples.* Sarasota, FL: Professional Resource Exchange.

Davidson, J. R. T. (1995). Posttraumatic stress disorder and acute stress disorder. In H. I. Kaplan & B. J. Sadock (Eds.), *Comprehensive textbook of psychiatry* (6th ed., Vol. 1, pp. 1227–1236). Baltimore: Williams & Wilkins.

Derogatis, L. R. (1977). *SCL-90: Administration, score and procedure manual—I for the R (Revised) Version.* Baltimore: Johns Hopkins University School of Medicine.

DeRubeis, R. J., Gelfand, L. A., Tang, T. Z., & Simons, A. D. (1999). Medications versus cognitive behavior therapy for severely depressed outpatients: Mega-analysis of four randomized comparisons. *American Journal of Psychiatry, 156,* 1007–1013.

DiGiuseppe, R., McGowan, L., Simon, K. S., & Gardner, F. (1990). A comparative outcome study of four cognitive therapies in the treatment of social anxiety. *Journal of Rational–Emotive and Cognitive-Behavior Therapy, 8*(3), 129–146.

DiNardo, P. A., & Barlow, D. H. (1988). *Anxiety Disorders Interview Schedule—Revised (ADIS-R).* Albany, NY: Phobia and Anxiety Disorders Clinic.

Donohue, B. C., Van Hasselt, V. B., & Hersen, M. (1994). Behavioral assessment and treatment of social phobia. *Behavior Modification, 18*(3), 262–288.

Durham, R. C. (1995). "Comparing treatments for generalised anxiety disorder": Reply. *British Journal of Psychiatry, 166,* 266–267.

Durham, R. C., Murphy, T., Allan, T., Richard, K., Treliving, L. R., & Genton, G. (1994). Cognitive therapy, analytic psychotherapy and anxiety management training for generalised anxiety disorder. *British Journal of Psychiatry, 165,* 315–323.

D'Zurilla, T. J. (1988). Problem-solving therapies. In K. Dobson (Ed.), *Handbook of cognitive-behavioral therapies* (pp. 85–135). New York: Guilford Press.

Eaton, W. W., Dryman, A., & Weissman, M. (1991). Panic and phobia. In L. N. Robins & D. A. Regier (Eds.), *Psychiatric disorders in America* (pp. 155–179). New York: Free Press.

Eibl-Eibesfeldt, I. (1972). *Love and hate: The natural history of behavior patterns.* New York: Holt, Rinehart & Winston.

Ellis, A. (1962). *Reason and emotion in psychotherapy.* New York: Lyle Stuart.

Epstein, N. (1997). Marital conflict. In R. L. Leahy (Ed.), *Practicing cognitive therapy: A guide to interventions* (pp. 249–276). Northvale, NJ: Jason Aronson.

Feske, U., & Chambless, D. L. (1995). Cognitive behavioral versus exposure only treatment for social phobia: A meta-analysis. *Behavior Therapy, 26,* 695–720.

Finlay-Jones, R., & Brown, G. W. (1981). Types of stressful life event and the onset of anxiety and depressive disorders. *Psychological Medicine, 11,* 803–815.

First, M. B., Spitzer, R. L., Gibbon, M., & Williams, J. B. W. (1995). The Structured Clinical Interview for DSM-III-R Personality Disorders (SCID-II): I. Description. *Journal of Personality Disorders, 9,* 83–91.

Fisher, R., & Ury, W. (1981). *Getting to yes: Negotiating agreement without giving in.* New York: Viking.

Foa, E. B., & Kozak, M. J. (1986). Emotional processing of fear: Exposure to corrective information. *Psychological Bulletin, 99*(1), 20–35.

Foa, E. B., & Kozak, M. J. (1991). Emotional processing: Theory, research, and clinical implications for anxiety disorders. In J. D. Safran & L. S. Greenberg (Eds.), *Emotion, psychotherapy, and change* (pp. 21–49). New York: Guilford Press.

Foa, E. B., & Kozak, M. J. (1997). Psychological treatment for obsessive–compulsive disorder. In M. R. Mavissakalian & R. G. Prien (Eds.), *Long-term treatments of anxiety disorders* (pp. 285–309). Washington, DC: American Psychiatric Press.

Foa, E. B., & Riggs, D. S. (1994). Posttraumatic stress disorder and rape. In R. S. Pynoos (Ed.), *Posttraumatic stress disorder: A clinical review* (pp. 133–163). Lutherville, MD: Sidran Press.

Foa, E. B., Rothbaum, B. O., & Molnar, C. (1995). Cognitive-behavioral therapy of post-traumatic stress disorder. In M. J. Friedman, D. S. Charney, & A. Y. Deutch (Eds.), *Neurobiological and clinical consequences of stress: From normal adaptation to PTSD* (pp. 483–494). Philadelphia: Lippincott–Raven.

Foa, E. B., Rothbaum, B. O., Riggs, D., & Murdock, T. B. (1991). Treatment of post-traumatic stress disorder in rape victims. *Journal of Consulting and Clinical Psychology, 59,* 715–723.

Foa, E. B., Steketee, G., & Rothbaum, B. O. (1989). Behavioral/cognitive conceptualizations of post-traumatic stress disorder. *Behavior Therapy, 20,* 155–176.

Foa, E., & Wilson, R. (1991). *Stop obsessing!: How to overcome your obsessions and compulsions.* New York: Bantam.

Foy, D. W. (1992). Introduction and description of the disorder. In D. W. Foy (Ed.), *Treating PTSD: Cognitive-behavioral strategies* (pp. 1–12). New York: Guilford Press.

Friedman, M. J., & Southwick, S. M. (1995). Towards pharmacotherapy for post-traumatic stress disorder. In M. J. Friedman, D. S. Charney, & A. Y. Deutch (Eds.), *Neurobiological and clinical consequences of stress: From normal adaptation to post-traumatic stress disorder* (pp. 465–481). Philadelphia: Lippincott-Raven.

Fyer, A. J., Mannuzza, S., Chapman, T. F., Liebowitz, M. R., & Klein, D. F. (1993). A direct interview family study of social phobia. *Archives of General Psychiatry, 50,* 286–293.

Fyer, A. J., Mannuzza, S., & Coplan, J. D. (1995). Panic disorders and agoraphobia In H. I. Kaplan & B. J. Sadock (Eds.), *Comprehensive textbook of psychiatry* (6th ed., Vol. 1, pp. 1191–1204). Baltimore: Williams & Wilkins.

Goodwin, F., & Jamison, K. R. (1991). *Manic–depressive illness.* New York: Oxford University Press.

Gorman, J., Liebowitz, M. R., Fyer, A. J., & Stein, J. (1989). A neuroanatomical hypothesis for panic disorder. *American Journal of Psychiatry, 146*(2), 148–161.

Guidano, V. F., & Liotti, G. (1983). *Cognitive processes and emotional disorders.* New York: Guilford Press.

Hamilton, N. (1959). The assessment of anxiety states by rating. *British Journal of Medical Psychology, 32, 50.*

Heckelman, L. R., & Schneier, F. R. (1995). Diagnostic issues. In R. G. Heimberg, M. R. Liebowitz, D. A. Hope, & F. R. Schneier (Eds.), *Social phobia: Diagnosis, assessment, and treatment* (pp. 3–20). New York: Guilford Press.

Heimberg, R. G., & Barlow, D. H. (1991). New developments in cognitive-behavioral therapy for social phobia. *Journal of Clinical Psychiatry, 52*(11, Suppl.), 21–30.

Heimberg, R. G., Dodge, C. S., Hope, D. A., Kennedy, C. R., & Zollo, L. J. (1990). Cognitive behavioral group treatment for social phobia: Comparison with a credible placebo control. *Cognitive Therapy and Research, 14*(1), 1–23.

Heimberg, R. G., & Juster, H. R. (1995). Cognitive-behavioral treatments: Literature review. In R. G. Heimberg, M. R. Liebowitz, D. A. Hope, & F. R. Schneier (Eds.), *Social phobia: Diagnosis, assessment, and treatment* (pp. 261–309). New York: Guilford Press.

Hiss, H., Foa, E. B., & Kozak, M. J. (1994). Relapse prevention program for treatment of obsessive–compulsive disorder. *Journal of Consulting and Clinical Psychology, 62*(4), 801–808.

Hodgson, R. J., & Rachman, S. (1977). Obsessional–compulsive complaints. *Behaviour Research and Therapy, 15,* 389–395.

Holland, S. J. (1997). Obsessive–compulsive disorder. In R. L. Leahy (Ed.), *Practicing cognitive therapy: A guide to interventions* (pp. 151–168). Northvale, NJ: Jason Aronson.

Jacobson, E. (1938). *Progressive relaxation.* Chicago: University of Chicago Press.

Jacobson, N., & Margolin, G. (1979). *Marital therapy: Strategies based on social learning and behavior exchange principles.* New York: Brunner/Mazel.

Jenike, M. A. (1995). Obsessive–compulsive disorder. In H. I. Kaplan & B. J. Sadock (Eds.), *Comprehensive textbook of psychiatry* (6th ed., Vol. 1, pp. 1218–1226). Baltimore: Williams & Wilkins.

Jenkins, S. C., & Hansen, M. R. (Eds.). (1995). *A pocket reference for psychiatrists* (2nd ed.). Washington, DC: American Psychiatric Press.

Judd, L. L. (1994). Social phobia: A clinical overview. *Journal of Clinical Psychiatry, 55*(6, Suppl.), 5–9.

Kaeler, C. T., Moul, D. E., & Farmer, M. E. (1995). Epidemiology of depression. In E. E. Beckham & W. R. Leber (Eds.), *Handbook of depression* (pp. 376–390). New York: Guilford Press.

Kaplan, H. I., & Sadock, B. J. (Eds.). (1988). *Synopsis of psychiatry* (5th ed.). Baltimore: Williams & Wilkins.

Karno, M., Golding, J. M., Sorenson, S. B., & Burnam, M. A. (1988). The epidemiology of obsessive-compulsive disorder in five U.S. communities. *Archives of General Psychiatry, 45,* 1094–1099.

Kendler, K. S., Kessler, R. C., Neale, M. C., Heath, A. C., & Eaves, L. J. (1993). The prediction of major depression in women: Toward an integrated etiologic model. *American Journal of Psychiatry, 150,* 1139–1148.

Kendler, K. S., Neale, M. C., Kessler, R. C., Heath, A. C., & Eaves, L. J. (1992). The genetic epidemiology of phobias in women: The interrelations of agoraphobia, social phobia, situational phobia, and simple phobia. *Archives of General Psychiatry, 49,* 273–281.

Kessler, R. C., McGonagle, K., Zhao, S., Nelson, C., Hughes, M., Eschlemann, S., Wittchen, H. U., & Kendler, K. S. (1994). Lifetime and 12-month prevalance of DSM-III-R psychiatric disorders in the United States: Results from the National Comorbidity Survey. *Archives of General Psychiatry, 51,* 8–19.

Klein, D. F., & Klein, H. M. (1989). The nosology, genetics, and theory of spontaneous panic and phobia. In P. Tyrer (Ed.), *Psychopharmacology of anxiety* (pp. 163–195). Oxford, England: Oxford University Press.

Klerman, G., Weissman, M., Rounsaville, B., & Chevron, E. (1984). *Interpersonal psychotherapy of depression.* New York: Basic Books.

Lazarus, A. (1984). *In the mind's eye.* New York: Guilford Press.

Lazarus, R. (1991). *Emotion and adaptation.* New York: Oxford University Press.

Lazarus, R., & Folkman, S. (1984). *Stress, appraisal and coping.* New York: Springer.

Leahy, R. L. (1985). The costs of development: Clinical implications. In R. L. Leahy (Ed.), *The development of the self.* San Diego: Academic Press.

Leahy, R. L. (1996). *Cognitive therapy: Basic principles and applications.* Northvale, NJ: Jason Aronson.

Leahy, R. L., & Beck, A. T. (1988). Cognitive therapy of depression and mania. In A. Georgotas & R. L. Cancro (Eds.), *Depression and mania* (pp. 517–537). New York: Elsevier.

Leary, M. R., & Kowalski, R. M. (1995). The self-presentation model of social phobia. In R. G. Heimberg, M. R. Liebowitz, D. A. Hope, & F. R. Schneier (Eds.), *Social phobia: Diagnosis, assessment, and treatment* (pp. 94–112). New York: Guilford Press.

Lewinsohn, P. M., Antonuccio, D. O., Steinmetz, J. L., & Teri, L. (1984). *The Coping with Depression course: A psychoeducational intervention for unipolar depression.* Eugene, OR: Castalia.

Lewinsohn, P. M., Mermelstein, R. M., Alexander, A., & MacPhillamy, D. J. (1985). The Unpleasant Events Scale: A scale for the measurement of aversive events. *Journal of Clinical Psychology, 41,* 483–498.

Lewinsohn, P. M., Munoz, R. F., Youngren, M. A., & Zeiss, A. M. (1986). *Control over depression* (2nd ed.). Englewood Cliffs, NJ: Prentice Hall.

Liebowitz, M. R. (1987). Social phobia. *Modern Problems of Pharmacopsychiatry, 22,* 141–173.

Liebowitz, M. R., & Marshall, R. D. (1995). Pharmacological treatments: Clinical applications. In R. G. Heimberg, M. R. Liebowitz, D. A. Hope, & F. R. Schneier (Eds.), *Social phobia: Diagnosis, assessment, and treatment* (pp. 366–385). New York: Guilford Press.

Litz, B. T., Penk, W. E., Gerardi, R. J., & Keane, T. M. (1992). Assessment of posttraumatic stress disorder. In P. A. Saigh (Ed.), *Posttraumatic stress disorder: A behavioral approach to assessment and treatment* (pp. 50–83). Boston: Allyn & Bacon.

Locke, H. J., & Wallace, K. M. (1959). Short marital-adjustment and prediction tests: Their reliability and validity. *Marriage and Family Living, 21,* 251–255.

Lorenz, K. (1966). *On aggression.* New York: Harcourt, Brace.

Lydiard, R. B., & Falsetti, S. A. (1995). Treatment options for social phobia. *Psychiatric Annals, 25*(9), 570–576.

MacPhillamy, D. J., & Lewinsohn, P. M. (1982). The Pleasant Events Schedule: Studies on reliability, validity and scale intercorrelations. *Journal of Consulting and Clinical Psychology, 50,* 363–380.

Markowitz, J., & Weissman, M. (1995). Interpersonal psychotherapy. In E. E. Beckham & W. R. Leber (Eds.), *Handbook of depression* (2nd ed., pp. 376–390). New York: Guilford Press.

Marks, I. M. (1985). Behavioral treatment of social phobia. *Psychopharmacology Bulletin, 21,* 615–618.

Marks, I. M. (1987). *Fears, phobia and rituals: Panic, anxiety and their disorders.* New York: Oxford University Press.

Marks, I. M., & Mathews, A. M. (1979). Brief standard self-rating for phobic patients. *Behaviour Research and Therapy, 17,* 263–267.

Marmar, C. R., Foy, D., Kagan, B., & Pynoos, R. S. (1994). An integrated approach for treating posttraumatic stress. In R. S. Pynoos (Ed.), *Posttraumatic stress disorder: A clinical review* (pp. 99–132). Lutherville, MD: Sidran Press.

Mavissakalian, M., & Hammen, M. S. (1986). DSM-III personality disorder in agoraphobia. *Comprehensive Psychiatry, 27,* 471–479.

May, R. (1950). *The meaning of anxiety.* New York: Ronald Press.

McNally, R. J. (1994). *Panic disorder: A critical analysis.* New York: Guilford Press.

Meichenbaum, D. H. (1974). *Cognitive behavior modification.* Morristown, NJ: General Learning Press.

Meichenbaum, D. H. (1977). *Cognitive behavior modification.* New York: Plenum Press.

Menzies, R. G., & Clarke, J. C. (1994). Retrospective studies of the origins of phobias: A review. *Anxiety, Stress and Coping, 7,* 305–318.

Menzies, R. G., & Clarke, J. C. (1995). The etiology of phobias: A nonassociative account. *Clinical Psychology Review, 15,* 23–48.

Meyer, V. (1966). Modification of expectations in cases with obsessional rituals. *Behaviour Research and Therapy, 4,* 273–280.

Mineka, S., & Zinbarg, R. (1995). Conditioning and ethological models of social phobia. In R. G. Heimberg, M. R. Liebowitz, D. A. Hope, & F. R. Schneier (Eds.), *Social phobia: Diagnosis, assessment, and treatment* (pp. 134–162). New York: Guilford Press.

Mowrer, O. (1947). On the dual nature of learning—A reinterpretation of "conditioning" and "problem-solving." *Harvard Educational Review, 17,* 102–148.

Mowrer, O. (1960). *Learning theory and behavior.* New York: Wiley.

Nezu, A. M., & Nezu, C. M. (1989a). Clinical decision making in the practice of behavior therapy. In A. M. Nezu & C. M. Nezu (Eds.), *Clinical decision making in behavior therapy: A problem-solving perspective* (pp. 57–113). Champaign, IL: Research Press.

Nezu, A. M., & Nezu, C. M. (1989b). Clinical prediction, judgment, and decision making: An overview. In A. M. Nezu & C. M. Nezu (Eds.), *Clinical decision making in behavior therapy: A problem-solving perspective* (pp. 9–34). Champaign, IL: Research Press.

Nezu, A. M., & Nezu, C. M. (1989c). Toward a problem-solving formulation of psychotherapy and clinical decision making. In A. M. Nezu & C. M. Nezu (Eds.), *Clinical decision making in behavior therapy: A problem-solving perspective* (pp. 35–56). Champaign, IL: Research Press.

Nezu, A. M., Nezu, C. M., & Perri, M. G. (1989). *Problem-solving therapy for depression: Theory, research and clinical guidelines.* New York: Wiley.

Novaco, R. W. (1978). Anger and coping with stress: Cognitive-behavioral interventions. In J. P. Foreyt & D. P. Rathjen (Eds.), *Cognitive-behavior therapy: Research and applications* (pp. 135–173). New York: Plenum Press.

Ohman, A., & Dimberg, U. (1978). Facial expressions as conditioned stimuli for electrodermal responses: A case of "preparedness"? *Journal of Personality and Social Psychology, 36,* 1251–1258.

Ost, L. (1987). Applied relaxation: Description of a coping technique and review of controlled studies. *Behaviour Research and Therapy, 25*(5), 397–409.

Ost, L. (1997). Rapid treatment of specific phobias. In G. C. L. Davey (Ed.), *Phobias: A handbook of theory, research and treatment* (pp. 227–246). New York: Wiley.

Ost, L. G., & Hugdahl, K. (1981). Acquisition of phobias and anxiety response patterns in clinical patients. *Behaviour Research and Therapy, 16,* 439–447.

Perry, P. J., Alexander, B., & Liskow, B. L. (1997). *Psychotropic drug handbook* (7th ed.). Washington, DC: American Psychiatric Press.

Persons, J. B., & Miranda, J. (1991). Treating dysfunctional beliefs: Implications of the mood-state hypothesis. *Journal of Cognitive Psychotherapy, 5,* 15–25.

Persons, J. B., & Miranda, J. (1992). Cognitive theories of vulnerability to depression: Reconciling negative evidence. *Cognitive Therapy and Research, 16,* 485–502.

Peterson, K. C., Prout, M. F., & Schwarz, R. A. (1991). *Post-traumatic stress disorder: A clinician's guide.* New York: Plenum Press.

Physician's desk reference (PDR). (1999). Montvale, NJ: Medical Economics Company.

Plomin, R., & Daniels, D. (1986). Genetics and shyness. In W. H. Hones, J. M. Cheek, & S. R. Briggs (Eds.), *Shyness: Perspectives on research and treatment* (pp. 63–80). New York: Plenum Press.

Potts, N. L. S., & Davidson, J. R. T. (1995). Pharmacological treatments: Literature review. In R. G. Heimberg, M. R. Liebowitz, D. A. Hope, & F. R. Schneier (Eds.), *Social phobia: Diagnosis, assessment, and treatment* (pp. 334–365). New York: Guilford Press.

Prince, S., & Jacobson, N. (1995). Couple and family therapy for depression. In E. E. Beckham & W. R. Leber (Eds.), *Handbook of depression* (pp. 404–424). New York: Guilford Press.

Rachman, S. J. (1978). *Fear and courage.* New York: W. H. Freeman.

Rapee, R. M. (1991a). Generalized anxiety disorder: A review of clinical features and theoretical concepts. *Clinical Psychology Review, 11,* 419–440.

Rapee, R. M. (1991b). Psychological factors involved in generalized anxiety. In R. M. Rapee & D. H. Barlow (Eds.), *Chronic anxiety: Generalized anxiety and mixed anxiety-depression* (pp. 76–94). New York: Guilford Press.

Rapee, R. M. (1995). Descriptive psychopathology of social phobia. In R. G. Heimberg, M. R. Liebowitz, D. A. Hope, & F. R. Schneier (Eds.), *Social phobia: Diagnosis, assessment, and treatment* (pp. 41–66). New York: Guilford Press.

Reich, J. H., & Yates, W. (1988). Family history of psychiatric disorders in social phobia. *Comprehensive Psychiatry, 29,* 72–75.

Rehm, L. P. (1977). A self-control model of depression. *Behavior Therapy, 8,* 787–804.

Rehm, L. P. (1990). Cognitive and behavioral theories. In B. B. Wolman & G. Stricker (Eds.), *Depressive disorders: Facts, theories and treatment methods* (pp. 64–91). New York: Wiley.

Reich, J., Noyes, R., & Troughton, E. (1987). Dependent personality disorder associated with phobic avoidance in patients with panic disorder. *American Journal of Psychiatry, 144,* 323–326.

Rounsaville, B. J., Weissman, M. M., Prusoff, B. A., & Herceg-Baron, R. L. (1979). Marital disputes and treatment outcome in depressed women. *Comprehensive Psychiatry, 20,* 483–490.

Roy, A. (1995). Psychiatric emergencies. In H. I. Kaplan & B. J. Sadock (Eds.), *Comprehensive textbook of psychiatry* (2nd ed., Vol. 2, pp. 1739–1751). Philadelphia: Williams & Wilkins.

Safran, J., & Inck, T. A. (1996). Psychotherapy integration: Implications for the treatment of depression. In E. E. Beckham & W. R. Leber (Eds.), *Handbook of depression* (2nd ed., pp. 425–434). New York: Guilford Press.

Salkovskis, P. M. (1989). Cognitive-behavioural factors and the persistence of intrusive thoughts in obsessive problems. *Behaviour Research and Therapy, 23,* 571–583.

Salkovskis, P. M. (1996). The cognitive approach to anxiety: Threat beliefs, safety-seeking behavior, and the special case of health anxiety and obsessions. In P. M. Salkovskis (Ed.), *Frontiers of cognitive therapy* (pp. 48–74). New York: Guilford Press.

Salkovskis, P. M., & Kirk, J. (1989). Obsessional disorders. In K. Hawton, P. M. Salkovskis, J. Kirk, & D. M. Clark (Eds.), *Cognitive behaviour therapy for psychiatric problems: A practical guide* (pp. 179–208). Oxford: Oxford University Press.

Salkovskis, P. M., & Kirk, J. (1997). Obsessive–compulsive disorder. In D. M. Clark & C. G. Fairburn

(Eds.), *Science and practice of cognitive behaviour therapy* (pp. 179–208). Oxford: Oxford University Press.

Sanderson, W. C., DiNardo, P. A., Rapee, R. M., & Barlow, D. H. (1990). Syndrome comorbidity in patients diagnosed with DSM-III-R anxiety disorder. *Journal of Abnormal Psychology, 99,* 308–312.

Sanderson, W., & Wetzler, S. (1991). Chronic anxiety and generalized anxiety disorder: Issues in comorbidity. In R. M. Rapee & D. H. Barlow (Eds.), *Chronic anxiety: Generalized anxiety disorder and mixed anxiety–depression* (pp. 119–135). New York: Guilford Press.

Saunders, B. E., Arata, C. M., & Kilpatrick, D. G. (1990). Development of a Crime-Related Post-Traumatic Stress Disorder Scale for women within the Symptom Checklist-90—Revised. *Journal of Traumatic Stress, 3*(3), 439–448.

Schneier, F. R., Johnson, J., Hornig, C. D., Liebowitz, M. R., & Weissman, M. M. (1992). Social phobia: Comorbitity and morbidity in an epidemiological sample. *Archives of General Psychiatry, 49,* 282–288.

Scholing, A., & Emmelkamp, P. M. G. (1993a). Exposure with and without cognitive therapy for generalized social phobia: Effects of individual and group treatment. *Behaviour Research and Therapy, 31*(7), 667–681.

Scholing, A., & Emmelkamp, P. M. G. (1993b). Cognitive and behavioural treatments of fear of blushing, sweating, or trembling. *Behaviour Research and Therapy, 31*(2), 155–170.

Schwartz, J. M., Stoessel, P. W., Baxter, L. R., Martin, K. M., & Phelps, M. E. (1996). Systematic changes in cerebral glucose metabolic rate after successful behavior modification treatment of obsessive–compulsive disorder. *Archives of General Psychiatry, 53,* 109–113.

Schwiezer, E., & Rickels, K. (1996). Developing psychological treatments for generalized anxiety disorder. In R. M. Rapee & D. H. Barlow (Eds.), *Chronic anxiety: Generalized anxiety disorder and mixed anxiety disorder* (pp. 172–186). New York: Guilford Press.

Seligman, M. (1971). Phobias and preparedness. *Behavior Therapy, 2,* 307–320.

Seligman, M. E. P. (1975). *Helplessness: On depression, development and death.* San Francisco: Freeman.

Shapiro, F. (1989). Eye movement desensitization procedure: A new treatment for post-traumatic stress disorder. *Psychotherapy, 4,* 591–595.

Speilberger, C. D., Gorsuch, R. L., & Lushene, R. (1970). *STAI manual.* Palo Alto, CA: Consulting Psychologists Press.

Spivak, G., Platt, J. J., & Shure, M. B. (1976). *The problem solving approach to adjustment.* San Francisco: Jossey-Bass.

Steketee, G. S. (1993). *Treatment of obsessive compulsive disorder.* New York: Guilford Press.

Steketee, G. S., & White, K. (1990). *When once is not enough.* Oakland, CA: New Harbinger Press.

Stravynski, A., Marks, I., & Yule, W. (1982). Social skills problems in neurotic outpatients: Social skills training with and without cognitive modification. *Archives of General Psychiatry, 39,* 1378–1385.

Suinn, R. M., & Richardson, F. (1971). Anxiety management training: A nonspecific behavior therapy program for anxiety control. *Behavior Therapy, 2,* 498–510.

Sullivan, H. S. (1953). *The interpersonal theory of psychiatry.* New York: Norton.

Taylor, C. B., Sheikh, J., Agras, W. S., Roth, W. T., Margraf, J., Ehlers, A., Maddock, R. J., & Gossard, D. (1986). Ambulatory heart-rate changes in patients with panic attacks. *American Journal of Psychiatry, 143,* 478–482.

Taylor, S. (1996). Meta-analysis of cognitive-behavioral treatments for social phobia. *Journal of Behavior Therapy and Experimental Psychiatry, 27*(1), 1–9.

Tinbergen, N. (1951). *The study of instinct.* London: Oxford University Press.

Turner, S. M., Beidel, D. C., Cooley, M. R., Woody, S. R., & Messer, S. C. (1994). A multicomponent behavioral treatment for social phobia: Social Effectiveness Training. *Behaviour Research and Therapy, 32*(4), 381–390.

van Etten, M. L., & Taylor, S. (1998). Comparative efficacy of treatments for posttraumatic stress disorder: A meta-analysis. *Clinical Psychology and Psychotherapy, 5,* 126–145.

van Oppen, P., & Arntz, A. (1994). Cognitive therapy for obsessive–compulsive disorder. *Behaviour Research and Therapy, 31*(1), 79–87.

Watson, J. B., & Rayner, R. (1920). Conditional emotional reactions. *Journal of Experimental Psychology.*

Wegner, D. M. (1989). *White bears and other unwanted thoughts: Suppression, obsession, and the psychology of mental control.* New York: Guilford Press.

Weissman, M. M. (1987). Advances in psychiatric epidemiology: Rates and risks for major depression. *American Journal of Public Health, 77,* 445–451.

Weissman, M. M., & Merikangas, K. R. (1986). The epidemiology of anxiety and panic disorders: An update. *Journal of Clinical Psychiatry, 47,* 11–17.

Wells, A. (1994a). A multidimensional measure of worry: Development and preliminary validation of the Anxious Thoughts Inventory. *Anxiety, Stress and Coping, 6,* 289–299.

Wells, A. (1994b). Attention and the control of worry. In G. C. L. Davey & F. Tallis (Eds.), *Worrying: Perspectives on theory, assessment and treatment.* Chichester, England: Wiley.

Wells, A. (1997). *Cognitive therapy of anxiety disorders: A practice manual and conceptual guide.* New York: Wiley.

Wells, A., & Butler, G. (1997). Generalized anxiety disorder. In D. M. Clark & C. G. Fairburn (Eds.), *Science and practice of cognitive behaviour therapy* (pp. 155–178). Oxford, England: Oxford University Press.

Williams, J. M. G., Watts, F. N., MacLeod, C., & Mathews, A. (1997). *Cognitive psychology and emotional disorders.* Chichester, England: Wiley.

Wilson, T. R. (1987). *Don't panic.* New York: HarperCollins.

Wolpe, J. (1958). *Psychotherapy by reciprocal inhibition.* Stanford, CA: Stanford University Press.

Young, J. E. (1990). *Cognitive therapy for personality disorders: A schema-focused approach.* Sarasota, FL: Professional Resource Exchange.

Zuckerman, E. L. (1995). *Clinician's thesaurus* (4th ed.). New York: Guilford Press.

Index

Note. Page numbers in italics indicate pages containing forms and figures.